HISTOCOMPATIBILITY

Edited by

Bahaa Kenawy Abuel-Hussien Abdel-Salam

Histocompatibility
Edited by Bahaa Kenawy Abuel-Hussien Abdel-Salam

Published by InTech
Janeza Trdine 9, 51000 Rijeka, Croatia

Publishing Process Manager Iva Simcic

Technical Editor Teodora Smiljanic

Cover Designer InTech Design Team

Additional hard copies can be obtained from orders@intechopen.com

Histocompatibility, Edited by Bahaa Kenawy Abuel-Hussien Abdel-Salam
p. cm.
ISBN 978-953-51-0589-3

For EU product safety concerns:
IN TECH d.o.o., Prolaz Marije Krucifikse Kozulić 3, 51000 Rijeka, Croatia,
info@intechopen.com or visit our website at intechopen.com.

Meet the editor

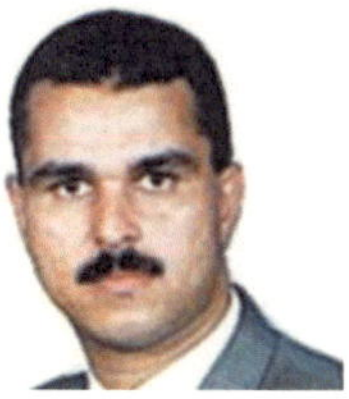

Dr Bahaa Kenawy Abuel-Hussien Abdel-Salam currently holds the position of Assistant Professor in Zoology Department, Minia University, El-Minia, Egypt. He received B.Sc. in Zoology, M.Sc. in Acarology and Ph.D in Immunology. Some of his previous positions on Minia University were Demonstrator, Assistant Lecture and Lecture in Zoology Department.

Contents

Preface

This book is intended as an introductory text for scientists who want to know more about the histocompatability. It attempts to present the field of immunology from a consistent viewpoint, that of the host's interaction with an environment containing many species of potentially harmful microbes.

The book includes the following topics: 1) HLA Polymorphism in Anthropology. 2) Distinctive Immunological Functions of HLA-G. 3) Immune Privilege Revisited: The Roles of Neuronal MHC Class I Molecules in Brain Development and Plasticity. 4) Human Leukocyte Antigen Class II in Stimulated Polymorphnuclear Neutrophils. 5) Dicer Regulates the Expression of Major Histocompatibility Complex (MHC) Class I Chain-Related Genes A and B. 6.) Killer Immunoglobulin-Like Receptors and Their Ligands. 7.) Sequence Analysis of MHC Class II Genes in Cetaceans. 8.) Regulation of MHC Class I by Viruses. 9.) Major and Minor Histocompatibility Antigens to Non-Inherited Maternal Antigens (NIMA). 10.) MHC Class I Quality Control.

This book would not exist without the efforts of the following authors - Sundararajulu Panneerchelvam and Mohd Nor Norazmi; Giada Amodio and Silvia Gregori; Adema Ribic; Bahaa K. A. Abdel-Salam; Kai-Fu Tang; Roberto Biassoni, Irene Vanni and Elisabetta Ugolotti; Wei-Cheng Yang, Lien-Siang Chou and Jer-Ming Hu; Shatrah Othman and Rohana Yusof; Masahiro Hirayama, Eiichi Azuma and Yoshihiro Komada; Gustav Røder, Linda Geironson, Elna Follin, Camilla Thuring and Kajsa Paulsson which were extremely helpful to all of us, and kept the book running.

Dr. Bahaa Kenawy Abuel-Hussien Abdel-Salam
Zoology Department, Faculty of Science
Minia University, El-Minia,
Egypt

1

HLA Polymorphism in Anthropology

Sundararajulu Panneerchelvam and Mohd Nor Norazmi
University Sains Malaysia
Malaysia

1. Introduction

Humans are the most adaptable species among living organisms. Adaptation is the sum of all processes which allows the organism to cope with environmental stresses, in particular climate and topography, for its survival. All living species continuing through time and space to the present day are endowed with innate biological adaptation. The whole gamut of biological adaptation of human species is dependent on the sum total of anatomical, physiological, immunological and genetic characteristics. But the human species, in addition to biological adaptation, also possess cultural adaptation. Cultures are customs and traditions which help shape the human body and mind. The quest for understanding diversity of his own species and the rest of the species through time and space has promoted the expansion of the science of biological/physical Anthropology [1].

The irresistible urge for understanding the phenomenon of evolution of *Homo sapiens* with a systematic scientific search to decipher the chronological events of the past led researchers to the objective reconstruction of the vanished past, postulating that anatomically similar modern humans had emerged in Africa 200,000 years ago and dispersed to all regions of the world. The accumulated evidences which led to such a suggestion encompasses research from several scientific disciplines viz., hierarchical taxonomy of primates displaying nested groupings; comparative anatomy of all primates exhibiting homologies such as arboreal adaptation and brachiating anatomy of apes and humans; comparative primate embryology exhibiting similar ontogeny; comparative molecular genetics of hominoid chromosome exhibiting 98% similarity between chimpanzees and humans; adaptive anatomical structures such as pelvic structure adapted to erect bipedalism and larynx adapted for speech; presence of vestigial structures mimicking ancient forms, nipples on males; paleogeographical evidences such as distribution of fossils of earlier and later forms of hominoids and their sequence and pattern and chronological sequence of ancient tools, overwhelmingly centred around the African origin of modern humans [2-7].

Biological anthropology, primarily deals with tracing the biological origins by analysing change in gene frequency in a population gene pool over a period of time leading to heritable genetic differences in subsequent generations and ultimately the genetic diversity of the human species. In the process, scientists undertake genetic analysis to find reasons behind the physical differences between people of various groups [1]. The genetic analysis assesses frequency of variant allele relating to genetic markers and comparing genetic variation among populations with a view to trace evolution. In this article a general appraisal of genetic diversity, the causative factors of genetic diversity, their impact on evolution [7], and the different molecular genetic markers with emphasis on the human leukocyte antigen (HLA) genetic markers, used in the study of tracing past events of human migrations are discussed.

2. Genetic diversity

Humans across the world exhibit remarkable phenotypic variations coupled with behavioural attributes. These variations are due to the combined effect of genetic and environmental factors. Researchers assess genetic variation by comparing variation between individuals in a group and by comparing variation between individuals in different groups (intra and inter population differences). The sources of individual variation are due to recombinant events in the genome and mutational events in meiosis leading to polymorphic alleles. Variation between groups is due to selective pressure on the genome due to differences in the environment and due to the combined outcome of founder effect and genetic drift. These differences are the source to trace/validate migration patterns in populations [8-15]. There are four major causes for genetic diversity in populations. They are (1) random sampling of gametes, (2) mutation, (3) subdivision, migration and genetic exchange and (4) natural selection.

3. Random sampling of gametes

In finite populations in the absence of any selection, random sampling of gametes effects a change in the gene frequency from the previous generation by chance. Random sampling is better visualised in finite populations. In real life, all populations are finite. For some populations (bacteria), the assumption of infinite size is a good approximation. For some, this is completely unrealistic. Hardy-Weinberg equilibrium (HW) assumes that the population is infinite. When a population is finite, random genetic drift produces a more pronounced effect. Random genetic drift is the random fluctuation of allele frequencies resulting in fixation or loss of an allele [10-16]. Wright-Fisher model explains the random change of frequency in finite populations. This model assumes a constant number of small panmictic populations producing infinite number of gametes evolving through non-overlapping discrete generations without mutation and without selection. This concept of random selection resulting in random genetic drift is explained in Fig.1. Consider that the parents are heterozygous for a locus, say, A and a. The parents produce a large number of gametes of which A and a will be 0.5 in proportion approximately. This proportion may not be 0.5 since reproductive cell death may occur at any stage of the gamete formation and besides, in females ¾ of the products are lost as polar bodies. In Fig. 1, the population is shown as consisting of 10 (3 AA homozygote; 4Aa heterozygotes and 3 aa homozygotes) individuals at t_0 generation with (allele frequency) of A = 0.5 and a = 0.5, producing infinite gametes and 10 individuals by random selection of gametes in each generation. At generation t_{20} (Fig.1) the gene frequency of A=0.55 and a=0.45 (3 Aa heterozygous 4 AA homozygous and 3 aa homozygous) and over generations, the finite sampling process erase the heterozygosity in the population. The end result of the random change will be that the frequency of A will eventually be 1 and a = 0; - that is the population is becoming homozygous [Fig.1].

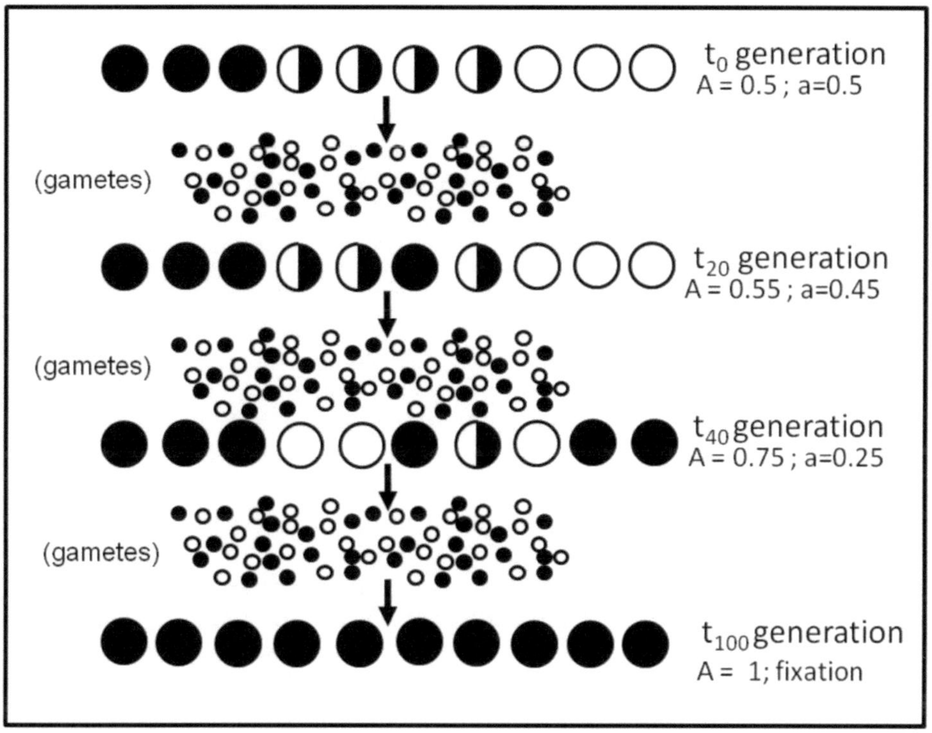

Fig. 1. Random Selection of Gametes
Illustration of random selection of gametes in a finite population represented by 10 circles, producing infinite number of gametes evolving through non-overlapping discrete generations without mutation and without selection. Solid circles (homozygous AA), open circle (homozygous a a) and semi-solid circles (heterozygous individuals A a)

The rate of genetic drift has an inverse relationship to the size of the population. This is to say that in an infinite population the loss of heterozygosity is extremely minimal. One reason for this is that the pool of reproductive individuals is always smaller than the total population. There are other reasons, including individual differences in expected fertility and changes in population size. Basic principles show that if the population size fluctuates, genetic diversity (heterozygosity) is lost at a rate related to the smallest size. There are two specific circumstances that greatly accelerate genetic drift. The first, called a bottleneck, occurs when a population size is reduced for a protracted period of time and then rebounds. The second, called a founder effect, occurs when all individuals in a population are traced back to a small number of founding individuals. Genetic diversity is lost very slowly in large populations. Like selection, drift is a process of differential reproductive success; however, the key element of genetic drift is that which individuals survive and reproduce is unrelated to their phenotype and genotype and it is random.

4. Mutation

Mutation is the ultimate source of all variations in a population. Mutations can be beneficial, neutral, or harmful for the organism, but mutations do not try to supply what the organism needs. In this respect, mutations are random. Many mutations are functionally silent either due to their presence outside the protein coding region of the genome or when present within the coding region does not alter the final protein product [17]. These silent mutations are used in deciphering genetic ancestry and demography of populations. Random genetic drift due to finite sample size which results in loss of genetic variation is offset by mutations generating genetic variation. The balance between these two opposing forces is assessed by using Coalescent modelling [18, 19].

Coalescent theory states that all genes or alleles in a given population are ultimately inherited from a single ancestor shared by all members of the population, known as the most recent common ancestor (MRCA) [19-21]. If the inheritance relationships are displayed in the form of a phylogenetic tree (termed a gene genealogy), the gene or allele of interest is said to undergo coalescence to the common ancestor (sometimes termed the coancestor to emphasize the coalescent relationship) [Fig 2]. Basic coalescence theory assumes that genes do not undergo recombination and models genetic drift as a stochastic process. Because the process of gene fixation due to genetic drift is a crucial component of coalescence theory, it is most useful when the genetic locus under study is not under natural selection. Coalescent modeling helps to understand the structure of whole population by assessing a small sample of descendents. It allows quantitating expected sequence diversity, the expected number of segregating sites, expected heterozygosity etc. Though the coalescent model addresses complex issues of population genetics there underlies the following basic components viz., the expected time back to the MRCA, the mutation rate and the outcome of the mutation [16-21].

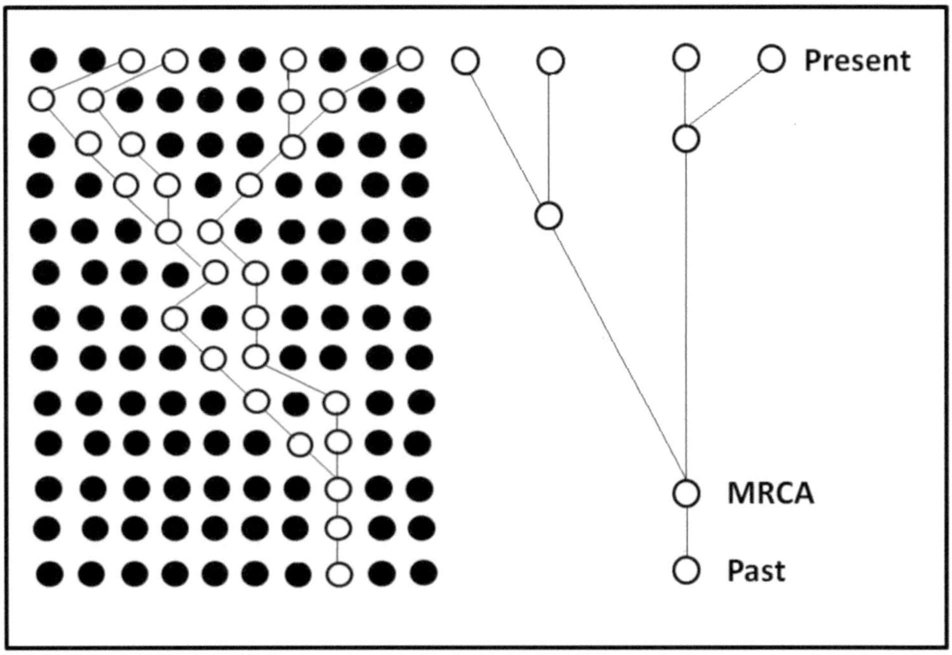

Fig. 2. Coalescent Model
Tracing the gene geneology of the four sub-divided present day population leading back to the MRCA.

5. Subdivision, migration and genetic exchange

The collection of genetically differentiated subpopulations is referred to as population substructure [22, 23]. In a large random mating population the genes with multiple alleles obey HW equilibrium in the absence of natural selection. Migration into and out of a population affects the population genetic structure [23-26]. Consider a hypothetical supposition that immigrants from a large population formed a new population in a different location. The parental population and the new population after hundreds of generations may again subdivide. This gives rise to two additional populations. All the four populations (ie. the parental plus the 3 sub-divided populations) will go through hundreds of generations. Eventually these populations are known as meta populations - regardless of whether they remain completely isolated or they may have been in communication with each other through the exchange of individuals.

Migration between two populations may have effect on genetic variation. However, it will be difficult to identify the boundaries of sub-populations and on genetic analyses one may confront with samples of individuals that may come from one sub-population or from more than one sub-population. The parental and the newly formed sub-populations may genetically be different from each other. Even if each of the subpopulations obeys HW and linkage equilibrium, a pooled sample from these populations may not match the expected and observed data. It is due to the fact that populations are more likely to choose mates living nearby and not in a random fashion. Since individuals that live close to one another tend to be more genetically similar than those that live far apart, the impacts of local mating will mimic those of inbreeding within a single well-mixed population. This is known as Walhund effect [27].

On genetic analysis the copies of a certain genetic locus coexisting in a sub-population do not always coalesce together. With reference to Fig. 3, sub-populations B and C, before coalescing at (MRCA), coalesce with D. If the subpopulations have high frequencies of certain alleles at a locus, the pooled population will show substantial linkage disequilibrium. If all the populations are in contact and random mating takes place it will take a considerable time for attaining linkage equilibrium since the reduction in linkage disequilibrium is by a factor of 1-r per generation, where r is the recombination fraction between two loci, that is the linkage disequilibrium between two linked loci will be reduced by ½ per generation. Continued random mating eventually result in linkage equilibrium. The genetic exchange between the local sub-populations is termed as gene flow.

6. F statistics

Walhund effect is the observation of excess homozygotes or deficiency of heterozygotes in a population of pooled subpopulations. Subpopulations fixed for a particular allele in a certain locus, is indicative of homozygous individuals in that population for that allele. Sewall Wright [11,12,28,29] expressed such effect by defining fixation index. Wright defined fixation index (F) as,

$$F=\frac{2\overline{p}(1-\overline{p})-\overline{p}}{2\overline{p}(1-\overline{p})}$$

$\overline{p}$ is the average allele frequency of homozygotes in sub-populations. Wright's F parameter values lies between 0 to 1. If there is no difference in allele frequency between

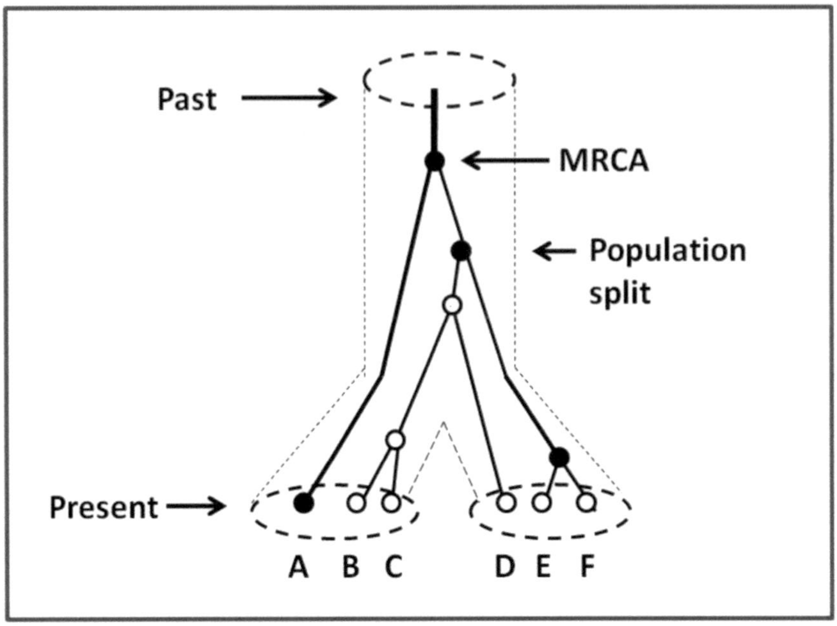

Fig. 3. Coalescent model in a subdivided population. Adapted from (16)
The present day sub-divided populations (also known as meta populations) represented by A, B, C, D, E and F tracing back to one single parent population in the past. Selected genetic locus coexisting in a sub-population do not always coalesce together. For example, the subdivided populations B and C coalesce with sub-divided population D before they coalesce with the MRCA despite sub-divided population D being in another group of sub-divided population. Solid circle represents unchanged allele within the selected gene locus of the parent while open circle represents the alternate allele in the selected locus.

subpopulations, then F = 0 (random population); alternatively if they are fixed for an allele then F = 1 (100% homozygosity). In the absence of selection and mutation, genetic drift is the primary evolutionary force causing differentiation of the population. Mutation and migration may prevent F from reaching 1 by introducing alternative alleles. Low levels of migration leads to moderately high level of F value. If the drift and migration is continuing through many generations and reaching equilibrium then F attains a constant value and can be deduced by the equation,

$$F=\frac{1}{4Nm+1}$$

Where N is the effective population size (often referred as N_e) and m is number of migration rate.

7. Natural selection

Natural selection is the fourth primary mechanism which acts as a whole on populations rather than individual organisms that produces changes in the genetic composition of a population from one generation to the next and in due course causes evolutionary change

[29,30]. Individuals in a population vary in genetic composition and some may have genetic variants conferring reproductive fitness making them more adaptable than others. In successive generations more offsprings will have better traits leading to changes in the frequency of that trait. Mutation often produces deleterious alleles. Selection removes deleterious alleles thereby providing stability of biological structures, and it is known as negative selection. Since negative selection confers stability by removing deleterious alleles it is also known as purifying selection or background selection. T cells which recognise self molecules and are eliminated in the thymus, is an example of negative selection. In some circumstances, a favorable allele may arise by mutation and may sweep through the entire population replacing all other alleles and such a selection is known as positive selection. The null allele at Duffy blood group locus conferring resistance to malaria parasite in African populations is a well known example for positive selection [26].

8. Genetic markers in the study of genetic diversity

Genetic variation is the fundamental prerequisite for evolution. Evolution is a continuous process and hence there should be processes to increase or decrease genetic variation. Genes mutate resulting in new alleles and they are the source of variation. Natural selection process acts on them furthering evolution. Genetic variation is the result of mutation and random association of alleles. Considerable variations are present in natural populations. The study of genetic variation assists us to understand the place and time of origin of modern humans and their dispersal pattern to all regions of the world. The study of migratory pattern using genetic variation requires extensive genetic marker based population data. The application of various genetic markers in assessing genetic diversity in populations paralleled the development and design of new genetic markers [30]. One can distinguish three phases in the use of various genetic markers [31-33]. Blood grouping and other serological characteristics based genetic polymorphism data formed the first phase of genetic diversity information. With the advent of electrophoresis to separate variant alleles in protein markers, the second phase utilized protein markers extending across all the populations. The third phase is marked with the use of DNA markers. The DNA marker based genetic diversity studies on populations completely replaced the use of serological/protein based genetic markers. In the subsequent paragraphs, an overview of the utility of DNA molecular genetic markers in Anthropological studies of human populations, with special emphasis on the HLA genetic marker is discussed.

DNA-based genetic diversity studies either use frequency data or direct sequence data. In general such studies involve three important steps in deciphering the phylogeography of populations. The three steps are (1) assessing inter and intra population differentiation; (2) ascertaining gene genealogies by constructing phylogenetic tree and (3) drawing inferences about dispersal pattern. The DNA-based molecular genetic markers routinely used in human population genetic diversity studies includes mitochondrial DNA (mtDNA), Y chromosome markers, single nucleotide polymorphism (SNPs), microsatellites and HLA markers.

9. Mitochondrial DNA

Human mtDNA is a single double-stranded circular DNA consisting of 16,569 basepairs in length. It is endowed with certain unique features such as high copy number per cell, maternal inheritance, lack of recombination and higher mutation rate than nuclear genes. The mtDNA behave as a haploid genome. The maternal inheritance and haploid nature of the genome facilitates in identifying relationships in a population. Using sequencing and RFLP-based high resolution mapping, Cann et al [34] suggested that Africa is the likely source of human mitochondrial gene pool and based on mtDNA sequence divergence suggested that the common ancestor of all surviving mtDNA types existed 140,000-200,000 years ago. Using a different method, Ingmann et al [35] estimated the time since most recent common ancestor (TMRCA) as 171 ± 50 thousand years ago (kya). Mitochondrial studies on various worldwide populations found further evidence for the African origin hypothesis and also estimated TMRCA at about 100,000-200,000 years. mtDNA studies on evolution is approached in two ways, namely, lineage based (haplogroups) and population based. However the recent trend is to use both haplogroup and population based studies to understand the pre-history of human populations.

10. Y chromosome

The Y chromosome in the human nuclear genome is haploid as that of mtDNA. The Y chromosome is paternally inherited. The human Y chromosome has now been sequenced [36]. It consists of the recombining segments, known as pseudoautosomal regions at the Yp and Yq ends. The Male sex determining region of Y (MSY) previously known as non-recombining region of Y (NRY) consists of euchromatic and heterochromatic regions accumulate changes due to insertions, deletions, base changes (SNPs) and Alu sequence insertions polymorphisms (YAP). The stable YAP and SNPs together are known as unique event polymorphisms (UEP) and many of them are bi-allelic markers. The microsatellites present in MSY region of Y chromosome accumulate changes, which either increase or decrease the copy number of core repeats faster than UEPs. The Y-linked loci in the MSY are haploid and the non-recombining nature of this region coupled with accumulated changes over thousands of generations are useful in delineating male lineages in populations and usefully exploited to study the prehistoric migrations of human populations [37]. Extensive genetic studies were undertaken on worldwide populations to ascertain male Y haplotype lineages, and their pattern of distribution suggest a recent origin between 60 and 150 thousand years ago in Africa for all the present day Y chromosomes [37-42].

11. Microsatellites

Microsatellites, also known as short tandem repeats (STRs) are arrays of 2-6 bp length tandem repeat motifs present throughout the genome. Changes in the repeat number take place due to replication slippage and the rate of change in repeat number is faster than SNPs. It is in the order of 10^{-3}. The change in repeat number follows most often stepwise mutation model (SMM) that is either increase or decrease by one repeat at a time. It is also reported that multistep changes or point mutations are also responsible for change in motif number. Being a neutral polymorphic marker, microsatellites are used in genetic mapping and studies of the evolutionary connections between species and populations. Microsatellites are the preferred markers for high resolution genetic mapping and useful in inferring relationships between closely related population groups. In a pilot study, Bowcock et al [43] studied 30 dinucleotide loci from 14 aboriginal populations and constructed a phylogenetic tree, in which the first split separated Africans from the rest of the populations and Goldstein [44] reanalyzed the data using a new genetic distance and estimated TMRCA 75,000 -287,000 years.

12. Single nucleotide polymorphism

Single nucleotide polymorphism (SNP) is defined as a single base change in the sequence of a segment of DNA occurring at a rate of >1% in a large population. SNPs occur in high frequency in the human genome and they can be found in coding and non-coding regions and they occur with very high frequencies - about 1 in 1,200 bases on average, which results in approximately 10 million SNPs in the human genome. SNPs are due to either base change or by deletion/insertion of a base. A base change in a coding region either alters the protein structure (synonymous mutation) or does not alter the protein structure (non-synonymous mutation). SNPs are the major cause of genetic diversity among different individuals facilitating large scale genetic association studies as genetic markers. With the advances in statistical methodologies in population genetics and the availability of large scale SNP data, this marker may facilitate in the study of prehistoric migration and demographic history of modern humans [45-47].

13. HLA polymorphic markers

The HLA is a multigene family and spans approximately 4 mega bases [48-50]. Currently there are at least 7,130 alleles in the class I and class II HLA loci described by the HLA nomenclature and included in the IMGT/HLA database (as of January 2012). The IMGT/HLA consortium directly receives the sequences for new alleles from researchers for checking and assignment of official name prior to publication to avoid confusion and multiple names. The polypeptides produced by these alleles differ by one or more amino acid substitutions. The polymorphic nature of the HLA class I and class II loci is a useful tool for the study of human evolution.

Serological and DNA based typing methods are used in HLA typing [51-53]. High resolution sequence specific primer (SSP) and sequence based typing (SBT) methods are more appropriate since both the methods are able to identify all the alleles so far defined, and for SBT, capable of identifying new alleles.

14. Significance of HLA diversity in evolution

The rate and number of nucleotide substitutions leading to new alleles in each of the functional HLA class I and II loci are quite high compared to neutral loci such as mtDNA and Y chromosome markers. Besides that the class I and class II loci exhibit high heterozygosity (80-90%) and hence are good genetic markers for phylogenetic study. Some of the lineages especially the DRB1 lineages are perpetuated more than 35 million years ago, the time of evolutionary divergence of the so-called hominoids (apes) from old world monkeys. Though the exact nature of mechanism for the high number of alleles and the perpetuation of alleles is not known, it is suggested that high mutation, inter locus genetic exchange (gene conversion) coupled with over dominant diversity results in the perpetuation of high number of alleles in the HLA locus. In such a selection, not only new alleles but old alleles have high selective advantage for perpetuation [54-67].

15. HLA polymorphism in phylogenetics

HLA markers are codominant SNP markers enabling heterozygotes to be distinguished from homozygotes, and allowing the determination of genotypes and allele frequencies. The class I and class II alleles in HLA are closely linked and occur jointly in individuals more often than by chance (linkage disequilibrium) [68]. Population migration and genetic drift can cause linkage disequilibrium. Linkage disequilibrium decreases by random mating over a period of time which is dependent on recombination fraction per generation. The study and analysis of remnant linkage disequilibrium, assuming that there is no selection shall provide information on the number of generations passed in-between two closely related populations from the time of their separation. Haplotype diversity, allele frequency variation and linkage disequilibrium analysis in HLA genetic markers are used to reflect the amount of variation between closely related populations. Comparison of variation is used to assess population genetic substructure. The analysis of variation in the HLA class I and II markers increase the power of detecting population substructure because each locus will contain an independent history of the population depending on the amounts of random drift, mutation, and migration that have occurred. The allele frequency based genetic distance help to construct phylogenetic tree to infer the relative estimate of the time that has passed since the populations have existed as single cohesive units [69-72]. The HLA marker allele frequencies of various populations are also used for cluster analysis using principal coordinate analysis (PCA).

Each population has unique HLA profile with reference to class I and class II HLA gene distributions. This has been reported in several studies compiling population data on HLA class I and class II genes from various populations of the world and it has significance in anthropological studies [73-108]. To highlight the effectiveness of HLA genetic markers in phylogenetics, a few studies relevant to genetic relationships among populations are described. Serjeantson et al [75] used allele frequency variation and linkage disequilibrium studies of HLA A and B loci in 16 Pacific Island populations to trace the phylogeogrphy of the populations to elucidate the interrelationships and migrations among peoples of the Pacific Islands. Shaw et al [89] used HLA-A, -B, -DR and -DQ allele frequency and haplotype frequency data to show that the aborigines in Taiwan has a distinct profile than the Chinese population groups and found Javanese closely related to Taiwan aborigines. Using HLA class I (A and B) and HLA class II (DRB1 and DQB1) allele distribution, linkage disequilibrium and cluster analysis it was shown that Amerindians are the very first American Natives that were already in America when Na Dene (Athabascans, Navajo, Apache) and Eskimo speaking people reached it [105]. Recently, Buhler and Sanchez-Mazas [108] used sequence based analysis on seven HLA genes in 23,500 individuals from 200 populations across the world to report on the significant correlation between genetics and geography which is in agreement with earlier HLA based studies using allele frequency data for population genetic diversity studies. They also concluded that geography plays a major role in shaping molecular variability among populations.

16. HLA genetic diversity studies and effective population size

The theory of African replacement model of evolution of modern humans generalize that the modern humans originated in Africa 200,000 years ago and the transition from archaic to modern humans was associated with a narrow bottleneck and the number of individuals in the bottleneck period was small. The theory of coalescence permits us to estimate the effective population size (N_e) and based on mtDNA and Y STR markers, the N_e at the time of divergence of modern humans is estimated to be 10^4 (10,000) individuals. In contrast, HLA based genetic diversity studies, taking into consideration the occurrence of large number of alleles and the perpetuation of HLA lineages more than 35 million years ago, previously estimated the effective population size to the order of 10^5 (100,000) individuals without bottleneck [61-63]. However subsequently this hypothesis was revised which included a bottleneck but spanning for a shorter period although the effective population size is maintained at 10^5 [64]. However Bergstrom et al (1998) on analysis of intron sequences of more than 135 contemporary human DRB1 alleles generated after the separation of hominoids from old world monkeys suggested that the coalescent time of alleles within these allelelic lineages indicate that the effective population size (N_e) is similar to estimates based on mtDNA that is 10^4 [66].

17. Conclusion

The high polymorphism, tight linkage, the random association of alleles and the perpetuation of allelic lineages over time make HLA genetic markers an invaluable tool in unravelling the human past. The vital information relating to amount, pattern and distribution of genetic variation of HLA genetic markers in different populations enable us to correlate genetic profile of populations and their past migrations in the determination of their origin.

18. Acknowledgements

The authors acknowledge the funds provided by the USM Research University Grant (1001/PPSK/813053) for the publication of this work.

19. References

[1] Kottak C P (Ed) (2006) Anthropology The exploration of Human Diversity. 11th edition, Mc Graw Hill company Inc., New York, PP: 3-23
[2] Smith F H (1992) Models and realities in modern human origins: The African fossil evidence, Phil Trans, R Soc Lond B (33): 243-250.
[3] Cartmill M and Smith F H (Ed) (2009) The human lineage, John Wiley & Sons, PP63-121
[4] Stringer C B and Andrews P (1988) Genetic and fossil evidence for the origin of modern humans, Science (239):1263-1268.
[5] Cavalli-Sforza L L, Piazza A, Menozzi P and Mountain J (1988) Reconstruction of human evolution bringing together genetic, archaeological and linguistic data (origin of modern humans/phylogenetic tree/paleoanthropology), Proc Natl Acad Sci USA (92): 6002-6006.
[6] Templeton A R (2002) Out of Africa again and again, Nature 416(7): 45-51
[7] Dobzhansky T. (1970) Genetics of the Evolutionary Process. Columbia University Press, New York.
[8] Cavalli-Sforza L L (1997). Genes, peoples, and languages. Proc Natl Acad Sci USA 94: 7719-7724.

[9] Amos W and Harwood J (1998) Factors affecting levels of genetic diversity in natural populations, Phil Trans. R. Soc. Lond B 353: 177-186.

[10] Long J C, Kittles R A (2003) Human genetic diversity and the non existence of biological races, Hum Biol. (75): 449-471.

[11] Wright S (1931) Evolution in Mendelian populations, Genetics 16: 97-159.

[12] Wright S (1948) On the roles of directed and random changes in gene frequency in the genetics of populations, Evolution 2: 279-294.

[13] Kimura M (1954) Process leading to quasi fixation of genes in natural populations due to random fluctuation of selection, Proc.Natl.Acad.Sci.USA.31: 382-389.

[14] Seneta E (1974) A note on the balance between random sampling and population size. Genetics 77: 607-610.

[15] Suzuki D T, Griffiths A J F, Miller J H and Lewontin R C(1989) In: An Introduction to genetic analysis 4th ed, W.H. Freeman p.704.

[16] Nei M (1987). Molecular Evolutionary Genetics. New York: Columbia University Press.

[17] Crow J F (1997) The high spontaneous mutation rate: is it a health risk? Proc. Natl. Acad.Sci.USA 94: 8380-8386.

[18] Hudson R R. (1990) Gene genealogies and the coalescent process, Oxford Surveys in Evolutionary Biology 7: 1-44.

[19] Griffiths R C and Tavere S (1998) The age of mutation in a general coalescent tree. Commun.Statist. Stochastic models, 14(1&2): 273-295.

[20] Nordborg M (2001) Coalescent theory. In Handbook of Statistical Genetics. M B D. Balding and Cannings C Eds. John Wiley & Sons, Chichester, UK PP: 179-212.

[21] Slatkin M. (1991). Inbreeding coefficients and coalescence times, Genetical Research 58: 167-75.

[22] Tuckwell H C (1976) The effects of random selection on gene frequency, Mathematical Biosciences 30:113-122.

[23] Bowcock A M, Kidd J R, J L Mountain J L, Hebert J M, Carotenuto L, Kidd K K and Cavalli-Sforza L L (1991) Drift, admixture and selection in human evolution: A study with DNA polymorphisms, Proc Natl Acad Sci USA. 88: 839-843.

[24] Slatkin M. (1993). Isolation by distance in equilibrium and non-equilibrium populations, Evolution 47: 264-279.

[25] Slatkin M (1995). A measure of population subdivision based on microsatellite allele frequencies, Genetics 139: 457-462.

[26] Excoffier L (2001) Analysis of population subdivision In Handbook of statistical genetics, M B D. Balding, and C. Cannings (Eds). pp. 271-302. John Wiley&Sons, Chichester, UK:

[27] Wahlund S (1928) Zusammensetzung von Populationen und Korrelation-Erscheinungen vom Standpunkt der Vererbungslehreaus betrachtet, Hereditas 11:65-106.

[28] Holsinger K E and Weir B S (2009) Genetics in geographically structured populations: defining, estimating and interpreting Fst, Nature Reviews Genetics 10: 639-650 http://digitalcommons.uconn.edu/eeb_articles.

[29] Balding M B D and Cannings C (Ed) (2001), Handbook of Statistical Genetics pp. 179-212.John Wiley&Sons Chichester, UK.

[30] Avise J C (2004) Molecular markers, Natural history and evolution, Sinuaer associates Inc., MA, USA.

[31] Cavalli-Sforza LL, Feldman, MW (2003) The application of molecular genetic approaches to the study of human evolution, Nat Genet.Suppl. 33: 266-275.

[32] Schlotterer C (2004) The evolution of molecular markers just a matter of fashion? Nature reviews, genetics 5: 63-69.

[33] Chenuil Anne (2006) Choosing a right molecular genetic marker for studying biodiversity from molecular evolution to practical aspects, Genetica (2006) 127:101-120.

[34] Cann R L, Stoneking M and Wilson A C (1987) Mitochondrial DNA and human evolution. Nature *325*:31–35.

[35] Ingmann M, Kaessmann H, Paabo S and Gyllensten U (2000) Mitochondrial genome variation and the origin of modern humans, Nature 408: 708–713.

[36] Hughes J F, Skaletsky H, Pyntikova T, Graves T A, van Daalen S K M, Minx PJ, Robert S. Fulton R S, Sean D. McGrath S D, Locke D P, Friedman C, Barbara J. Trask BJ, Elaine R. Mardis E R, Warren W C, Repping S, Rozen S, Richard K, Wilson RK and Page DC,(2010)1. Chimbanzee and human Y chromosome are remarkably divergent in structure and content Nature 463: 536 -543.

[37] Jobling M A, Williams G, Schiebel K, Pandya A, Mc Elreavey K, Salas L,Rappold G A, Affara NA, Tyler-Smith C (1998). A selective difference between human Y-chromosomal DNA haplotypes, Curr. Biol. 8:1391–1394.

[38] Shen P, Wang F, Underhill P A, Franco C, YangW-H, Roxas A, Sun R, Lin A A, Hyman R W, Vollrath D, Davis R W, Cavalli-Sforza L. L and Oefner P J (2000). Population genetic implications from sequence variation in four Y chromosome genes, Proc Natl Acad Sci USA 97: 7354-7359.

[39] Underhill P A, Li Jin, Lin A A, Qasim Mehdi S, Jenkins T, Vollrath D, Davis R W, Cavalli-Sforza L L, Peter J and Oefner P J (1997) Detection of Numerous Chromosome biallelic Polymorphisms by Denaturing High-Performance Liquid Chromatography, Genome Res. 7: 996-1000.

[40] Stoneking M, Fontius J J, Clifford S L, Soodyall H and Arcot S S (1997) Alu insertion polymorphisms and human evolution: evidence for a larger population size in Africa, Genome Res. 7: 1061–1071.

[41] Underhill P A, Shen P and Lin A (2000) Y chromosome sequence variation and the history of human populations. Nature Genetics 26: 358–361.

[42] Jobling MA, Tyler-Smith C. 2003. The human Y chromosome: an evolutionary marker comes of age. Nat Rev Genet 4(8):598-612.

[43] Bowcock A M, Ruiz-Linares A, Tomfohrde J, Minch E, Kidd JR, Cavalli-Sforza L L (1994) High resolution of human evolutionary history trees with polymorphic microsatellites. Nature 368: 455–457.

[44] Goldstein DB, Ruiz Linares A, Cavalli-Sforza LL, Feldman MW.1995. Genetic absolute dating based on microsatellites and the origin of modern humans, Proc Natl Acad Sci USA 92:6723–6727.

[45] Cargill M, Altshuler D, Ireland J, Sklar P and Ardlie K (1999) Nucleotide diversity in Eurasians is essentially a subset characterization of single-nucleotide polymorphisms in coding regions of human genes, Nat. Genet. 22: 231–238.
[46] International SNP Working Group, (2001) A map of human genome sequence variation containing 1.42 million single nucleotide polymorphisms, Nature 409: 928–933.
[47] Ning Yu, Feng-Chi Chen, Satoshi Ota, Jorde L B, Pamilo P, Laszlo Patthy, Michele Ramsay, Trefor Jenkins, Song-Kun Shyue and Wen-Hsiung Li, (2002) Larger genetic differences within Africans than between Africans and Eurasians, Genetics 161: 269–274.
[48] Duquesnoy R J and Trucco M (1988). Genetic basis of cell surface polymorphisms encoded by the major histocompatibility complex in humans, Crit Rev Immunol 8:103-145.
[49] Halloran P F, Wadgymar A and Autenried P (1986) The regulation of expression of major histocompatibility complex products. Transplantation 41:413-420.
[50] Parham P and Ohta T (1996) Population biology of antigen presentation by MHC class I molecules, Science 272:67-74.
[51] Kurz B, Steiert I, Heuchert G and Mu¨ller C A (1999) New high resolution typing strategy for HLA-A locus alleles based on dye terminator sequencing of haplotypic group-specific PCR-amplicons of exon 2 and exon 3. Tissue Antigens 53: 81–96.
[52] American Association of Blood Banks. Technical Manual (1999). 13th ed., Bethesda, MD: American Association of Blood Banks.
[53] Bunce M, Fanning G C and Welsh K I (1995) Comprehensive, serologically equivalent DNA typing for HLA-B by PCR using sequence-specific primers (PCAR-SSP), Tissue Antigens. 45: 81-90.
[54] Hedrick P W and Thomson G (1983) Evidence for balancing selection at HLA, Genetics 104:449-456.
[55] Klein J and Figueroa F (1986) Evolution of the major histocompatibility complex, Crit Rev Immunol. 6(4):295–386.
[56] Klitz W, Thomson G and Baur M P (1986) Contrasting evolutionary histories among tightly linked HLA loci, Am J Hum Genet. 39:340-349.
[57] Klein J (1987) Origin of major histocompatibility complex polymorphism: the trans-species hypothesis. Hum Immunol.19 (3):155–162.
[58] Hughes A L and Nei M (1988): Pattern of nucleotide substitution at major histocompatibility complex class I loci reveals over dominant selection, Nature. 335:1
[59] Hughes A L and Nei M 1989) Nucleotide substitution at major histocompatibility complex class II loci: evidence for overdominant selection, Proc Natl Acad Sci.USA. 86:958-962.
[60] Gyllensten U, Sundvall M, Ezcurra I and Erlich H A (1991) Genetic diversity at class II DRB loci of the primate MHC, J Immunol.146 (12):4368–4376.
[61] Takahata N (1993) Allelic Genealogy and Human Evolution. Mol.Biol.Evol. 10(1):2-22
[62] Ayala F J (1995) The myth of Eve: molecular biology and human origins, Science. 270 (5244): 1930–1936.

[63] Ayala F J and Escalante A A (1996) The evolution of human populations: a molecular perspective, Mol Phylogenet Evol 5(1):188–201.
[64] Tkahata N, Satta Y, and Klein J (1995) Divergence time and population size in the lineage leading to Modern humans, Theoretical population Biology. 48:198-221.
[65] Parham P, Arnett K L, Adams E J, Little A M, Tees K, Barber L D, Marsh S G, Ohta T, Markow T and Petzl-Erler M L (1997) Episodic evolution and turnover of HLA-B in the indigenous human populations of the Americas, Tissue Antigens. 50:219, 1997.
[66] Bergström T F, Josefsson A, Erlich H A and Gyllensten U (1998) Recent origin of HLA-DRB1 alleles and implications for human evolution, Nat Genet. 18 (3):237–242.
[67] Takahata N and Satta Y (1998) Footprints of intragenic recombination at HLA loci, Immunogenetics.
[68] Hudson R R (2001) Analysis of population subdivision in Handbook of statistical genetics, M B D. BaldingM.B D and C. Cannings (Eds). pp. 309-324. John Wiley&Sons Chichester, UK.
[69] Nei M (1973). Analysis of gene diversity in subdivided populations. Proc Natl Acad Sci USA. 70: 3321–3323.
[70] Nei M, Tajima Y and Tateno Y (1983) Accuracy of estimated phylogenetic trees from molecular data, J Mol Evol. 19: 153–70.
[71] Saito N and Nei M (1987) The neighbor-joining method: a new method for reconstructing phylogenetic trees, Mol Biol Evol. 4: 406–425.
[72] Excoffier L and Slatkin M (1995). Maximum likelihood estimation of molecular haplotype frequencies in a diploid population, Mol Biol Evol. 12: 921–927.
[73] Cohen N, Mickelson E, Amar A, Battat S, Hansen J A and Brautbar C (1987) HLA-Dw clusters associated with DR4 in Israeli Jew s and the definition of a new DR4 associated Dw subtype:Dw 'SHA'. Hum Immunol 19:179-183.
[74] Bouali M, Dehay C, Benajam A, Poirier J C, Degos L, Marcelli-Barge A (1981) HLA-A, B, C, Bf and glyoxalase I polymorphisms in a sample of the Kabyle population (Algeria), Tissue Antigens 17:501-506.
[75] Serjeantson D, Ryan D P, Thompson A R (1982) The Colonization of the Pacific: The Story According to Human Leukocyte Antigens. Am J Hum Genet 34: 904-909.
[76] Mercier P, Vallo J J, Vialettes B and Vague Ph (1985) HLA-A, B, DR antigens and insulin-dependent diabetes in Algerians, Tissue Antigens 26:20-24.
[77] Imanishi T, Akaza T, Kimura A, Tokunaga K and Gjobori T (1992a) Estimation of Allele and haplotype frequencies for HLA and complement loci in various ethnic groups. In: HLA 1991, Vol 1 (Eds. Tsuji K, Aizawa M and Sasazuki T) pp 76-79 Oxford: Oxford University Press, Oxford, UK.
[78] Morales P, Martinez-Laso J, Martin-Villa JM, Corell A, Vicario JL, Varela P, Arnaiz-Villena A (1991) High frequency of the DRB 1*0405-(Dw 15)-DQw8 haplotype in Spaniards and its relationship to diabetes susceptibility, Hum Immunol 32: 170-175.
[79] Fernandez-Viiia M A, Gao X, Moraes M E, Moraes J R, Salatiel I, Miller S, Tsai J, Sun Y, An J, Layrisse Z, Gazit E, Brautbar C and Stastny P(1991) Alleles at four HLA class

II loci determined by oligonucleotide hybridization and their associations in five ethnic groups, Immunogenetics 34:299-312.

[80] Vilches C, De Pablo R, Moreno M, Solis R and Kreisler M (1992),Characterization of an HLA-DR15 DQS haplotype found in the Spanish Caucasoid population, Hum Immunol 35:223-229.

[81] Williams R C and McAuley J E (1992) HLA Class I variation controlled for genetic admixture in the Gila River Indian community of Arizona: A model for the Paleo-Indians, Hum Immunol 33: 39-46.

[82] Hmida S, Gauthier A and Dridi A (1995) HLA class II gene polymorphism in Tunisians, Tissue Antigens 45: 63–68.

[83] Arnaiz-Villena A, Benmamar D and Alvarez M (1995) HLA allele and haplotype frequencies in Algerians. Relatedness to Spaniards and Basques.,Hum Immunol. 43: 259–268.

[84] Roitberg-Tambour A, Witt CS and Friedmann A (1995).Comparative analysis of HLA polymorphism at the serologic and molecular level in Moroccan and Ashkenazi Jews, Tissue Antigens 46: 104–110.

[85] Clayton J, Lonjou C. (1997) Allele and Haplotype frequencies for HLA loci in various ethnic groups. In: Charron D, ed. Genetic Diversity of HLA. Functional and medical implications, Vol. 1. Paris: EDK, 665–820.

[86] Arnaiz-Villena A, Martinez-Laso J and Gomez-Casado E (1997) Relatedness among Basques Portuguese, Spaniards, and Algerians studied by HLA allelic frequencies and haplotypes, Immunogenetics. 47: 37–43.

[87] Comas D, Mateu E and Calafell F (1998). HLA class I and class II DNA typing and the origin of Basques, Tissue Antigens 51: 30–40.

[88] Izaabel H, Garchon H J and Caillat-Zucman S (1998) HLA Class II DNA polymorphism in a Moroccan population from the Souss Agadir area, Tissue Antigens. 51: 106–110.

[89] Shaw C K, Chen L L, Lee A and Lee TD (1999) Distribution of HLA gene and haplotype frequencies in Taiwan: a comparative study among Minnan, Hakka, Aborigines and Mainland Chinese, Tissue Antigens. 53: 51–64.

[90] Arnaiz-Villena A, Iliakis P, Gonzalez-Hevilla M, Longas J, Gomez-Casado E, Sfyridaki K, Trapaga J, Silvera-Redondo C, Matsouka C and Martinez-Laso J (1999) The origin of Cretan population as determined by characterization of HLA alleles, Tissue Antigens 53: 213–226.

[91] Gomez-Casado E, Del Moral P, Martinez-Laso J, Garcia-Gomez A, Allende L and Silvera-Redondo C (2000) HLA genes in Arabic-speaking Moroccans: close relatedness to Berbers and Iberians, Tissue Antigens. 55: 239–249.

[92] Middleton D, Williams F, Meenagh A, Daar A S, Gorodezky C, Hammond M, Nascimento E, Briceno I and Perez M P (2000) Analysis of the Distribution of HLA-A alleles in populations from five continents, Hum Immunol. 61: 1048–1052

[93] Williams F, Meenagh A, Darke C, Acosta A, Daar A S Gorodezky C, Hammond M, Nascimento E, Middleton D (2001) Analysis of the Distribution of HLA-B alleles in populations from five Continents Hum Immunol. 62: 645-650.

[94] Main P (2001) The Peopling of New Guinea: Evidence from Class I Human Leukocyte Antigen, Human Biology, 73(3): 365-383.

[95] Chu C C, NLaiknajima F M, Lee H L, Chang S L, Juji T and Tokunaga K (2001) Diversity of HLA among Taiwan's indigenous tribes and the Ivatans in the Philippines. Tissue Antigens. 58: 9–18.

[96] Arnaiz-Villena A, Dimitroski K, Pacho A, Moscoso J, Gómez-Casado E, Silvera-Redondo C, Varela P, Blagoevska M, Zdravkovska V and Martínez-Laso J. (2001) HLA genes in Macedonians and the Sub-Saharan origin of the Greeks, Tissue Antigens. 57: 118–127.

[97] Grimaldi M C, Crouau-Roy B and Amoros J P (2001). West Mediterranean islands (Corsica, Balearic islands, Sardinia) and the Basque population: contribution of HLA class I molecular markers to their evolutionary history, Tissue Antigens 58: 281–292.

[98] Arnaiz-Villena A ,Karin M, Bendikuze N, Gomez-Casado E, Moscoso J, Silvera C, Oguz F S , Sarper Diler A, De Pacho A[1],Allende L, Guillen J and Martinez Laso J (2001) HLA alleles and haplotypes in the Turkish population: relatedness to Kurds, Armenians and other Mediterraneans. Tissue Antigens 57: 308–317.

[99] Sanchez-Velasco P, Gomez-Casado E, and Martinez-Laso J (2003) HLA allele in isolated populations from North Spain: origin of the Basques and the ancient Iberians. Tissue Antigens 61: 384–392.

[100] Tsuneto L T, Pros C M, Hutz M H, Salzano F M, Rodriguez-Delving L A, Zago M A, Hill K, Hurtado A M, Ribeiro-dos-Santos A K and Petzl-Erler M L (2003) HLA class II diversity in seven Amerindian populations. Clues about the origins of the Ache, Tissue Antigens 62: 512–526.

[101] Ayed K, Ayed-Jendoubi S, Sfar I, Labonne M P, Gebuhrer L(2004) HLA class-I and HLA class-II phenotypic, gene and haplotypic frequencies in Tunisians by using molecular typing data, Tissue Antigens 64: 520–532.

[102] Piancatelli D, Canossi A, and Aureli A (2004) Human leukocyte antigen -A-B and -Cw polymorphism in a Berber population from North Morocco using sequence-based typing, Tissue Antigens 63: 158–72.

[103] Middleton D, Hawkins BR and Williams F Meenagh A, Moscoso J, Zamora J, and Arnaiz-Villena A (2004) HLA class I allele distribution of a Hong Kong Chinese population based on high-resolution PCR-SSOP typing, Tissue Antigens 63: 555–561.

[104] Hong w, Fu Y, Chen S, Wang F, Ren X and Xu A (2005) Distributions of HLA class I alleles and haplotypes in Northern Han Chinese, Tissue Antigens. 66 (2005) 297–304.

[105] Arnaiz-Villena A, Moscoso J, Serrano-VelaJ I and Martinez-Laso J (2006) The uniqueness of Amerindians according to HLA genes and the peopling of the Americas, Inmunología / Enero-Marzo 25(1): 13-24.

[106] Hajjej A, Ka^ abi H, Sellami M H, Dridi A, Jeridi A, El borg W, Cherif G and Elgaaied, Almawi W Y, Boukef K and Hmida S (2006) The contribution of HLA class I and II alleles and haplotypes to the investigation of the evolutionary history of Tunisians, Tissue Antigens 68: 153–162.

[107] Edinur HA, Zafarina Z,Spínola H,Nurhaslindawaty A R, Panneerchelvam S, Norazmi M N (2009) HLA polymorphism in six Malay subethnic groups in Malaysia, Human Immunology 70(7): 518-526.

[108] Ste´phane Buhler and Alicia Sanchez-Mazas (2011) HLA DNA Sequence Variation among Human Populations: Molecular Signatures of Demographic and Selective Events. PLoS ONE 6(2):1-16.

2

Distinctive Immunological Functions of HLA-G

Giada Amodio and Silvia Gregori
San Raffaele Telethon Institute for Gene Therapy (HSR-TIGET), Division of Regenerative Medicine, Stem Cells and Gene Therapy, San Raffaele Scientific Institute, Milan, Italy

1. Introduction

HLA-G is a non-classical HLA class Ib molecule belonging to the Major Histocompatibility Complex (MHC) located on the short arm of chromosome 6. The tissue-restricted distribution of HLA-G, the low polymorphism in the coding region, the fact that HLA-G primary transcript is alternatively spliced in seven isoforms, and the inhibitory action on immune cells, constitute four hallmarks of HLA-G, which distinguish it from other HLA class I molecules (Carosella et al., 1999). In healthy conditions, a basal level of HLA-G gene transcription is observed in most cells and tissues. However, translation into HLA-G protein is restricted to trophoblasts at the fetal-maternal interface (Carosella et al., 2003), and in adults, to thymic epitelial, cornea, mesenchymal stem cells (MSCs), nail matrix, pancreatic-β cells, erythroid and endothelial precursors. HLA-G can be also neo-expressed in pathological conditions including malignant transformation, viral infections, inflammatory and autoimmune diseases, and allogeneic transplantation (Carosella, 2011).

HLA-G locus is very low polymorphic and, due to its structure, HLA-G molecule can recognize and present only a restricted peptide repertoire compared to classical HLA class I molecules (Clements et al., 2005). These peculiarities render HLA-G exclusively oriented towards immune inhibition and tolerance. In the late ninety, Rouas-Freiss et al. showed that HLA-G expressing trophoblasts were protected from maternal NK cell-mediated cytolysis, indicating for the first time HLA-G as a key molecule in fetal-maternal tolerance (Rouas-Freiss et al., 1997). From this first observation, several groups have worked to define the mode of action of HLA-G and in which settings it is involved in promoting tolerance. It is now generally accepted that HLA-G is a unique molecule with several immuno-modulatory properties: it plays an important role not only in fetal-maternal tolerance, but also in modulating immune responses and promoting and maintaining peripheral tolerance in healthy and pathological conditions. HLA-G can indeed act on both the innate and the adaptive branches of immunity and regulate short- and long-term immune-responses.

2. HLA-G molecule

The alternative splicing of HLA-G primary transcript results in seven different isoforms, four of which are membrane bound (HLA-G1 to –G4) and three are soluble (HLA-G5 to –G7) forms (Fujii et al., 1994; Ishitani and Geraghty, 1992) (Fig. 1A).

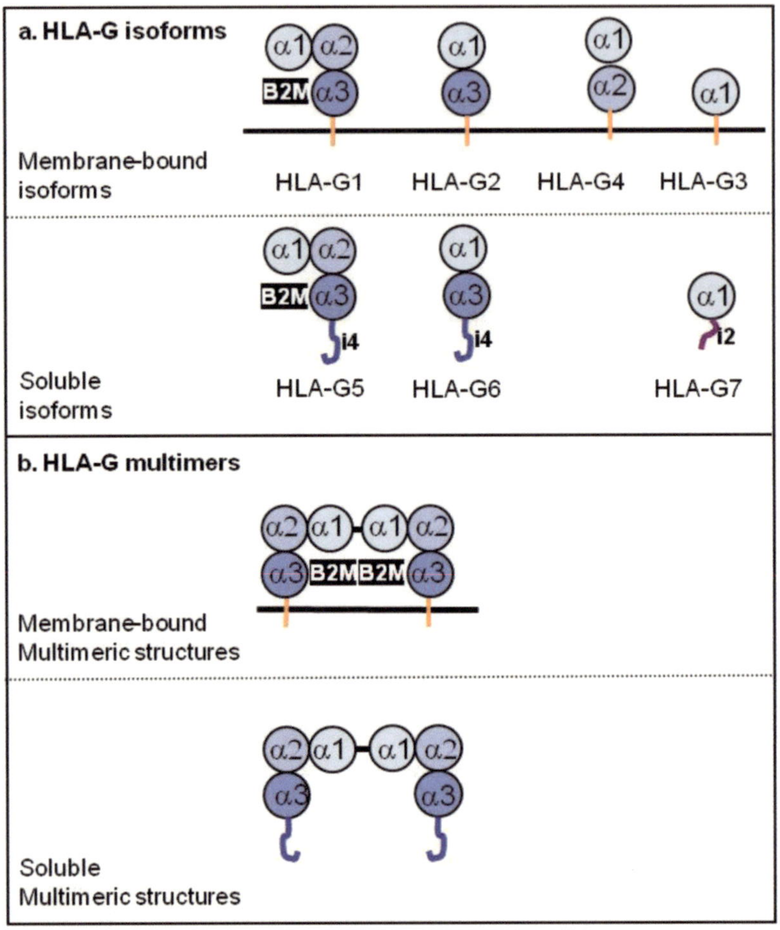

Fig. 1. HLA-G isoforms, monomers and dimers

A. The alternative splicing of a unique primary transcript yields 7 protein isoforms: truncated isoforms are generated by excision of one or two exons encoding globular (α) domains, whereas translation of intron 4 (i4) or intron 2 (i2) yields soluble isoforms that lack the transmembrane domain. **B**. HLA-G molecules can form homodimers through the generation of Cys42-Cys42 disulfide bonds.

In addition, a soluble HLA-G1 isoform (shed HLA-G1) can be generated by the membrane HLA-G1 proteolytic cleavage that is dependent on metalloproteinase activity (Park et al., 2004), and is regulated by Nitric Oxide (NO) concentration (Diaz-Lagares et al., 2009) and Tumor Necrosis Factor (TNF)-α/NFkB pathway activation (Zidi et al., 2006). Soluble and membrane-bound HLA-G isoforms have similar functions. HLA-G1, HLA-G5, and shed HLA-G1 are the most described isoforms in healthy tissues (Paul et al., 2000) and their structure is similar to that of classical HLA class I molecules: a heavy chain of three globular domains non-covalently associated with β2-microglobulin (β2m) and a nona-peptide (Clements et al., 2005). The other HLA-G isoforms contain the α1 domain but lack one or two of the other globular domains, and are not associated with β2m and the peptide. The presence of the α3 domain is important to HLA-G functions since it represents a binding site for HLA-G receptors (Clements et al., 2005; Clements et al., 2007).

HLA-G possesses two unique cysteine residues, in position 42 of the α1 domain and in position 147 of the α2 domain. Through these residues, HLA-G may dimerize by intra-molecular disulfide bonds (Boyson et al., 2002). Membrane-bound or soluble HLA-G dimers were detected both *in vitro* and *in vivo* (Apps et al., 2007; Boyson et al., 2002; Gonen-Gross et al., 2005) (Fig. 1B). Dimerization of HLA-G is one of its key features since dimers bind to HLA-G receptors with higher affinity and slower dissociation rates compared to monomers (Shiroishi et al., 2006a) and, as a consequence, dimers, but not monomers, carry most of the HLA-G functions (Gonen-Gross et al., 2003; Li et al., 2009).

HLA-G acts through three inhibitory receptors: immunoglobulin-like transcript (ILT)2 (CD85j/LILRB1), ILT4 (CD85d/LILRB2), the killer cell immunoglobulin-like receptor (KIR)2DL4 (CD158d), and the co-receptor CD8 (Colonna et al., 1997; Colonna et al., 1998; Rajagopalan and Long, 1999) (Fig. 2).

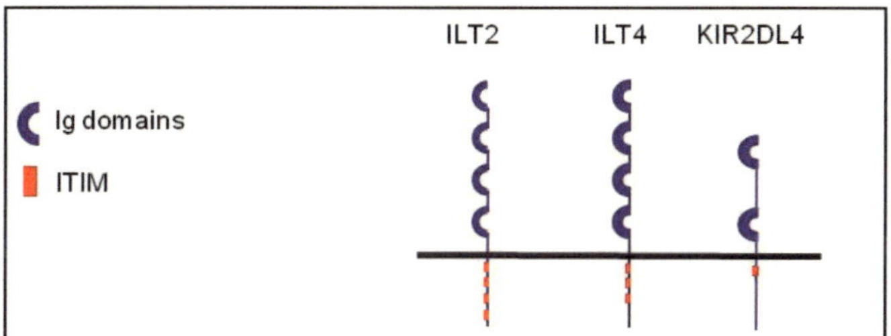

Expression	ILT2	ILT4	KIR2DL4
NK	+/-	-	+
CD8+ T cells	+/-	-	+/-
CD4+ T cells	+/-	-	+/-
B cells	+	-	-
Monocytes/MΦ	+	+	-
DC	+	+	-

Fig. 2. HLA-G receptors

Inhibitory receptors known to bind HLA-G. Basic structural organization and expression patterns are shown. The HLA-G structural configuration that these receptors are known to bind are indicated as '+' (reported binding) and '–' (reported absence of binding or minor binding).

ILT2 is expressed by B cells, some T cells (both CD4⁺ and CD8⁺), a sub-population of NK cells, and all monocytes/Dendritic Cells (DCs) (Colonna et al., 1997), whereas ILT4 is only expressed by mono/macrophages and DCs (Colonna et al., 1998). KIR2DL4 is expressed by some CD8⁺ T and NK cells (Goodridge et al., 2003).

Even if ILT2 and ILT4 recognize other HLA Class I molecules, HLA-G is their ligand of highest affinity and they bind HLA-G dimers even more strongly (Shiroishi et al., 2006a; Shiroishi et al., 2003). ILT2 and ILT4 can recognize different HLA-G structures: ILT2 binds only β2m-associated HLA-G1/G5 isoforms, whereas ILT4 also recognizes their β2m-free counterparts (Gonen-Gross et al., 2005; Shiroishi et al., 2006b). Finally, significantly higher expression of ILT2 was necessary for efficient HLA-G tetramer binding, suggesting that this interaction may have relatively lower affinity compared to that of ILT4 (Allan et al., 1999). Interestingly, HLA-G can directly influence the expression rate of its receptors both at mRNA level and at the protein level (LeMaoult et al., 2005). Thus, HLA-G is unique in its ability to be expressed in different isoforms and to act through inhibitory receptors.

3. Mechanisms underlying HLA-G expression

Even if theoretically any tissue might express HLA-G, its physiological expression is restricted to few tissues such as trophoblasts, thymic epithelium, cornea, MSC and pancreatic β-cells (Carosella, 2011). Nonetheless, in pathological conditions, HLA-G expression can be induced and/or up-regulated. So far the reason why HLA-G can be expressed in some, but not in all tissues has not been fully elucidated. However, several factors such as immune-modulatory cytokines and hormones, were described to potentially affect transcriptional mechanisms responsible for HLA-G expression (Moreau et al., 2009). In contrast to classical HLA class I molecules, HLA-G expression is not influenced by the transcription factor NF-*k*B (Gobin et al., 1998) or by classical pro-inflammatory cytokines such as Interferon (IFN)-γ (Gobin et al., 1999), since responsive elements for IFN-γ are missed in HLA-G promoter (Gobin et al., 1999; Steimle et al., 1995). In contrast, HLA-G transcriptional rate is increased by the presence of a number of anti-inflammatory cytokines including IFN-β (Lefebvre et al., 2001), Interleukin (IL)-4, IL-5, IL-6 (Deschaseaux et al., 2011), and IL-10 (Moreau et al., 1999) and can be modulated by Granulocyte Macrophage Colony-Stimulating Factor (GM-CSF) (Onno et al., 2000; Yang et al., 1996), Transforming Growth Factor (TGF)-β, or Granulocyte Colony-Stimulating Factor (G-CSF).

In addition to cytokines, hormones like glucocorticoids (dexamethasone) and progesterone were shown to increase the secretion of both HLA-G5 and HLA–G6 by trophoblasts (Akhter et al., 2011; Moreau et al., 2001; Yie et al., 2006a; Yie et al., 2006b). HLA-G expression can be also influenced by Adenosine Triphosphate (ATP) and by the tryptophan catalayzing enzyme indoleamine 2 3-dioxygenase (IDO). ATP acts as a potent inhibitor of HLA-G1 and HLA–G5 production from LPS-activated PBMCs *via* down-regulation of IL-10 (Rizzo et al., 2009). IDO, known to be involved in the generation of tolerogenic microenvironments by tryptophan depletion and in the generation of T regulatory (Treg) cells (Chung et al., 2009; Munn et al., 2002), was shown to differentially modulate HLA-G expression in monocytes and myeloid DCs. IDO blocked HLA-G cell-surface expression on monocytes (Gonzalez-Hernandez et al., 2005), but it induced HLA-G expression and shedding in myeloid DCs (Lopez et al., 2006). Overall, a number of immune mediators can influence HLA-G expression. It has to be taken in account that these molecules can be up-regulated in conditions, such as inflammation, in which HLA-G expression is needed to control or dampen the immune response.

In addition to soluble factors, it has been recently reported that "transient" HLA-G expression can be acquired *via* trogocytosis, a cell-to-cell contact-dependent uptake of membranes and associated molecules from one cell by another (reviewed in (Davis, 2007; LeMaoult et al., 2007a). Trogocytosis of HLA-G was shown for activated $CD4^+$ and $CD8^+$ T cells (LeMaoult et al., 2007b), activated NK cells (Caumartin et al., 2007), and monocytes (HoWangYin et al., 2011). For $CD4^+$ T cells, the most important consequence of HLA-G acquisition, is that the newly-expressing cells became transiently tolerogenic (LeMaoult et al., 2007a), as discussed below. Thus, trogocytosis generates HLA-G positive cells, which display, but do not express HLA-G. The ability of different cells to transiently acquire HLA-G expression broadens the immuno-modulatory activity of HLA-G.

4. HLA-G immunological function

The functions of HLA-G are exclusively oriented towards immune inhibition and tolerance. HLA-G exerts its inhibitory functions on several immune cells through direct binding to the inhibitory receptors ILT2, ILT4, and KIR2DL4 (Shiroishi et al., 2006b).

4.1 Short-term immuno-modulation mediated by HLA-G

HLA-G:ILT2 interaction modulates NK cell activity (Rouas-Freiss et al., 1997). HLA-G-expressing target cells are indeed resistant to the lysis mediated by NK cells (Riteau et al., 2001). Although the mechanisms underlying this effect are not completely elucidated, it has been recently defined that HLA-G:ILT2 interaction disrupts the immunological synapse (IS), a supramolecular structure responsible for both T and NK cell activation and function (Favier et al., 2010), leading to inhibition of NK cytolysis. HLA-G binds to KIR2DL4 on NK cells (Shiroishi et al., 2006b). However, it still remains unclear which are the effects mediated by this interaction. Ligation of KIR2DL4 activates cytokine production but not cytotoxicity (Rajagopalan et al., 2001), and it has been recently proposed that activation of KIR2DL4 by soluble HLA-G activates a pro-inflammatory/pro-angigenic responses, consistent with a role in promoting vascularization during early pregnancy (Rajagopalan et al., 2006). HLA-G can also bind CD8, which is expressed by a subpopulation of NK cells leading to Fas ligand expression, and induction of apoptosis (Contini et al., 2003).

The interaction between HLA-G and $CD8^+$ T cells impairs the antigen-specific cytotoxic T lymphocyte (CTLs) activity (Le Gal et al., 1999). HLA-G has a dose-dependent effect on the generation of allo-CTL responses, while it seems to not affect pre-existing allo-CTLs (Kapasi et al., 2000). Furthermore, during later stages of T cell activation, HLA-G:CD8 interaction promotes TCR-independent apoptosis of $CD8^+$ T cells through the same mechanisms described for NK cells (Fournel et al., 2000).

During the early phase of $CD4^+$ T cell activation, HLA-G:ILT2 interaction induces a cell cycle blockade at the G1 phase (Bahri et al., 2006), and inhibits allo-reactive T-cell proliferation (Naji et al., 2007a). Interestingly, it has been proposed that HLA-G isoforms have different impact on the cytokine secretion profile of $CD4^+$ T cells. HLA-G1 was indeed shown to promote T helper (h)2 polarization of naïve T cells (Kanai et al., 2001b; Kapasi et al., 2000) whereas HLA-G5 induces tumor necrosis factor (TNF)-α, IFN-γ, and IL-10 (Kanai et al., 2001a). Morandi et al. recently described that HLA-G5 has an additional effect on $CD4^+$ T cells since it down-regulates expression and function of CCR2, CXCR3, and CXCR4 on different subsets of activated $CD4^+$ T cells, impairing their migratory capability (Morandi et al., 2010).

The immunological functions of HLA-G on B cells are poorly described. It has been shown that in patients who underwent renal transplantation, serum levels of soluble HLA-G are negatively associated with anti-HLA antibodies and with graft rejection, suggesting that soluble HLA-G may possibly act to inhibit the immune humoral responses against HLA (Qiu et al., 2006). Further investigation is needed to better highlight the role of HLA-G in modulating B cell responses.

Myeloid antigen presenting cells (APCs) express both ILT2 and ILT4, which render them targets of HLA-G-mediated modulation. In the presence of HLA-G, myeloid APCs fail to stimulate allo-proliferative T cell responses *in vitro* (LeMaoult et al., 2004) and reduce NK-mediated cytotoxicity (Gros et al., 2008). Moreover, HLA-G inhibits the up-regulation of HLA Class II, CD80 and CD86 on myeloid DCs in response to LPS or allo-activation signals *in vitro* (Ristich et al., 2007) (Gros et al., 2008). Thus, HLA-G inhibits the functions and differentiation of myeloid APCs, leading to improper T lymphocyte activation and to impair NK cytotoxic activity. However, HLA-G does not block myeloid APCs functions, but induces them to differentiate into tolerogenic cells. Several reports indeed show that HLA-G treatment up-regulates the expression of cytokines, chemokines, and chemokine receptors by myeloid APCs (Apps et al., 2007; Gros et al., 2008; Li et al., 2009; Liang et al., 2008). The first evidence that HLA-G promotes the induction of tolerogenic APCs comes from studies conducted by the group of Horuzsko demonstrating that HLA-G treatment of monocyte-derived DCs that highly express ILT2 and ILT4 results in cells with tolerogenic-like phenotype and the potential to induce T-cell anergy (Ristich et al., 2005). Results obtained in a murine model support this notion by showing that HLA-G inhibited maturation of DCs (Horuzsko et al., 2001) and that in ILT4 transgenic mice, the HLA-G:ILT4 interaction impaired DC maturation *in vivo*, leading to delayed skin allograft rejection (Liang et al., 2002). Thereby, HLA-G by interacting with ILT receptors present on myeloid APCs induces their differentiation into regulatory cells.

4.2 Long-term tolerogenic properties of HLA-G

Myeloid APCs are not only the cells more sensitive to HLA-G-mediated modulation, but they also commonly express HLA-G. Myeloid APCs may express all HLA-G isoforms (Le Friec et al., 2004), but cell-surface HLA-G1 and secreted HLA-G5 have been described the most. In pathological contexts including transplantation, cancer, viral infections, and inflammatory diseases, the expression of HLA-G on myeloid cells can be up-regulated (Carosella et al., 2008). Recently, in liver-transplanted patients, the presence of HLA-G-expressing myeloid DCs has been correlated with tolerance and graft acceptance (Castellaneta et al., 2011). Similarly, in cancer (reviewed in (Amiot et al., 2011) as well as in viral infections (reviewed in (Fainardi et al., 2011), myeloid APCs expressing HLA-G were reported, and often correlated with poor clinical outcomes. Myeloid APCs not only express membrane-bound HLA-G1 but they may also secrete or shed HLA-G molecules, contributing to the generation of a tolerogenic microenvironment. Such a microenvironment may alter the functions not only of lymphocytes, but also of the HLA-G-expressing myeloid APCs themselves, in a tolerogenic feedback loop. HLA-G can indeed directly promote its expression and the expression of its receptors on myeloid APCs (LeMaoult et al., 2005). Thus, myeloid APCs may be viewed as suppressor cells capable of inhibiting other immune effectors, and also of generating regulatory cells including Treg cells.

Treg cells are critical players for preservation of immune homeostasis and for establishment and maintenance of peripheral tolerance. Treg cells belonging to different T cell subsets, including $CD4^+$ and $CD8^+$, NKT, and γδ T cells. The best characterized Treg populations are the forkhead box P3 (FOXP3)-expressing, $CD4^+CD25^+$ Tregs ($FOXP3^+$ Tregs) (Sakaguchi et al., 2010), and the $CD4^+$ IL-10-producing Tr1 cells (Akdis et al., 2004; Barrat et al., 2002; Groux et al., 1997; Roncarolo et al., 2006). $FOXP3^+$ Tregs and Tr1 cells are distinct populations of Treg cells that play a non-redundant role in maintaining tolerance, and are distinguished from one another by their distinct phenotype and cytokine profiling. FOXP3+ Treg cells are characterized by the constitutively-high expression of CD25 and the transcription factor FOXP3 (Sakaguchi, 2005), and their development and function is strictly dependent on FOXP3 (Bacchetta et al., 2007; Gavin et al., 2007). Tr1 cells can be induced in the periphery upon chronic antigen (Ag) stimulation in the presence of IL-10 (Roncarolo et al., 2006), and are currently identified by their unique cytokine profile consisting of high levels of IL-10, TGF-β, and low levels of IL-2 and IFN-γ and the absence of IL-4 after stimulation (Bacchetta et al., 1994; Groux et al., 1997). Once activated through their specific TCR, Tr1 cells secrete IL-10 and TGF-β that directly inhibit effector T cell proliferation and expression of HLA class II and co-stimulatory molecules on APCs, which indirectly suppress effector T-cell activation. More recently, we demonstrated that Tr1 cells specifically kill myeloid cells *via* a Granzyme B-dependent mechanism (Magnani et al., 2011).

HLA-G-expressing APCs were shown to be capable of priming naïve T cells to become Treg cells. Indeed, APC lines over-expressing membrane-bound HLA-G1 induced the differentiation of $CD4^{+}$ and $CD8^{+}$ T cells able to inhibit allogeneic responses (LeMaoult et al., 2004). Resulting HLA-G-induced Treg cells included $CD4^{low}$ and $CD8^{low}$ T cells that suppress *via* soluble factors (Naji et al., 2007a; Naji et al., 2007b). These results are in agreement with those obtained in patients who received a combined liver-kidney transplant, in which high plasma levels of HLA-G5 correlated with an increased percentage of suppressor T cells (Le Rond et al., 2004; Naji et al., 2007b). They are also in line with results showing that high HLA-G5 plasma levels in the peripheral blood of stem cell-transplanted patients are associated with the expansion in peripheral blood of $CD4^{+}CD25^{+}CD152^{+}$ T cells with suppressive activity (Le Maux et al., 2008).

We recently identified and characterized a new subset of human DCs that arises in the presence of IL-10 and endogenously expresses cell-surface HLA-G (Gregori et al., 2010). DC-10 are characterized by the outstanding ability to produce IL-10 and by the expression of high levels of membrane-bound HLA-G1 and other tolerogenic signaling molecules such as ILT2, ILT3, and ILT4 (Fig. 3).

DC-10 are potent inducers of adaptive allo-specific Tr1 cells (Gregori et al., 2010). Furthermore, allergen-specific Tr1 cells can be generated *in vitro* by stimulating human T cells with autologous tolerogenic DC-10 pulsed with allergen (Pacciani et al., 2010). Interestingly, the expression of membrane-bound HLA-G1 and that of its receptors are up-regulated by IL-10 on both DC-10 and T cells, and the expression of high levels of membrane-bound HLA-G1, ILT4, and IL-10 by DC-10 is critical to the generation of Tr1 cells by DC-10 (Rossetti et al., 2011).

5. HLA-G expressing regulatory cells

In addition to myeloid cells that can constitutively or transiently express HLA-G, T cells or other immune cells can express or secrete HLA-G.

A subpopulation of $CD4^{+}$ $HLA\text{-}G1^{+}$ and $CD8^{+}$ $HLA\text{-}G1^{+}$ T cells has been described (Feger et al., 2007). They represent a small subset of peripheral blood cells in healthy individuals, but

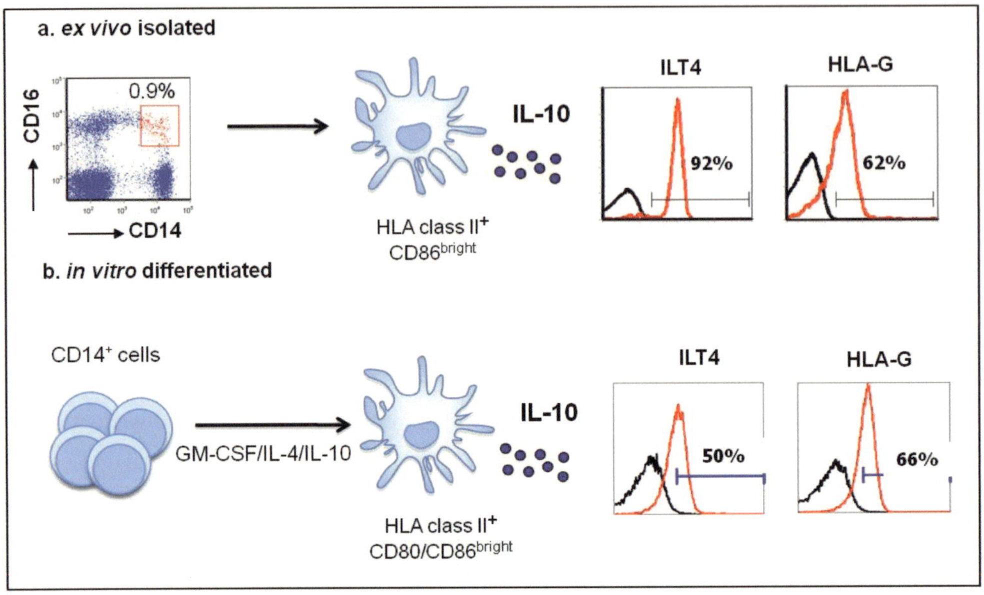

Fig. 3. A unique subset of human tolerogenic DC: DC-10

A. DC-10 are present *in vivo* and characterized by the expression of the surface markers CD14, CD16, CD83. They also express high levels of HLA-G1 and its receptor ILT4. **B.** DC-10 can be differentiated *in vitro* starting from the CD14+ fraction of PBMCs cultured for 7 days in the presence of GM-CSF, IL-4 and IL-10.

are increased at sites of inflammation, such as in the central nervous system of patients with neuro-inflammatory disorders and in muscle tissue in patients with idiopathic myositis (Feger et al., 2007; Huang et al., 2009a; Wiendl et al., 2005). $CD4^+$ HLA-$G1^+$ T cells represent a population of naturally occurring Treg cells distinct from nTreg cells, since they lack CD25 and FOXP3 expression. HLA-G^+ Treg cells showed reduced proliferation in response to allogeneic (mDCs) and polyclonal stimulation (αCD3/CD28), and have a cytokine profiling different from Tr1 cells. $CD4^+$ HLA-G^+ and $CD8^+$ HLA-G^+ Treg cells inhibit the proliferation of autologous HLA-G^- T cells through HLA-G1/sHLA-G1 (Feger et al., 2007) and soluble factors, including IL-10 (Huang et al., 2009b). A population of induced HLA-G^+ T cells has been also described, these allo-specific $CD4^+$ and $CD8^+$ T cells were shown to express HLA-G1 and to secrete HLA-G5 (Le Rond et al., 2004; Lila et al., 2001). Moreover, we demonstrated that up-regulation of HLA-G on $CD4^+$ T cells is critically required for DC-10 mediated induction of adoptive Tr1 cells (Gregori et al., 2010).

Adult bone marrow MSCs can also express HLA-G and have been included in the list of regulatory cells. MSCs are multipotent cells that play an important role in tissue regeneration and also have strong immuno-modulatory properties (reviewed in (Uccelli et al., 2008)). MSCs express low levels of HLA Class I molecules, do not express HLA class II or co-stimulatory molecules, and therefore do not induce T-cell activation. It has been demonstrated that MSCs constitutively express HLA-G5 (Selmani et al., 2009). Even though HLA-G expression decrease during MSCs expansion *in vitro*, recent studies clearly identified it as a key contributor to MSCs immune-tolerogenic functions (Nasef et al., 2007; Rizzo et al.,

2008; Selmani et al., 2008). In addition to a direct suppressive function through HLA-G5, MSCs can induce *via* a cell-to-cell contact mechanism CD4+ CD25high Foxp3+ Treg cells (Selmani et al., 2008).

6. HLA-G and its polymorphisms

Very few polymorphisms have been identified in the coding region of the HLA-G locus. The heavy chain encoding region exhibits 33 Single Nucleotide Polymorphisms (SNPs) but only 13 amino acid variations are observed. This peculiarity is important in determining the biological function of HLA-G, since a reduced variability leads to a limited peptide repertoire and presentation capability (Clements et al., 2005), and can influence the polymerization rate. Moreover, the 5′ Up-stream Regulatory Region (5′ URR), containing the promoter, and the 3′ untranslated region (UTR) exhibit numerous nucleotide variations that may influence HLA-G expression (Donadi et al., 2011; Larsen and Hviid, 2009) and consequently its tissue distribution in healthy and pathological conditions (Fig. 4).

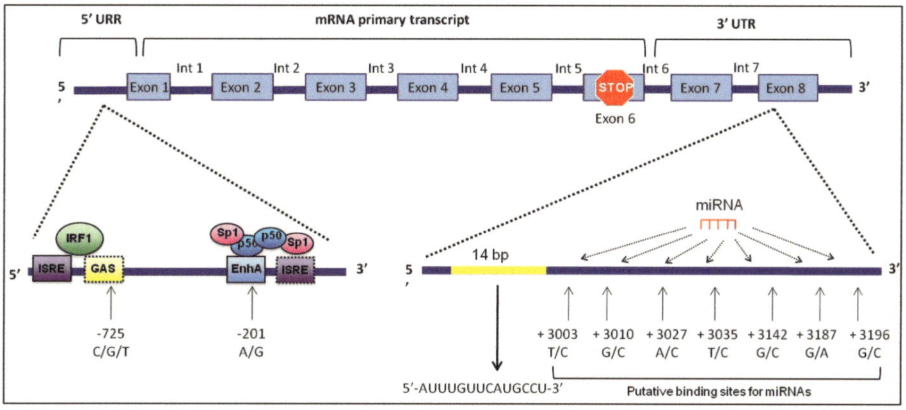

Fig. 4. HLA-G locus and its polymorphisms

Schematic representation of HLA-G locus. The major polymorphisms observed at the 5′URR and at 3′UTR regions are indicated. URR: Up-stream regulatory region; UTR: Untraslated region.

6.1 5′ up-stream regulatory region (URR)

Because of the presence of regulatory elements, polymorphisms at the 5′ URR might have a relevant impact in the regulation of HLA-G expression (Fig. 4). The region up-stream from the transcriptional start site of HLA-G contains 27 different polymorphisms but only 13 of them are within or very close to known transcription factor binding sites or regulatory elements (Hviid et al., 1999; Ober et al., 2003; Tan et al., 2005). Interestingly, all the 27 polymorphisms are in strong linkage disequilibrium (LD) and define 13 unique promoter haplotypes (Ober et al., 2003; Tan et al., 2005). Among the 5′ URR polymorphisms, only the -725C/G/T single nucleotide polymorphism (SNP) has been associated with HLA-G expression. Ober et al. demonstrated that the presence of G in position -725 significantly increases HLA-G transcription rate in JEG-3 cell line (Ober et al., 2006) and, when it is present in both parents, it is significantly associated with fetal loss rate (Ober et al., 2003).

An additional interesting SNP located in 5' URR is the -201 A/G SNP since it resides into the enhancer A region (Hviid et al., 1999). However, it still remains to be clarified if this polymorphism has any impact on the expression of certain HLA-G alleles.

6.2 3'untraslated region (UTR)

The exon 7 of the HLA-G locus is always absent in the mature messenger(m)RNA. Moreover, due to the presence of a stop codon in the exon 6 of HLA-G, the exon 8 is not translated. Thus, exon 8 is considered the 3' UTR of the mature RNA. This region contains several regulatory elements (Kuersten and Goodwin, 2003), including polyadenylation signals, AU-rich elements (Alvarez et al., 2009), and several polymorphic sites that may potentially influence mRNA stability, turnover, mobility and splicing pattern. 3'UTR polymorphisms that can influence HLA-G expression are: i) the insertion (INS) or deletion (DEL) of a 14bp fragment (14bp INS/DEL) that has been associated with mRNA stability; ii) the SNP at position +3142, which may be a target for certain microRNAs (miRNAs), small RNA sequences which once bound to a complementary mRNA lead to its translational repression or degradation and gene silencing (Bartel, 2009); iii) additional six SNPs landed in putative binding sites for miRNAs (Castelli et al., 2009) (Fig.4).

The first identified 3'UTR HLA-G polymorphism is the 14bp INS/DEL and has been studied the most. The insertion of the 14bp fragment, results in the formation of a cryptic breakpoint in the mRNA that loose the first 92bp of exon 8 (Hviid et al., 2003). Rousseau et al. demonstrated that HLA-G transcript with the 92bp deleted seems to be more stable than the complete mRNA fragment generated by the 14bp DEL (Rousseau et al., 2003), suggesting that 14bp INS might be associated with high levels of HLA-G expression. Nonetheless, several groups have demonstrated that 14 bp INS/INS genotype is associated with lower serum and plasma level of sHLA-G1/HLA-G5 compared to those observed in 14bp INS/DEL and 14bp DEL/DEL genotypes (Chen et al., 2008; Hviid et al., 2004; Hviid et al., 2006), an observation that constitutes the "14bp paradox". Consistently, conflicting results have been obtained in different studies concerning the association of the 14bp HLA-G genotypes with autoimmune diseases, pathological pregnancy, recurrent spontaneous abortions, and pre-eclampsia. Notably, the presence of 14bp DEL has been found to be predictive for the incidence of GvHD after unrelated (La Nasa et al., 2007) and HLA-identical sibling (Sizzano et al., in press) Human Stem Cell Transplantation (HSCT) for beta-thalassemia.

Several SNPs at 3'UTR of HLA-G locus have been identified (Castelli et al., 2009). Among them, the +3142 C/G SNP has been proposed to be critically involved in HLA-G regulation since it is associated with asthma (Tan et al., 2005). The G variant of a G/C SNP at position +3142 of the 3'UTR has been hypothesized to increase the affinity of the resulting mRNA for miR-148a, miR-148b and miR-152 (Veit and Chies, 2009). Among these miRNAs, only miR-152 has been demonstrated responsible for HLA-G post-transcriptional regulation. Indeed, over-expression of miR-152 in JEG-3 cell lines resulted in decreasing HLA-G expression and increased susceptibility to NK cell-mediated cytolysis (Zhu et al., 2010).

In silico analysis of the 3'UTR of the HLA-G locus revealed the presence of additional six SNPs that are landed in putative binding sites for miRNAs (Castelli et al., 2009). Interestingly the 14bp INS/DEL and the 7 SNPs arrange in different combinations to generate eight distinct haplotypes of 3'UTR HLA-G region (Castelli et al., 2010) (Table 1).

Therefore, it has been hypothesized that the expression of HLA-G might be influenced by a combination of specific polymorphisms. Our group is currently investigating the impact of the HLA-G 3'UTR haplotypes on HLA-G expression. Preliminary results indicate that different 3'UTR HLA-G haplotypes are associated with variable levels of HLA-G1 expression on myeloid APCs.

Haplotype	14-bp	+3003	+3010	+3027	+3035	+3142
UTR-1	Del	T	G	C	C	C
UTR-2	Ins	T	C	C	C	G
UTR-3	Del	T	C	C	C	G
UTR-4	Del	C	G	C	C	C
UTR-5	Ins	T	C	C	T	G
UTR-6	Del	T	G	C	C	C
UTR-7	Ins	T	C	A	T	G
UTR-8	Ins	T	G	C	C	G

Table 1. 3'UTR HLA-G haplotypes

7. Conclusions and perspectives

Since the discovery of HLA-G, research has established its role in modulating immune responses and inducing tolerance. While a great deal of progress has been made in understanding the mechanisms underlying immune modulation by HLA-G, several questions remain to be clarified. First, HLA-G can promote the differentiation of regulatory cells and HLA-G-expressing cells act as regulatory cells, however additional studies are required to better define their role in promoting tolerance. Second, although it is generally accepted that 5' URR and 3' UTR are involved in HLA-G expression, further investigation are needed to elucidate the molecular mechanisms involved in HLA-G regulation. Third, 3'UTR HLA-G haplotypes have been identified, future studies are warranted to define whether they can influence the transcriptional rate of HLA-G isoforms and their functions. Answering these questions will not only bring us closer to understanding how HLA-G function, but also how to exploit or modulate its suppressive activity for targeted therapy against a wide variety of diseases.

8. Acknowledgement

This work was supported by Telethon Foundation, the Associazione Italiana per la Ricerca sul Cancro (AIRC) IG 8978, and the Italian Ministry of Health.

9. References

Akdis, M., Verhagen, J., Taylor, A., Karamloo, F., Karagiannidis, C., Crameri, R., Thunberg, S., Deniz, G., Valenta, R., Fiebig, H., *et al.* (2004). Immune responses in healthy and allergic individuals are characterized by a fine balance between allergen-specific T regulatory 1 and T helper 2 cells. The Journal of experimental medicine *199*, 1567-1575.

Akhter, A., Das, V., Naik, S., Faridi, R.M., Pandey, A., and Agrawal, S. (2011). Upregulation of HLA-G in JEG-3 cells by dexamethasone and hydrocortisone. Archives of gynecology and obstetrics.

Allan, D.S., Colonna, M., Lanier, L.L., Churakova, T.D., Abrams, J.S., Ellis, S.A., McMichael, A.J., and Braud, V.M. (1999). Tetrameric complexes of human histocompatibility leukocyte antigen (HLA)-G bind to peripheral blood myelomonocytic cells. The Journal of experimental medicine *189*, 1149-1156.

Alvarez, M., Piedade, J., Balseiro, S., Ribas, G., and Regateiro, F. (2009). HLA-G 3'-UTR SNP and 14-bp deletion polymorphisms in Portuguese and Guinea-Bissau populations. Int J Immunogenet *36*, 361-366.

Amiot, L., Ferrone, S., Grosse-Wilde, H., and Seliger, B. (2011). Biology of HLA-G in cancer: a candidate molecule for therapeutic intervention? Cell Mol Life Sci *68*, 417-431.

Apps, R., Gardner, L., Sharkey, A.M., Holmes, N., and Moffett, A. (2007). A homodimeric complex of HLA-G on normal trophoblast cells modulates antigen-presenting cells via LILRB1. Eur J Immunol *37*, 1924-1937.

Bacchetta, R., Bigler, M., Touraine, J.L., Parkman, R., Tovo, P.A., Abrams, J., de Waal Malefyt, R., de Vries, J.E., and Roncarolo, M.G. (1994). High levels of interleukin 10 production in vivo are associated with tolerance in SCID patients transplanted with HLA mismatched hematopoietic stem cells. The Journal of experimental medicine *179*, 493-502.

Bacchetta, R., Gambineri, E., and Roncarolo, M.G. (2007). Role of regulatory T cells and FOXP3 in human diseases. J Allergy Clin Immunol *120*, 227-235; quiz 236-227.

Bahri, R., Hirsch, F., Josse, A., Rouas-Freiss, N., Bidere, N., Vasquez, A., Carosella, E.D., Charpentier, B., and Durrbach, A. (2006). Soluble HLA-G inhibits cell cycle progression in human alloreactive T lymphocytes. J Immunol *176*, 1331-1339.

Barrat, F.J., Cua, D.J., Boonstra, A., Richards, D.F., Crain, C., Savelkoul, H.F., de Waal-Malefyt, R., Coffman, R.L., Hawrylowicz, C.M., and O'Garra, A. (2002). In vitro generation of interleukin 10-producing regulatory CD4(+) T cells is induced by immunosuppressive drugs and inhibited by T helper type 1 (Th1)- and Th2-inducing cytokines. The Journal of experimental medicine *195*, 603-616.

Bartel, D.P. (2009). MicroRNAs: target recognition and regulatory functions. Cell *136*, 215-233.

Boyson, J.E., Erskine, R., Whitman, M.C., Chiu, M., Lau, J.M., Koopman, L.A., Valter, M.M., Angelisova, P., Horejsi, V., and Strominger, J.L. (2002). Disulfide bond-mediated dimerization of HLA-G on the cell surface. Proc Natl Acad Sci U S A *99*, 16180-16185.

Carosella, E.D. (2011). The tolerogenic molecule HLA-G. Immunol Lett.

Carosella, E.D., Favier, B., Rouas-Freiss, N., Moreau, P., and Lemaoult, J. (2008). Beyond the increasing complexity of the immunomodulatory HLA-G molecule. Blood *111*, 4862-4870.

Carosella, E.D., Moreau, P., Le Maoult, J., Le Discorde, M., Dausset, J., and Rouas-Freiss, N. (2003). HLA-G molecules: from maternal-fetal tolerance to tissue acceptance. Adv Immunol *81*, 199-252.

Carosella, E.D., Rouas-Freiss, N., Paul, P., and Dausset, J. (1999). HLA-G: a tolerance molecule from the major histocompatibility complex. Immunol Today *20*, 60-62.

Castellaneta, A., Mazariegos, G.V., Nayyar, N., Zeevi, A., and Thomson, A.W. (2011). HLA-G level on monocytoid dendritic cells correlates with regulatory T-cell Foxp3 expression in liver transplant tolerance. Transplantation *91*, 1132-1140.

Castelli, E.C., Mendes-Junior, C.T., Deghaide, N.H., de Albuquerque, R.S., Muniz, Y.C., Simoes, R.T., Carosella, E.D., Moreau, P., and Donadi, E.A. (2010). The genetic structure of 3'untranslated region of the HLA-G gene: polymorphisms and haplotypes. Genes Immun *11*, 134-141.

Castelli, E.C., Moreau, P., Oya e Chiromatzo, A., Mendes-Junior, C.T., Veiga-Castelli, L.C., Yaghi, L., Giuliatti, S., Carosella, E.D., and Donadi, E.A. (2009). In silico analysis of microRNAS targeting the HLA-G 3' untranslated region alleles and haplotypes. Human immunology *70*, 1020-1025.

Caumartin, J., Favier, B., Daouya, M., Guillard, C., Moreau, P., Carosella, E.D., and LeMaoult, J. (2007). Trogocytosis-based generation of suppressive NK cells. EMBO J *26*, 1423-1433.

Chen, X.Y., Yan, W.H., Lin, A., Xu, H.H., Zhang, J.G., and Wang, X.X. (2008). The 14 bp deletion polymorphisms in HLA-G gene play an important role in the expression of soluble HLA-G in plasma. Tissue Antigens *72*, 335-341.

Chung, D.J., Rossi, M., Romano, E., Ghith, J., Yuan, J., Munn, D.H., and Young, J.W. (2009). Indoleamine 2,3-dioxygenase-expressing mature human monocyte-derived dendritic cells expand potent autologous regulatory T cells. Blood *114*, 555-563.

Clements, C.S., Kjer-Nielsen, L., Kostenko, L., Hoare, H.L., Dunstone, M.A., Moses, E., Freed, K., Brooks, A.G., Rossjohn, J., and McCluskey, J. (2005). Crystal structure of HLA-G: a nonclassical MHC class I molecule expressed at the fetal-maternal interface. Proc Natl Acad Sci U S A *102*, 3360-3365.

Clements, C.S., Kjer-Nielsen, L., McCluskey, J., and Rossjohn, J. (2007). Structural studies on HLA-G: implications for ligand and receptor binding. Human immunology *68*, 220-226.

Colonna, M., Navarro, F., Bellon, T., Llano, M., Garcia, P., Samaridis, J., Angman, L., Cella, M., and Lopez-Botet, M. (1997). A common inhibitory receptor for major histocompatibility complex class I molecules on human lymphoid and myelomonocytic cells. The Journal of experimental medicine *186*, 1809-1818.

Colonna, M., Samaridis, J., Cella, M., Angman, L., Allen, R.L., O'Callaghan, C.A., Dunbar, R., Ogg, G.S., Cerundolo, V., and Rolink, A. (1998). Human myelomonocytic cells express an inhibitory receptor for classical and nonclassical MHC class I molecules. J Immunol *160*, 3096-3100.

Contini, P., Ghio, M., Poggi, A., Filaci, G., Indiveri, F., Ferrone, S., and Puppo, F. (2003). Soluble HLA-A,-B,-C and -G molecules induce apoptosis in T and NK CD8+ cells and inhibit cytotoxic T cell activity through CD8 ligation. Eur J Immunol *33*, 125-134.

Davis, D.M. (2007). Intercellular transfer of cell-surface proteins is common and can affect many stages of an immune response. Nat Rev Immunol *7*, 238-243.

Deschaseaux, F., Delgado, D., Pistoia, V., Giuliani, M., Morandi, F., and Durrbach, A. (2011). HLA-G in organ transplantation: towards clinical applications. Cell Mol Life Sci *68*, 397-404.

Diaz-Lagares, A., Alegre, E., LeMaoult, J., Carosella, E.D., and Gonzalez, A. (2009). Nitric oxide produces HLA-G nitration and induces metalloprotease-dependent shedding creating a tolerogenic milieu. Immunology *126*, 436-445.

Donadi, E.A., Castelli, E.C., Arnaiz-Villena, A., Roger, M., Rey, D., and Moreau, P. (2011). Implications of the polymorphism of HLA-G on its function, regulation, evolution and disease association. Cell Mol Life Sci *68*, 369-395.

Fainardi, E., Castellazzi, M., Stignani, M., Morandi, F., Sana, G., Gonzalez, R., Pistoia, V., Baricordi, O.R., Sokal, E., and Pena, J. (2011). Emerging topics and new perspectives on HLA-G. Cell Mol Life Sci *68*, 433-451.

Favier, B., Lemaoult, J., Lesport, E., and Carosella, E.D. (2010). ILT2/HLA-G interaction impairs NK-cell functions through the inhibition of the late but not the early events of the NK-cell activating synapse. FASEB J *24*, 689-699.

Feger, U., Tolosa, E., Huang, Y.H., Waschbisch, A., Biedermann, T., Melms, A., and Wiendl, H. (2007). HLA-G expression defines a novel regulatory T-cell subset present in human peripheral blood and sites of inflammation. Blood *110*, 568-577.

Fournel, S., Aguerre-Girr, M., Huc, X., Lenfant, F., Alam, A., Toubert, A., Bensussan, A., and Le Bouteiller, P. (2000). Cutting edge: soluble HLA-G1 triggers CD95/CD95 ligand-mediated apoptosis in activated CD8+ cells by interacting with CD8. J Immunol *164*, 6100-6104.

Fujii, T., Ishitani, A., and Geraghty, D.E. (1994). A soluble form of the HLA-G antigen is encoded by a messenger ribonucleic acid containing intron 4. J Immunol *153*, 5516-5524.

Gavin, M.A., Rasmussen, J.P., Fontenot, J.D., Vasta, V., Manganiello, V.C., Beavo, J.A., and Rudensky, A.Y. (2007). Foxp3-dependent programme of regulatory T-cell differentiation. Nature *445*, 771-775.

Gobin, S.J., Keijsers, V., van Zutphen, M., and van den Elsen, P.J. (1998). The role of enhancer A in the locus-specific transactivation of classical and nonclassical HLA class I genes by nuclear factor kappa B. J Immunol *161*, 2276-2283.

Gobin, S.J., van Zutphen, M., Woltman, A.M., and van den Elsen, P.J. (1999). Transactivation of classical and nonclassical HLA class I genes through the IFN-stimulated response element. J Immunol *163*, 1428-1434.

Gonen-Gross, T., Achdout, H., Arnon, T.I., Gazit, R., Stern, N., Horejsi, V., Goldman-Wohl, D., Yagel, S., and Mandelboim, O. (2005). The CD85J/leukocyte inhibitory receptor-1 distinguishes between conformed and beta 2-microglobulin-free HLA-G molecules. J Immunol *175*, 4866-4874.

Gonen-Gross, T., Achdout, H., Gazit, R., Hanna, J., Mizrahi, S., Markel, G., Goldman-Wohl, D., Yagel, S., Horejsi, V., Levy, O., *et al.* (2003). Complexes of HLA-G protein on the cell surface are important for leukocyte Ig-like receptor-1 function. J Immunol *171*, 1343-1351.

Gonzalez-Hernandez, A., LeMaoult, J., Lopez, A., Alegre, E., Caumartin, J., Le Rond, S., Daouya, M., Moreau, P., and Carosella, E.D. (2005). Linking two immuno-suppressive molecules: indoleamine 2,3 dioxygenase can modify HLA-G cell-surface expression. Biol Reprod *73*, 571-578.

Goodridge, J.P., Witt, C.S., Christiansen, F.T., and Warren, H.S. (2003). KIR2DL4 (CD158d) genotype influences expression and function in NK cells. J Immunol *171*, 1768-1774.

Gregori, S., Tomasoni, D., Pacciani, V., Scirpoli, M., Battaglia, M., Magnani, C.F., Hauben, E., and Roncarolo, M.G. (2010). Differentiation of type 1 T regulatory cells (Tr1) by tolerogenic DC-10 requires the IL-10-dependent ILT4/HLA-G pathway. Blood *116*, 935-944.

Gros, F., Cabillic, F., Toutirais, O., Maux, A.L., Sebti, Y., and Amiot, L. (2008). Soluble HLA-G molecules impair natural killer/dendritic cell crosstalk via inhibition of dendritic cells. Eur J Immunol *38*, 742-749.

Groux, H., O'Garra, A., Bigler, M., Rouleau, M., Antonenko, S., de Vries, J.E., and Roncarolo, M.G. (1997). A CD4+ T-cell subset inhibits antigen-specific T-cell responses and prevents colitis. Nature *389*, 737-742.

Horuzsko, A., Lenfant, F., Munn, D.H., and Mellor, A.L. (2001). Maturation of antigen-presenting cells is compromised in HLA-G transgenic mice. Int Immunol *13*, 385-394.

HoWangYin, K.Y., Alegre, E., Daouya, M., Favier, B., Carosella, E.D., and LeMaoult, J. (2011). Different functional outcomes of intercellular membrane transfers to monocytes and T cells. Cell Mol Life Sci *67*, 1133-1145.

Huang, Y.H., Zozulya, A.L., Weidenfeller, C., Metz, I., Buck, D., Toyka, K.V., Bruck, W., and Wiendl, H. (2009a). Specific central nervous system recruitment of HLA-G(+) regulatory T cells in multiple sclerosis. Ann Neurol *66*, 171-183.

Huang, Y.H., Zozulya, A.L., Weidenfeller, C., Schwab, N., and Wiendl, H. (2009b). T cell suppression by naturally occurring HLA-G-expressing regulatory CD4+ T cells is IL-10-dependent and reversible. Journal of leukocyte biology.

Hviid, T.V., Hylenius, S., Rorbye, C., and Nielsen, L.G. (2003). HLA-G allelic variants are associated with differences in the HLA-G mRNA isoform profile and HLA-G mRNA levels. Immunogenetics *55*, 63-79.

Hviid, T.V., Rizzo, R., Christiansen, O.B., Melchiorri, L., Lindhard, A., and Baricordi, O.R. (2004). HLA-G and IL-10 in serum in relation to HLA-G genotype and polymorphisms. Immunogenetics *56*, 135-141.

Hviid, T.V., Rizzo, R., Melchiorri, L., Stignani, M., and Baricordi, O.R. (2006). Polymorphism in the 5' upstream regulatory and 3' untranslated regions of the HLA-G gene in relation to soluble HLA-G and IL-10 expression. Human immunology *67*, 53-62.

Hviid, T.V., Sorensen, S., and Morling, N. (1999). Polymorphism in the regulatory region located more than 1.1 kilobases 5' to the start site of transcription, the promoter region, and exon 1 of the HLA-G gene. Human immunology *60*, 1237-1244.

Ishitani, A., and Geraghty, D.E. (1992). Alternative splicing of HLA-G transcripts yields proteins with primary structures resembling both class I and class II antigens. Proc Natl Acad Sci U S A *89*, 3947-3951.

Kanai, T., Fujii, T., Kozuma, S., Yamashita, T., Miki, A., Kikuchi, A., and Taketani, Y. (2001a). Soluble HLA-G influences the release of cytokines from allogeneic peripheral blood mononuclear cells in culture. Mol Hum Reprod *7*, 195-200.

Kanai, T., Fujii, T., Unno, N., Yamashita, T., Hyodo, H., Miki, A., Hamai, Y., Kozuma, S., and Taketani, Y. (2001b). Human leukocyte antigen-G-expressing cells differently modulate the release of cytokines from mononuclear cells present in the decidua versus peripheral blood. Am J Reprod Immunol *45*, 94-99.

Kapasi, K., Albert, S.E., Yie, S., Zavazava, N., and Librach, C.L. (2000). HLA-G has a concentration-dependent effect on the generation of an allo-CTL response. Immunology *101*, 191-200.

Kuersten, S., and Goodwin, E.B. (2003). The power of the 3' UTR: translational control and development. Nat Rev Genet *4*, 626-637.

La Nasa, G., Littera, R., Locatelli, F., Lai, S., Alba, F., Caocci, G., Lisini, D., Nesci, S., Vacca, A., Piras, E., *et al.* (2007). The human leucocyte antigen-G 14-basepair polymorphism correlates with graft-versus-host disease in unrelated bone marrow transplantation for thalassaemia. Br J Haematol *139*, 284-288.

Larsen, M.H., and Hviid, T.V. (2009). Human leukocyte antigen-G polymorphism in relation to expression, function, and disease. Human immunology *70*, 1026-1034.

Le Friec, G., Gros, F., Sebti, Y., Guilloux, V., Pangault, C., Fauchet, R., and Amiot, L. (2004). Capacity of myeloid and plasmacytoid dendritic cells especially at mature stage to express and secrete HLA-G molecules. Journal of leukocyte biology *76*, 1125-1133.

Le Gal, F.A., Riteau, B., Sedlik, C., Khalil-Daher, I., Menier, C., Dausset, J., Guillet, J.G., Carosella, E.D., and Rouas-Freiss, N. (1999). HLA-G-mediated inhibition of antigen-specific cytotoxic T lymphocytes. Int Immunol *11*, 1351-1356.

Le Maux, A., Noel, G., Birebent, B., Grosset, J.M., Vu, N., De Guibert, S., Bernard, M., Semana, G., and Amiot, L. (2008). Soluble human leucocyte antigen-G molecules in peripheral blood haematopoietic stem cell transplantation: a specific role to prevent acute graft-versus-host disease and a link with regulatory T cells. Clin Exp Immunol *152*, 50-56.

Le Rond, S., Le Maoult, J., Creput, C., Menier, C., Deschamps, M., Le Friec, G., Amiot, L., Durrbach, A., Dausset, J., Carosella, E.D., *et al.* (2004). Alloreactive CD4+ and CD8+ T cells express the immunotolerant HLA-G molecule in mixed lymphocyte reactions: in vivo implications in transplanted patients. Eur J Immunol *34*, 649-660.

Lefebvre, S., Berrih-Aknin, S., Adrian, F., Moreau, P., Poea, S., Gourand, L., Dausset, J., Carosella, E.D., and Paul, P. (2001). A specific interferon (IFN)-stimulated response element of the distal HLA-G promoter binds IFN-regulatory factor 1 and mediates enhancement of this nonclassical class I gene by IFN-beta. J Biol Chem *276*, 6133-6139.

LeMaoult, J., Caumartin, J., and Carosella, E.D. (2007a). Exchanges of membrane patches (trogocytosis) split theoretical and actual functions of immune cells. Human immunology *68*, 240-243.

LeMaoult, J., Caumartin, J., Daouya, M., Favier, B., Le Rond, S., Gonzalez, A., and Carosella, E.D. (2007b). Immune regulation by pretenders: cell-to-cell transfers of HLA-G make effector T cells act as regulatory cells. Blood *109*, 2040-2048.

LeMaoult, J., Krawice-Radanne, I., Dausset, J., and Carosella, E.D. (2004). HLA-G1-expressing antigen-presenting cells induce immunosuppressive CD4+ T cells. Proc Natl Acad Sci U S A *101*, 7064-7069.

LeMaoult, J., Zafaranloo, K., Le Danff, C., and Carosella, E.D. (2005). HLA-G up-regulates ILT2, ILT3, ILT4, and KIR2DL4 in antigen presenting cells, NK cells, and T cells. FASEB J *19*, 662-664.

Li, C., Houser, B.L., Nicotra, M.L., and Strominger, J.L. (2009). HLA-G homodimer-induced cytokine secretion through HLA-G receptors on human decidual macrophages and natural killer cells. Proc Natl Acad Sci U S A *106*, 5767-5772.

Liang, S., Baibakov, B., and Horuzsko, A. (2002). HLA-G inhibits the functions of murine dendritic cells via the PIR-B immune inhibitory receptor. Eur J Immunol *32*, 2418-2426.

Liang, S., Ristich, V., Arase, H., Dausset, J., Carosella, E.D., and Horuzsko, A. (2008). Modulation of dendritic cell differentiation by HLA-G and ILT4 requires the IL-6--STAT3 signaling pathway. Proc Natl Acad Sci U S A *105*, 8357-8362.

Lila, N., Rouas-Freiss, N., Dausset, J., Carpentier, A., and Carosella, E.D. (2001). Soluble HLA-G protein secreted by allo-specific CD4+ T cells suppresses the allo-proliferative response: a CD4+ T cell regulatory mechanism. Proc Natl Acad Sci U S A *98*, 12150-12155.

Lopez, A.S., Alegre, E., LeMaoult, J., Carosella, E., and Gonzalez, A. (2006). Regulatory role of tryptophan degradation pathway in HLA-G expression by human monocyte-derived dendritic cells. Mol Immunol *43*, 2151-2160.

Magnani, C.F., Alberigo, G., Bacchetta, R., Serafini, G., Andreani, M., Roncarolo, M.G., and Gregori, S. (2011). Killing of myeloid APCs via HLA class I, CD2 and CD226 defines a novel mechanism of suppression by human Tr1 cells. Eur J Immunol *41*, 1652-1662.

Morandi, F., Ferretti, E., Bocca, P., Prigione, I., Raffaghello, L., and Pistoia, V. (2010). A novel mechanism of soluble HLA-G mediated immune modulation: downregulation of T cell chemokine receptor expression and impairment of chemotaxis. PLoS One *5*, e11763.

Moreau, P., Adrian-Cabestre, F., Menier, C., Guiard, V., Gourand, L., Dausset, J., Carosella, E.D., and Paul, P. (1999). IL-10 selectively induces HLA-G expression in human trophoblasts and monocytes. Int Immunol *11*, 803-811.

Moreau, P., Faure, O., Lefebvre, S., Ibrahim, E.C., O'Brien, M., Gourand, L., Dausset, J., Carosella, E.D., and Paul, P. (2001). Glucocorticoid hormones upregulate levels of HLA-G transcripts in trophoblasts. Transplant Proc *33*, 2277-2280.

Moreau, P., Flajollet, S., and Carosella, E.D. (2009). Non-classical transcriptional regulation of HLA-G: an update. J Cell Mol Med *13*, 2973-2989.

Munn, D.H., Sharma, M.D., Lee, J.R., Jhaver, K.G., Johnson, T.S., Keskin, D.B., Marshall, B., Chandler, P., Antonia, S.J., Burgess, R., *et al.* (2002). Potential regulatory function of human dendritic cells expressing indoleamine 2,3-dioxygenase. Science *297*, 1867-1870.

Naji, A., Durrbach, A., Carosella, E.D., and Rouas-Freiss, N. (2007a). Soluble HLA-G and HLA-G1 expressing antigen-presenting cells inhibit T-cell alloproliferation through ILT-2/ILT-4/FasL-mediated pathways. Human immunology *68*, 233-239.

Naji, A., Le Rond, S., Durrbach, A., Krawice-Radanne, I., Creput, C., Daouya, M., Caumartin, J., LeMaoult, J., Carosella, E.D., and Rouas-Freiss, N. (2007b). CD3+CD4low and CD3+CD8low are induced by HLA-G: novel human peripheral blood suppressor T-cell subsets involved in transplant acceptance. Blood *110*, 3936-3948.

Nasef, A., Mathieu, N., Chapel, A., Frick, J., Francois, S., Mazurier, C., Boutarfa, A., Bouchet, S., Gorin, N.C., Thierry, D., *et al.* (2007). Immunosuppressive effects of mesenchymal stem cells: involvement of HLA-G. Transplantation *84*, 231-237.

Ober, C., Aldrich, C.L., Chervoneva, I., Billstrand, C., Rahimov, F., Gray, H.L., and Hyslop, T. (2003). Variation in the HLA-G promoter region influences miscarriage rates. Am J Hum Genet *72*, 1425-1435.

Ober, C., Billstrand, C., Kuldanek, S., and Tan, Z. (2006). The miscarriage-associated HLA-G -725G allele influences transcription rates in JEG-3 cells. Hum Reprod *21*, 1743-1748.

Onno, M., Le Friec, G., Pangault, C., Amiot, L., Guilloux, V., Drenou, B., Caulet-Maugendre, S., Andre, P., and Fauchet, R. (2000). Modulation of HLA-G antigens expression in myelomonocytic cells. Human immunology *61*, 1086-1094.

Pacciani, V., Gregori, S., Chini, L., Corrente, S., Chianca, M., Moschese, V., Rossi, P., Roncarolo, M.G., and Angelini, F. (2010). Induction of anergic allergen-specific suppressor T cells using tolerogenic dendritic cells derived from children with allergies to house dust mites. J Allergy Clin Immunol *125*, 727-736.

Park, G.M., Lee, S., Park, B., Kim, E., Shin, J., Cho, K., and Ahn, K. (2004). Soluble HLA-G generated by proteolytic shedding inhibits NK-mediated cell lysis. Biochem Biophys Res Commun *313*, 606-611.

Paul, P., Cabestre, F.A., Ibrahim, E.C., Lefebvre, S., Khalil-Daher, I., Vazeux, G., Quiles, R.M., Bermond, F., Dausset, J., and Carosella, E.D. (2000). Identification of HLA-G7 as a new splice variant of the HLA-G mRNA and expression of soluble HLA-G5, -G6, and -G7 transcripts in human transfected cells. Human immunology *61*, 1138-1149.

Qiu, J., Terasaki, P.I., Miller, J., Mizutani, K., Cai, J., and Carosella, E.D. (2006). Soluble HLA-G expression and renal graft acceptance. Am J Transplant *6*, 2152-2156.

Rajagopalan, S., Bryceson, Y.T., Kuppusamy, S.P., Geraghty, D.E., van der Meer, A., Joosten, I., and Long, E.O. (2006). Activation of NK cells by an endocytosed receptor for soluble HLA-G. PLoS Biol *4*, e9.

Rajagopalan, S., Fu, J., and Long, E.O. (2001). Cutting edge: induction of IFN-gamma production but not cytotoxicity by the killer cell Ig-like receptor KIR2DL4 (CD158d) in resting NK cells. J Immunol *167*, 1877-1881.

Rajagopalan, S., and Long, E.O. (1999). A human histocompatibility leukocyte antigen (HLA)-G-specific receptor expressed on all natural killer cells. The Journal of experimental medicine *189*, 1093-1100.

Ristich, V., Liang, S., Zhang, W., Wu, J., and Horuzsko, A. (2005). Tolerization of dendritic cells by HLA-G. Eur J Immunol *35*, 1133-1142.

Ristich, V., Zhang, W., Liang, S., and Horuzsko, A. (2007). Mechanisms of prolongation of allograft survival by HLA-G/ILT4-modified dendritic cells. Human immunology *68*, 264-271.

Riteau, B., Menier, C., Khalil-Daher, I., Martinozzi, S., Pla, M., Dausset, J., Carosella, E.D., and Rouas-Freiss, N. (2001). HLA-G1 co-expression boosts the HLA class I-mediated NK lysis inhibition. Int Immunol *13*, 193-201.

Rizzo, R., Campioni, D., Stignani, M., Melchiorri, L., Bagnara, G.P., Bonsi, L., Alviano, F., Lanzoni, G., Moretti, S., Cuneo, A., *et al.* (2008). A functional role for soluble HLA-G antigens in immune modulation mediated by mesenchymal stromal cells. Cytotherapy *10*, 364-375.

Rizzo, R., Ferrari, D., Melchiorri, L., Stignani, M., Gulinelli, S., Baricordi, O.R., and Di Virgilio, F. (2009). Extracellular ATP acting at the P2X7 receptor inhibits secretion of soluble HLA-G from human monocytes. J Immunol *183*, 4302-4311.

Roncarolo, M.G., Gregori, S., Battaglia, M., Bacchetta, R., Fleischhauer, K., and Levings, M.K. (2006). Interleukin-10-secreting type 1 regulatory T cells in rodents and humans. Immunological reviews *212*, 28-50.

Rossetti, M., Gregori, S., and Roncarolo, M.G. (2011). Granulocyte-colony stimulating factor drives the in vitro differentiation of human dendritic cells that induce anergy in naive T cells. Eur J Immunol *40*, 3097-3106.

Rouas-Freiss, N., Goncalves, R.M., Menier, C., Dausset, J., and Carosella, E.D. (1997). Direct evidence to support the role of HLA-G in protecting the fetus from maternal uterine natural killer cytolysis. Proc Natl Acad Sci U S A *94*, 11520-11525.

Rousseau, P., Le Discorde, M., Mouillot, G., Marcou, C., Carosella, E.D., and Moreau, P. (2003). The 14 bp deletion-insertion polymorphism in the 3' UT region of the HLA-G gene influences HLA-G mRNA stability. Human immunology *64*, 1005-1010.

Sakaguchi, S. (2005). Naturally arising Foxp3-expressing CD25+CD4+ regulatory T cells in immunological tolerance to self and non-self. Nat Immunol *6*, 345-352.

Sakaguchi, S., Miyara, M., Costantino, C.M., and Hafler, D.A. (2010). FOXP3+ regulatory T cells in the human immune system. Nat Rev Immunol *10*, 490-500.

Selmani, Z., Naji, A., Gaiffe, E., Obert, L., Tiberghien, P., Rouas-Freiss, N., Carosella, E.D., and Deschaseaux, F. (2009). HLA-G is a crucial immunosuppressive molecule secreted by adult human mesenchymal stem cells. Transplantation *87*, S62-66.

Selmani, Z., Naji, A., Zidi, I., Favier, B., Gaiffe, E., Obert, L., Borg, C., Saas, P., Tiberghien, P., Rouas-Freiss, N., *et al.* (2008). Human leukocyte antigen-G5 secretion by human mesenchymal stem cells is required to suppress T lymphocyte and natural killer function and to induce CD4+CD25highFOXP3+ regulatory T cells. Stem Cells *26*, 212-222.

Shiroishi, M., Kuroki, K., Ose, T., Rasubala, L., Shiratori, I., Arase, H., Tsumoto, K., Kumagai, I., Kohda, D., and Maenaka, K. (2006a). Efficient leukocyte Ig-like receptor signaling and crystal structure of disulfide-linked HLA-G dimer. J Biol Chem *281*, 10439-10447.

Shiroishi, M., Kuroki, K., Rasubala, L., Tsumoto, K., Kumagai, I., Kurimoto, E., Kato, K., Kohda, D., and Maenaka, K. (2006b). Structural basis for recognition of the nonclassical MHC molecule HLA-G by the leukocyte Ig-like receptor B2 (LILRB2/LIR2/ILT4/CD85d). Proc Natl Acad Sci U S A *103*, 16412-16417.

Shiroishi, M., Tsumoto, K., Amano, K., Shirakihara, Y., Colonna, M., Braud, V.M., Allan, D.S., Makadzange, A., Rowland-Jones, S., Willcox, B., *et al.* (2003). Human inhibitory receptors Ig-like transcript 2 (ILT2) and ILT4 compete with CD8 for MHC class I binding and bind preferentially to HLA-G. Proc Natl Acad Sci U S A *100*, 8856-8861.

Steimle, V., Durand, B., Barras, E., Zufferey, M., Hadam, M.R., Mach, B., and Reith, W. (1995). A novel DNA-binding regulatory factor is mutated in primary MHC class II deficiency (bare lymphocyte syndrome). Genes Dev *9*, 1021-1032.

Tan, Z., Shon, A.M., and Ober, C. (2005). Evidence of balancing selection at the HLA-G promoter region. Hum Mol Genet *14*, 3619-3628.

Uccelli, A., Moretta, L., and Pistoia, V. (2008). Mesenchymal stem cells in health and disease. Nat Rev Immunol *8*, 726-736.

Veit, T.D., and Chies, J.A. (2009). Tolerance versus immune response -- microRNAs as important elements in the regulation of the HLA-G gene expression. Transpl Immunol *20*, 229-231.

Wiendl, H., Feger, U., Mittelbronn, M., Jack, C., Schreiner, B., Stadelmann, C., Antel, J., Brueck, W., Meyermann, R., Bar-Or, A., *et al.* (2005). Expression of the immune-tolerogenic major histocompatibility molecule HLA-G in multiple sclerosis: implications for CNS immunity. Brain *128*, 2689-2704.

Yang, Y., Chu, W., Geraghty, D.E., and Hunt, J.S. (1996). Expression of HLA-G in human mononuclear phagocytes and selective induction by IFN-gamma. J Immunol *156*, 4224-4231.

Yie, S.M., Li, L.H., Li, G.M., Xiao, R., and Librach, C.L. (2006a). Progesterone enhances HLA-G gene expression in JEG-3 choriocarcinoma cells and human cytotrophoblasts in vitro. Hum Reprod *21*, 46-51.

Yie, S.M., Xiao, R., and Librach, C.L. (2006b). Progesterone regulates HLA-G gene expression through a novel progesterone response element. Hum Reprod *21*, 2538-2544.

Zhu, X.M., Han, T., Wang, X.H., Li, Y.H., Yang, H.G., Luo, Y.N., Yin, G.W., and Yao, Y.Q. (2010). Overexpression of miR-152 leads to reduced expression of human leukocyte antigen-G and increased natural killer cell mediated cytolysis in JEG-3 cells. Am J Obstet Gynecol *202*, 592 e591-597.

Zidi, I., Guillard, C., Marcou, C., Krawice-Radanne, I., Sangrouber, D., Rouas-Freiss, N., Carosella, E.D., and Moreau, P. (2006). Increase in HLA-G1 proteolytic shedding by tumor cells: a regulatory pathway controlled by NF-kappaB inducers. Cell Mol Life Sci *63*, 2669-2681.

3

Immune Privilege Revisited: The Roles of Neuronal MHC Class I Molecules in Brain Development and Plasticity

Adema Ribic
Yale University
Department of Molecular Biophysics and Biochemistry, New Haven, CT
USA

1. Introduction

1.1 MHC class I molecules: Molecular hallmarks of individuality

Ever since its initial discovery in 1948 by George Snell, major histocompatibility (MHC) complex became the focus of intense research that, due to its diverse roles, gradually extended far beyond transplantation biology. MHC class I molecules are found on virtually all nucleated cells of jawed vertebrates and are the most polymorphic molecules described to date (Cresswell et al. 2005, Solheim 1999). Their polymorphism is so high that, with the exception of identical twins, two individuals with the exact same set of MHC molecules (both class I and II) do not exist.

1.2 Structure, function and properties of MHC class I molecules

MHC class I molecules are normally composed of three subunits: transmembrane heavy chain, small β-2-microglobulin subunit and the presenting antigenic peptide [Figure 1; (Cresswell et al. 2005, Solheim 1999)]. MHC class I molecules are assembled in the endoplasmatic reticulum and are generally dependent on the presence of all three subunits for proper cell surface expression. The MHC class I heavy chain is a glycoprotein with reported molecular weight of 42-48 kDa. It consists of three extracellular domains (α1-3), and short transmembrane and cytoplasmic regions (Figure 1). α1 and α2 domains form the peptide binding groove and are the regions responsible for the high polymorphism of MHC class I molecules. α3 domain carries the signature of the immunoglobulin superfamily, the immunoglobulin fold.

β-2-microglobulin is the smaller, 11-13 kDa subunit, without a transmembrane domain. It is non-covalently attached to the MHC class I heavy chain on the cell surface. β-2-microglobulin is encoded by a gene settled outside of the MHC cluster and it is structurally also immunoglobulin-like (Figure 1). MHC class I molecules are divided in two groups: classical and non-classical MHC class I. Classical MHC class I molecules are highly polymorphic, usually form trimers on the cell surface and are mainly associated with antigen presentation. Non-classical MHC class I molecules are still somewhat of an enigma.

They are not as polymorphic as the classical MHC class I and some of them do not require β-2-microglobulin or the binding of peptide in order to reach the cell surface (Arosa et al. 2007). Non-classical MHC class I are also implicated in a wide range of immune and non-immune processes, from presentation of glycolipids to regulation of pheromone signalling (Arosa et al. 2007, Fishman et al. 2004).

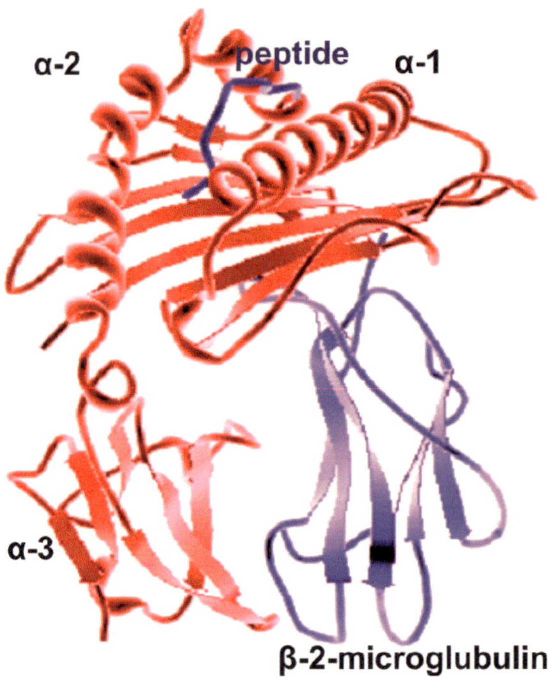

Fig. 1. Structure of MHC class I molecules.
Ribbon structure of MHC class I molecule: MHC class I molecule (HLA-A2, in this case) is composed of heavy chain (red), β-2-microglobulin (violet blue) and the presenting peptide (dark blue). Immunoglobulin fold structure of the α3 domain of the heavy chain and the β-2-microglubulin is visible. Image courtesy of Wikimedia Commons.

1.3 MHC class I signaling in immune and non-immune systems

The main function of classical MHC class I molecules is the presentation of foreign, "non-self" peptides to cytotoxic T-cells. This process initiates the canonical MHC class I/T-cell receptor signaling pathway (Figure 2). Cytotoxic T-cells become activated through this pathway after they recognize the MHC class I-presented peptide as foreign and potentially hazardous. The signalling cascade brought about by MHC class I/TCR interaction induces cytoskeletal rearrangements and cytokine production in T-cells activated by it (for more details, the reader should refer to general immunology textbooks). Although this is the canonical MHC class I signalling pathway, the TCR complex is not the only receptor for the MHC class I molecules. MHC class I proteins are able to interact with a large number of receptors within the immune system, both in *cis* and in *trans*, such as killer-cell immunoglobulin-like receptors (KIRs), leukocyte immunoglobulin-like receptors (LILRs), etc., causing a wide range of responses (Parham 2005).

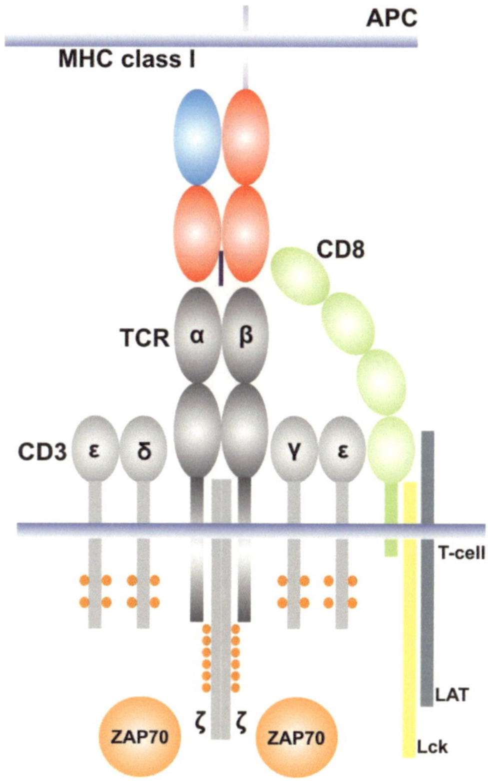

Fig. 2. Canonical MHC class I/T-cell receptor pathway.
TCR receptor complex is depicted with its main components: T-cell receptor (TCR) and accessory CD3 molecules (ε,γ,ζ and δ). CD8 is a co-receptor specific for MHC class I molecules. After T-cell receptor (TCR) complex recognizes the peptide presented by MHC class I as foreign, TCR receptor complex subunits rearrange within the membrane in a more spatially constricted configuration. CD3 subunits become phosphorylated (orange circles) by lymphocyte-specific protein kinase (Lck) and zeta-chain associated protein kinase 70 (ZAP70). ZAP70 also phosphorylates linker of activated T-cell kinase (LAT) before T-cell activation.

Outside of the immune system, MHC class I molecules have been implicated mainly in regulation of trafficking and internalization of hormone receptors. Interactions with insulin receptor (IR), γ-endorphin receptor, luteinizing hormone receptor and many others have been reported (Arosa et al. 2007). The best characterized non-immune interaction of MHC class I is with the IR. It has been suggested that MHC class I molecules are involved in glycosylation of IR and its proper transport to the cell surface, but most evidence has been provided for the role of MHC class I in insulin-induced IR internalization (Olsson et al. 1994, Ramalingam et al. 1997, Stagsted 1998, Stagsted et al. 1993a, Stagsted et al. 1990, Stagsted et al. 1993b). A number of studies have suggested that MHC class I associates with IR after insulin binding thereby causing its internalization and removal from the cell surface. Functional significance of these findings is still debated; however, certain MHC class I genes have been implicated in the aetiology of type I diabetes (Fernando et al. 2008).

1.4 Immune privilege and neuronal expression of MHC class I molecules

The concept of immune privilege refers to the ability of certain organs (eyes, brain, testicles and the uterus while harbouring a foetus) to evade inflammatory responses during antigen presentation (Hong and Van Kaer 1999). Tissues transplanted to the central nervous system (CNS) show prolonged survival compared to tissues grafted to other locations in the body, such as skin (Carson et al. 2006, Galea et al. 2007). Furthermore, a number of pathogens are able to evade the immune responses by "hiding" in the CNS structures (Carson et al. 2006, Galea et al. 2007). This immune privilege of the CNS is thought to be a consequence of the blood-brain barrier (BBB), considered impermeable to the cells of the immune system (Carson et al. 2006, Galea et al. 2007). A classical inflammatory response would be devastating for immune privileged structures due to their special properties and it is believed that immune privilege is an active process that has developed throughout the evolution (Hong and Van Kaer 1999). However, the concept of CNS immune privilege has been extensively challenged in the last few decades. Increasing evidence suggests not only that immune cells are able to cross the blood-brain barrier under normal conditions, but that they might be indispensable to normal functioning of the CNS (Kipnis et al. 2004). Furthermore, the notion of the CNS being completely devoid of neuronal MHC class I expression due its immune privileged status has been questioned with strong experimental evidence over the past decade. The new line of research on the interactions between the immune and the nervous system is slowly debunking the myth of classical CNS immune privilege. Strong experimental evidence is pointing to a novel concept: CNS functions highly depend on its proper interactions with the immune system.

2. Neuronal MHC class I molecules in brain development and plasticity

Based on the immune privileged status of the CNS, expression of MHC class I by neurons has always been considered either low or non-existent. Based on experimental evidence, it was believed that neurons were able to express MHC class I only after induction by cytokines (Neumann et al. 1995). However, a study by Corriveau et al. in 1998 demonstrated high neuronal MHC class I expression in normal, developing and adult brains. Since then, a number of studies confirmed that neurons do express MHC class I molecules in normal, non-pathological conditions (Datwani et al. 2009, Goddard et al. 2007, Huh et al. 2000, McConnell et al. 2009, Ribic et al. 2010, Rolleke et al. 2006). Furthermore, MHC class I have been implicated in proper development and maintenance of neuronal circuitry in various brain regions, especially in the development of the visual system (Huh et al. 2000, Ribic et al. 2011), and in modulation of synaptic plasticity in hippocampus and the cerebellum (Goddard et al. 2007, Huh et al. 2000, McConnell et al. 2009, Ribic et al. 2010).

2.1 MHC class I molecules and the mammalian visual system development

2.1.1 Mammalian visual system

Synaptic plasticity is the ability of neurons to change the strength of their synaptic connections in response to various stimuli. Plasticity is one of the fundamental properties of CNS. This process occurs in various forms with distinct properties and is thought to be essential for development and maintenance of brain circuits. The developing visual system is one of the main models of two forms of plasticity: visual activity-independent and visual input-driven or activity-dependent plasticity. There are two main stages of visual system development. The early stage encompasses the development of the eyes and the brain and the initial development of the neuronal connections between them. It is believed that at this early stage, both growth of neuronal processes and pathfinding are independent of retinal activity, as opposed to the later stage. The second stage involves proper development of connections in and between the thalamus and the visual cortex, regions responsible for the processing of the visual input. The thalamic dorsal lateral geniculate nucleus (LGN) is the first relay structure of visual input and is organized into segregated, eye-specific, neuronal layers that form upon early spontaneous activity from retinal ganglion cells in the eye [Figure 3, (Shatz 1996)].

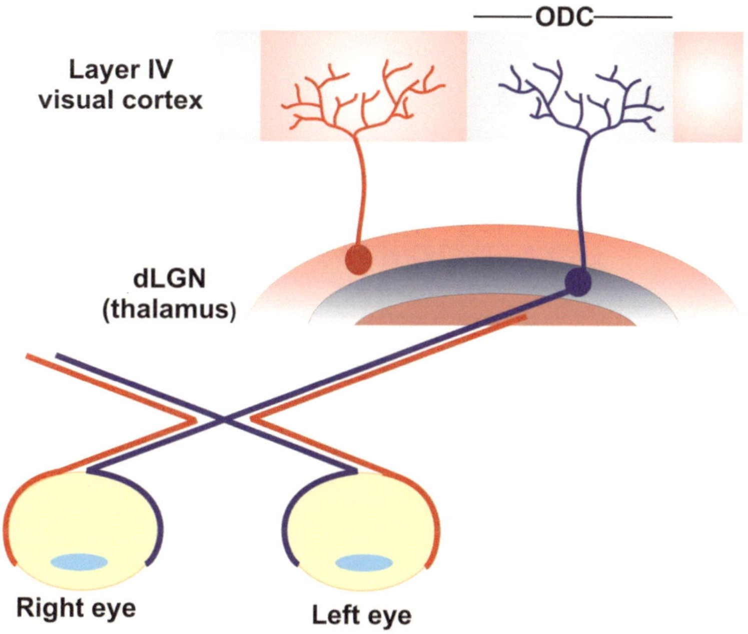

Fig. 3. Schematic structure of the mammalian visual system.
Retinal ganglion cells from both eyes project to the thalamic dorsal lateral geniculate nucleus (dLGN). Partial crossing of the two pathways occurs in the optic chiasm. Neurons of the lateral geniculate nucleus project to the visual cortex in the occipital lobes where neurons form eye-specific patches, ocular dominance columns (ODCs).
Neurons of the LGN send their projections to the primary visual cortex (V1), where their activity is required for the development of eye-specific patches of neurons in layer IV, i.e., the ocular dominance columns (ODCs) (Sur and Rubenstein 2005).

Although the development of both LGN and V1 is dependent on spontaneous retinal activity, visual activity is also required for their proper maturation. Blocking retinal activity of one eye during the development of the visual circuits while leaving the other one intact leads to the perturbation of the segregation of LGN neurons into eye-specific layers (Shatz 1996). In the visual cortex, ODCs do not form properly if one eye is deprived of input. As a consequence of visual deprivation, the ODCs increase the fraction of neurons responsive to the intact eye at the expense of neurons receiving afferents from the deprived eye (Berardi et al. 2003, Sur and Rubenstein 2005). Furthermore, neurons receiving afferents from the intact eye tend to expand their synaptic space and occupy more territory within the visual cortex. On the other hand, neurons receiving afferents from the deprived eye shrink their territory [Figure 4; (Berardi et al. 2003)].

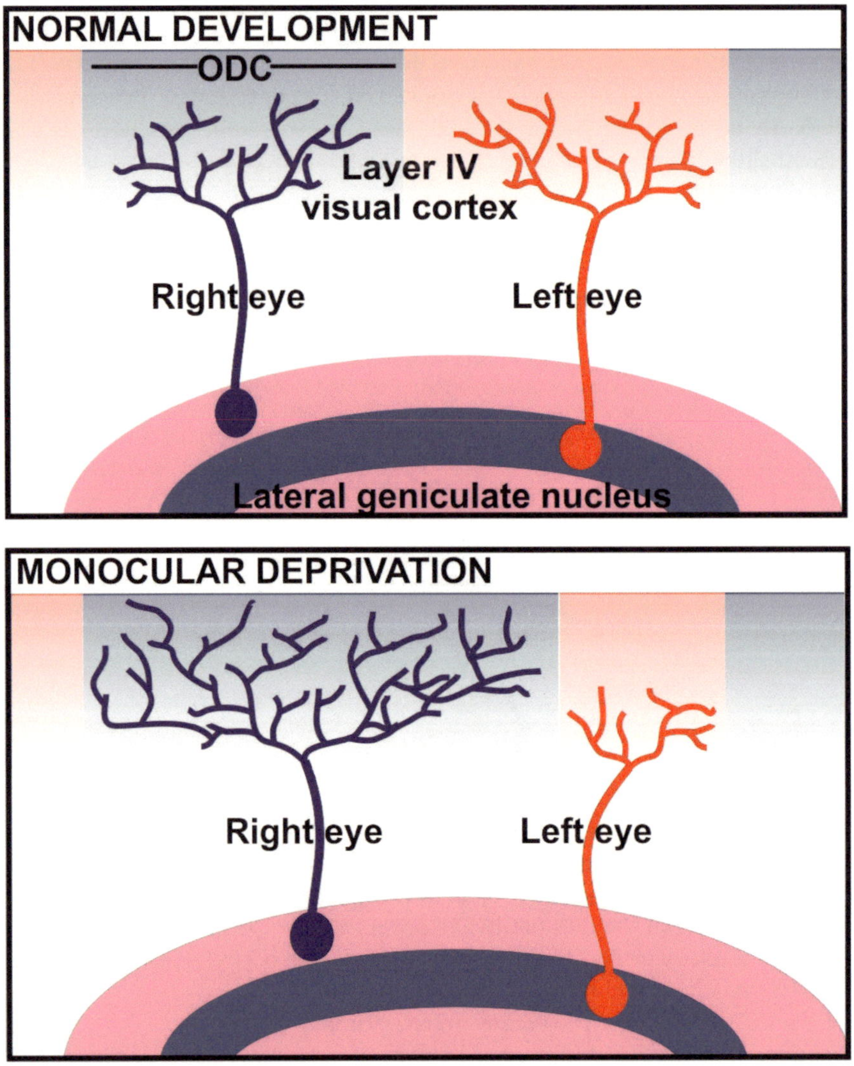

Fig. 4. Effects of monocular deprivation on visual cortex development.
Normal development of the visual cortex is based on the competition between the two eyes which confers balanced development of LGN neurons and their connections with the visual cortex neurons in ODCs (upper panel). If one eye is deprived of visual input throughout the development of the visual system, LGN neurons receiving afferents from the deprived eye shrink and prune their connections in the visual cortex (lower panel). This also causes shrinkage of ODCs in the visual cortex that receive input from the deprived eye (in the figure: left eye). On the other hand, ODCs receiving input from the intact eye, expand their territory within the visual cortex (in the figure: right eye).

2.1.2 The roles of MHC class I molecules in visual system development

In the mouse dLGN and visual cortex, MHC class I molecules are associated with mainly excitatory, glutamate-activated synapses (Datwani et al. 2009, Glynn et al. 2011, Needleman et al. 2010). Immunoelectron microscopy of mouse visual cortex has demonstrated that MHC class I molecules may be situated on both sides of the synapse (Needleman et al. 2010). Expression levels of MHC class I proteins decrease with development of mouse cortex, being very prominent in the early stages of cortical development (Needleman et al. 2010). First studies dealing with neuronal expression of MHC class I revealed an essential role for MHC class I genes in the segregation of retinal inputs and proper formation of neuronal layers within the LGN (Corriveau et al. 1998, Huh et al. 2000). MHC class I-deficient mice display an aberrant development of retinal projections and impairments in the formation of eye-specific regions in the LGN, caused by an excess of inappropriate synapses that are normally removed during LGN development in wild-type mice (Huh et al. 2000). These studies implicated MHC class I in weakening, removal and pruning of synapses, and it is believed that MHC class I molecules limit plasticity in the developing visual system (Syken et al. 2006). β-2-microglobulin deficient mice show an increased density of synapses in the visual cortex, consistent with the role of MHC class I in synapse pruning (Glynn et al. 2011). A recent study has shown that classical MHC class I molecules are mediating these effects (Datwani et al. 2009). Mutant mice lacking two classical MHC class I genes ($H2\text{-}K^b$ and $H2\text{-}D^b$) replicate the phenotype observed in the visual system of β-2-microglubulin/TAP-deficient mice used in previous studies (Datwani et al. 2009). Interestingly, mice that lack the expression of TCR complex subunit CD3-ζ also display similar defects in visual system development (Corriveau et al. 1998, Huh et al. 2000, Xu et al. 2010). Furthermore, a study that investigated the retinal phenotype of CD3-ζ knock-out mice revealed an important observation-the phenotype observed in the dLGN and visual cortex of both CD3-ζ and MHC class I-deficient mice may be just a consequence of retinal defects observed in these mice (Xu et al. 2010).MHC class I genes are also expressed in the retina (Huh et al. 2000) and time will show if this assumption holds true.

Majority of the above mentioned studies have been performed in mice and cats (Corriveau et al. 1998, Huh et al. 2000). The number of class I genes is highly variable between species; moreover, orthologous relationships are found only within same order of mammals such as within primates, but never between primates and rodents (Kumanovics et al. 2003, Gunther and Walter 2001). Mouse and rat MHC clusters are comprised of over 30 functional classical and non-classical genes (Gunther and Walter 2001, Kumanovics et al. 2003). Despite the orthologous relationship, MHC class I genes are still very variable between primates. Strict orthologues of classical human MHC class I genes are present only in the great apes, whereas orthologues of the non-classical genes are found in Old World (baboons, macaques) and New World monkeys. This, coupled with known differences in CNS anatomy and function between rodents and primates, poses a question of possible interspecies differences in the function of neuronal MHC class I genes. It is known that MHC class I genes are highly expressed in the visual cortex of the marmoset monkey (a New World primate) and that their expression closely follows the synapse development in the visual cortex, increasing with postnatal age (Ribic et al. 2011). Neuronal MHC class I gene expression appears activity-dependent in all species examined (Corriveau et al. 1998, Huh et al. 2000, Ribic et al. 2011), but the expression profile seems to be highly dependent on both the experimental paradigm and the model organism used (Corriveau et al. 1998, Ribic et al. 2011).

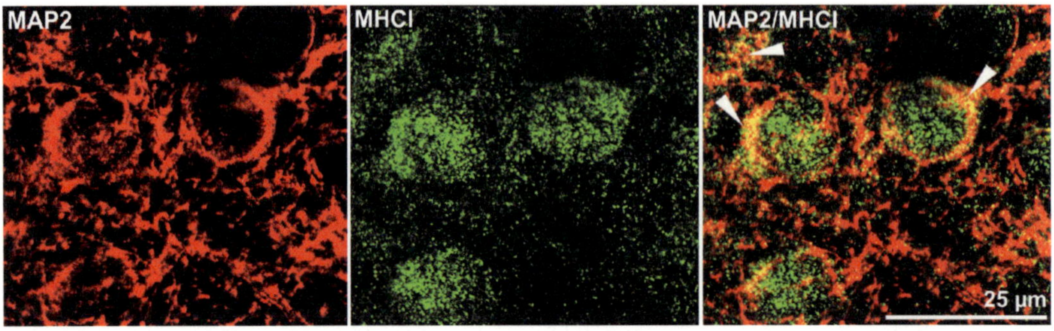

Fig. 5. Expression of MHC class I proteins in the visual cortex of the common marmoset. MHC class I proteins (green) colocalize with the neuronal marker MAP2 (red) in layer IV neuronal cell bodies of the common marmoset primary visual. Image adapted from Ribic et al., 2011.

Unavailability of transgenic non-human primate models has hindered the answers to the question of potential interspecies variability in neuronal MHC class I function. However, having in mind the high evolution rate of these molecules, differential interspecies function seems highly plausible.

2.2 MHC class I molecules and hippocampal plasticity

2.2.1 The hippocampus

Hippocampus is a part of the brain situated in the medial temporal lobe and implicated in learning and memory processes. It is organized as a series of connected cell layers: the dentate gyrus, hilus, and cornu ammonis 1, 2 and 3 (CA1-3, Figure 6), which form the so called "trisynaptic circuit". Due to its relatively simple structure, hippocampus is one of the best studied circuits within the brain. The dentate gyrus is composed of granule cells that receive input from the entorhinal cortex and send projections to the hilus and the CA3 pyramidal neurons region. The dentate gyrus to hilus and CA3 projections are known as the mossy fiber pathway (Figure 6). The CA3 pyramidal neurons innervate the CA1 cell layer, and the CA1 pyramidal neurons in turn send their axons to the entorhinal cortex. The CA3 to CA1 connections are also called Schaffer collaterals. Both mossy fiber pathway and Schaffer collaterals have received a great deal of attention over the past decades due to neuronal long-term plasticity properties within these two hippocampal regions. Prolonged correlated presynaptic (neurotransmitter release) and postsynaptic (activation of neurotransmitter receptors) activity is thought to underlie one form of long-term plasticity, long-term potentiation [LTP; (Cooke and Bliss 2006, Malenka and Bear 2004)]. LTP results in increased synapse strength between participating neurons (Cooke and Bliss 2006, Malenka and Bear 2004). In contrast to LTP, prolonged uncorrelated presynaptic and postsynaptic activity results in long-term depression (LTD), a form of plasticity thought to precede the weakening of synapses and their pruning (Collingridge et al. 2010, Malenka and Bear 2004). Although both LTP and LTD are experimental phenomena, they are considered cellular mechanisms of memory formation and storage and both have been extensively studied using hippocampus as a model system (Collingridge et al. 2010, Malenka and Bear 2004).

LTP and LTD in Schaffer collaterals are considered the classical examples of long term plasticity (Malenka and Bear 2004). Both LTP and LTD have various forms of induction and maintenance, but the most investigated forms are dependent on the activation of NMDAR (N-methyl D-aspartate receptors), as well as changes in Ca^{2+} concentrations (Malenka and Bear 2004). Both LTP and LTD occur in the visual cortex during developmental activity-dependent plasticity, where they regulate the strengthening of appropriate and removal of inappropriate synapses (Berardi et al. 2003, Heynen et al. 2003, Katz and Crowley 2002, Thompson 2000).

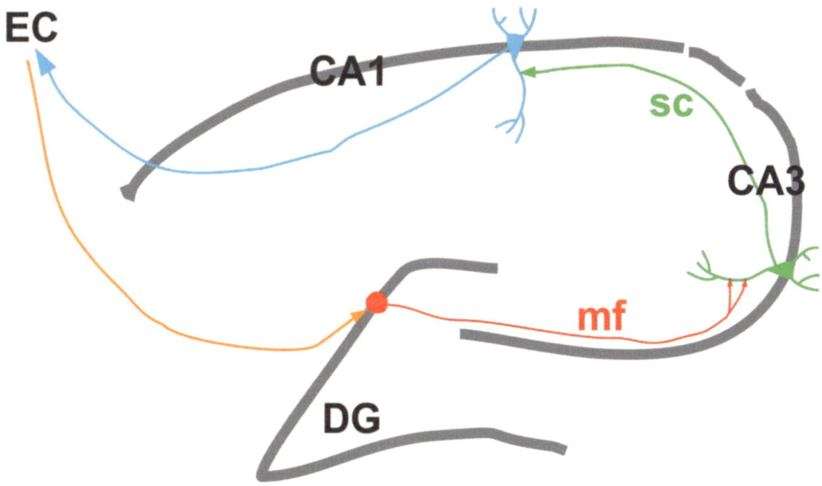

Fig. 6. Schematic structure of the hippocampus.
Granule cells in the dentate gyrus receive input from the entorhinal cortex (EC, orange) and send their projections to the CA3 pyramidal neurons [mossy fiber pathway (mf), red]. CA3 neurons innervate CA1 pyramidal neurons [Schaffer collaterals (sc), green], which in turn send their projections back to the entorhinal cortex (blue).

2.2.2 The roles of MHC class I proteins in hippocampal plasticity

MHC class I proteins in mice have been shown to localize postsynaptically on the somata and dendrites of the dentate gyrus granule neurons and the CA1-CA3 pyramidal neurons (Corriveau et al. 1998, Goddard et al. 2007). Both LTP and LTD at the Schaffer collaterals are aberrant in mice lacking MHC class I molecules (Huh et al., 2000). Schaffer collateral LTP in these mice is significantly enhanced, while LTD is completely absent (Huh et al. 2000). These findings parallel the effects of MHC class I in the visual system: LTP reflects strengthening of the neuronal connections and the absence of MHC class I causes strengthening of synapses that would otherwise be weakened by LTD. However, the enhancement of LTP in MHC class I deficient mice is not dependent on NMDAR receptors (Huh et al. 2000). In primates, at least a subset of neuronal MHC class I molecules is presynaptic and expressed exclusively in the mossy fibers within the hippocampal formation (Ribic et al. 2010). Blocking their function in vitro interferes with normal synaptic transmission (Ribic et al. 2010).

So far, presynaptic localization of neuronal MHC class I molecules in mice has only been detected in the spinal cord and at the neuromuscular junction (Oliveira et al. 2004, Thams et al. 2009). Future studies will no doubt reveal if there are any functional differences stemming from different localization of neuronal MHC class I molecules in different species.

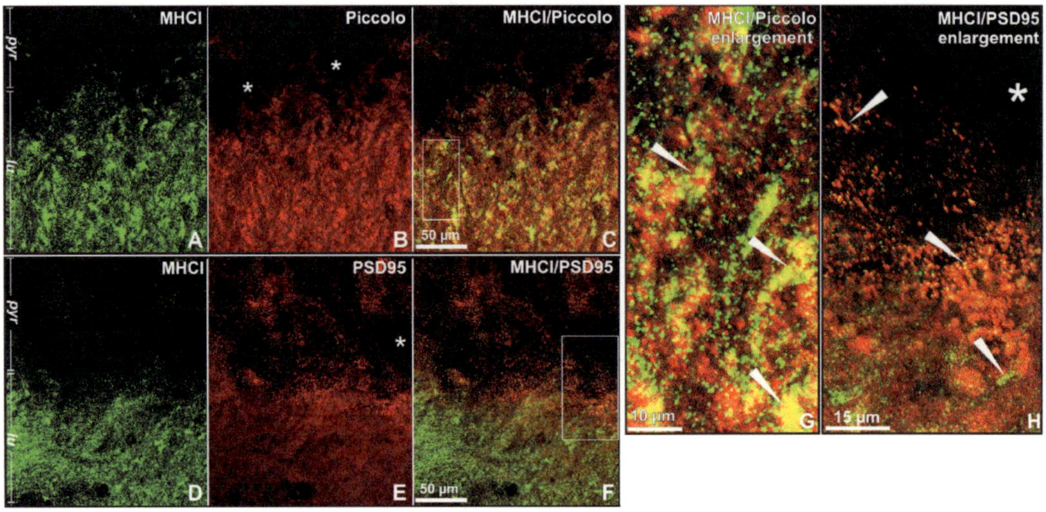

Fig. 7. MHC class I (MHCI) protein is localized to the presynaptic side of the mossy fiber-CA3 synapse in the common marmoset monkey hippocampus.
MHC class I signal (A, green) significantly overlaps with that of piccolo (B, red), a marker of the presynaptic active zone (C and G, white arrowheads). Almost no overlap is detected between MHC class I (D) and the postsynaptic marker PSD95 (E, F and H).

2.3 Molecular mechanisms of neuronal MHC class I action

The main unanswered question is how are neuronal MHC class I molecules mediating all these effects? A few studies have shown that MHC class I may recruit receptors other than TCR in the CNS. Mice lacking PirB, known interaction partner of MHC class I molecules in the immune system, also show similar defects in developmental synapse removal (Syken et al).

It has been hypothesized that MHC class I may engage in trans-synaptic interactions and hence exert presynaptic effects that have been observed (Goddard et al. 2007, Syken et al. 2006). As the phenotype of CD3ζ knock-out mice resembles the phenotype of MHC class I deficient mice, it is safe to assume that they may be involved in the same signaling pathway (Xu et al. 2010, Huh et al. 2000). Furthermore, MHC class I molecules may affect the function of synapses through their effects on neurotransmitter receptors, such as glutamate receptors (Fourgeaud et al. 2010). A recent study indicated that MHC class I proteins may regulate trafficking of NMDAR receptors, which parallels their previously described roles in insulin receptor signaling (Arosa et al. 2007, Fishman et al. 2004, Fourgeaud et al. 2010). Interestingly enough, insulin is mediating a non-NMDAR dependent form of LTD in the hippocampus (Ahmadian et al. 2004, Collingridge et al. 2010, Ge et al. 2010, Wang and Linden 2000). Receptor internalization seems to be the main role of MHC class I in the vomeronasal organ of mice, where non-classical MHC class I molecules appear to be involved in internalization of vomeronasal receptors (Olson et al. 2006, Dulac and Torello 2003, Loconto et al. 2003). In the primate hippocampus, blockade of neuronal MHC class I in vitro slows down basal synaptic transmission at the mossy fiber-CA3 synapses (Ribic et al. 2010). The mossy fiber-CA3 synapse displays a number of peculiarities in comparison to the majority of CNS synapses. It is e.g. characterized by a low basal transmission which is maintained by activation of a number of receptors that have inhibitory effects on synaptic transmission (Nicoll and Schmitz 2005). As previously mentioned, given that the best characterized non-immune function of MHC class I is regulation of trafficking and internalization of various receptors (Olsson et al. 1994, Stagsted 1998, Stagsted et al. 1990, Ramalingam et al. 1997), it is likely that neuronal MHC class I molecules in the marmoset hippocampus are needed for proper internalization of one or several of those receptors (Figure 8). One may speculate that blocking the interaction of MHC class I with such

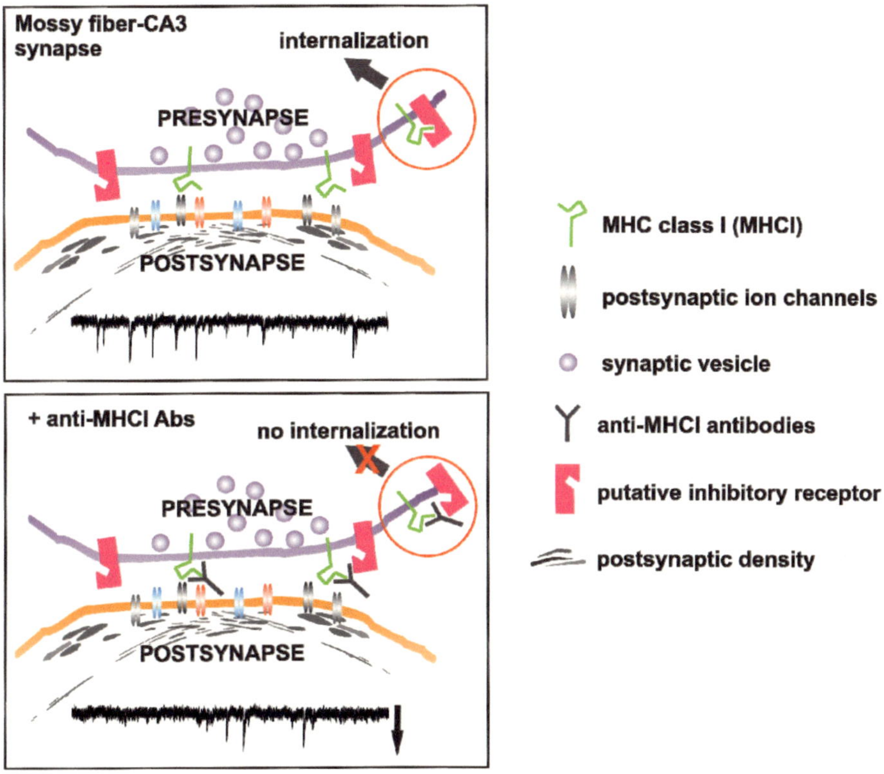

Fig. 8. Schematic representation of potential mode of action of MHC class I at the mossy fiber-CA3 synapse.

Mossy fiber-CA3 synapse normally displays lower levels of basal activity compared to other synapses in the central nervous system (representative electrophysiological trace of recorded spontaneous excitatory postsynaptic currents (EPSCs) of a marmoset CA3 neuron is shown in the lower part of the image). This is mainly due to large number of receptors (magenta) that have inhibitory effect on synaptic transmission (Nicoll and Schmitz, 2005). It is possible that MHC class I is needed for proper internalization and removal of one of these receptors from the cell surface. MHC class I would presumably bind to the receptor with its α1 and α2 domains. (D) If anti-MHC class I antibodies that bind to α1 and α2 domains are applied in the vicinity of the cell while the cell's activity is recorded using patch clamp technique, frequency of spontaneous EPSCs is decreased (trace in the lower part of the image). It is possible that antibodies block interaction of MHC class I with putative inhibitory receptor, which prolongs inhibitory signaling thereby decreasing the frequency of spontaneous EPSCs.

receptors by application of anti-MHC class I antibodies would prolong inhibitory signaling and exert the inhibitory effects on synaptic transmission. Future studies need to elucidate the exact molecular pathways that neuronal MHC class I molecules are involve in, as well as their potential involvement in insulin-induced hippocampal LTD.

3. Nervous and immune systems-shared molecules and mechanisms

A vast number of studies in the past decades have shown that the immune and the nervous system are interconnected more than previously thought. Recent discoveries have highlighted a number of roles performed by immune molecules in the CNS-molecules and pathways previously thought to be exclusively acting within the immune system. From MHC class I molecules in synapse development (Corriveau et al. 1998, Huh et al. 2000, Ribic et al. 2010), CD3ζ in retinal function and dendrite development (Baudouin et al. 2008, Xu et al. 2010), to DAP12 in astrocyte-neuron signaling (Roumier et al. 2004), a new picture of immune privilege emerges-a picture in which the immune system is actively involved in proper brain development and maintenance of neuronal circuitry. This concept has important implications for a number of diseases associated with MHC cluster, such as schizophrenia and autism (Torres et al. 2006, Kipnis et al. 2004, Needleman et al. 2010). Current research efforts are focused on elucidating the consequences of prenatal immune insult on the brain development, so called "maternal immune activation". Both schizophrenia and autism have been genetically linked to MHC cluster and to prenatal immune insult (Soumiya et al. 2011, Buehler 2011, Escobar et al. 2011, Patterson 2011, Fatemi et al. 2011, Parker-Athill and Tan 2010, Boksa 2010, Currenti 2010, Li et al. 2009, Patterson 2009, Smith et al. 2007, Cohly and Panja 2005, Patterson 2002, Stubbs and Magenis 1980). Future studies will no doubt elucidate the interactions between the nervous and immune systems in more detail, as well as shed more light on the vast polymorphism of MHC class I molecules, especially in the light of their neuronal functions.

4. References

Ahmadian, G., Ju, W., Liu, L., Wyszynski, M., Lee, S.H., Dunah, A.W., Taghibiglou, C., Wang, Y., Lu, J., Wong, T.P., Sheng, M. & Wang, Y.T. (2004) Tyrosine phosphorylation of GluR2 is required for insulin-stimulated AMPA receptor endocytosis and LTD. *EMBO J*, 23(5), 1040-50.

Arosa, F.A., Santos, S.G. & Powis, S.J. (2007) Open conformers: the hidden face of MHC-I molecules. *Trends Immunol*, 28(3), 115-23.

Baudouin, S.J., Angibaud, J., Loussouarn, G., Bonnamain, V., Matsuura, A., Kinebuchi, M., Naveilhan, P. & Boudin, H. (2008) The signaling adaptor protein CD3zeta is a negative regulator of dendrite development in young neurons. *Mol Biol Cell*, 19(6), 2444-56.

Berardi, N., Pizzorusso, T., Ratto, G.M. & Maffei, L. (2003) Molecular basis of plasticity in the visual cortex. *Trends Neurosci*, 26(7), 369-78.

Boksa, P. (2010) Effects of prenatal infection on brain development and behavior: a review of findings from animal models. *Brain Behav Immun*, 24(6), 881-97.

Buehler, M.R. (2011) A proposed mechanism for autism: an aberrant neuroimmune response manifested as a psychiatric disorder. *Med Hypotheses,* 76(6), 863-70.

Carson, M.J., Doose, J.M., Melchior, B., Schmid, C.D. & Ploix, C.C. (2006) CNS immune privilege: hiding in plain sight. *Immunol Rev,* 213, 48-65.

Cohly, H.H. & Panja, A. (2005) Immunological findings in autism. *Int Rev Neurobiol,* 71, 317-41.

Collingridge, G.L., Peineau, S., Howland, J.G. & Wang, Y.T. (2010) Long-term depression in the CNS. *Nat Rev Neurosci,* 11(7), 459-73.

Cooke, S.F. & Bliss, T.V. (2006) Plasticity in the human central nervous system. *Brain,* 129(Pt 7), 1659-73.

Corriveau, R.A., Huh, G.S. & Shatz, C.J. (1998) Regulation of class I MHC gene expression in the developing and mature CNS by neural activity. *Neuron,* 21(3), 505-20.

Cresswell, P., Ackerman, A.L., Giodini, A., Peaper, D.R. & Wearsch, P.A. (2005) Mechanisms of MHC class I-restricted antigen processing and cross-presentation. *Immunol Rev,* 207, 145-57.

Currenti, S.A. (2010) Understanding and determining the etiology of autism. *Cell Mol Neurobiol,* 30(2), 161-71.

Datwani, A., McConnell, M.J., Kanold, P.O., Micheva, K.D., Busse, B., Shamloo, M., Smith, S.J. & Shatz, C.J. (2009) Classical MHCI molecules regulate retinogeniculate refinement and limit ocular dominance plasticity. *Neuron,* 64(4), 463-70.

Dulac, C. & Torello, A.T. (2003) Molecular detection of pheromone signals in mammals: from genes to behaviour. *Nat Rev Neurosci,* 4(7), 551-62.

Escobar, M., Crouzin, N., Cavalier, M., Quentin, J., Roussel, J., Lante, F., Batista-Novais, A.R., Cohen-Solal, C., De Jesus Ferreira, M.C., Guiramand, J., Barbanel, G. & Vignes, M. (2011) Early, Time-Dependent Disturbances of Hippocampal Synaptic Transmission and Plasticity After In Utero Immune Challenge. *Biol Psychiatry.*

Fatemi, S.H., Folsom, T.D., Rooney, R.J., Mori, S., Kornfield, T.E., Reutiman, T.J., Kneeland, R.E., Liesch, S.B., Hua, K., Hsu, J. & Patel, D.H. (2011) The viral theory of schizophrenia revisited: Abnormal placental gene expression and structural changes with lack of evidence for H1N1 viral presence in placentae of infected mice or brains of exposed offspring. *Neuropharmacology.*

Fernando, M.M., Stevens, C.R., Walsh, E.C., De Jager, P.L., Goyette, P., Plenge, R.M., Vyse, T.J. & Rioux, J.D. (2008) Defining the role of the MHC in autoimmunity: a review and pooled analysis. *PLoS Genet,* 4(4), e1000024.

Fishman, D., Elhyany, S. & Segal, S. (2004) Non-immune functions of MHC class I glycoproteins in normal and malignant cells. *Folia Biol (Praha),* 50(2), 35-42.

Fourgeaud, L., Davenport, C.M., Tyler, C.M., Cheng, T.T., Spencer, M.B. & Boulanger, L.M. (2010) MHC class I modulates NMDA receptor function and AMPA receptor trafficking. *Proc Natl Acad Sci U S A.*

Galea, I., Bechmann, I. & Perry, V.H. (2007) What is immune privilege (not)? *Trends Immunol,* 28(1), 12-8.

Ge, Y., Dong, Z., Bagot, R.C., Howland, J.G., Phillips, A.G., Wong, T.P. & Wang, Y.T. (2010) Hippocampal long-term depression is required for the consolidation of spatial memory. *Proc Natl Acad Sci U S A,* 107(38), 16697-702.

Glynn, M.W., Elmer, B.M., Garay, P.A., Liu, X.B., Needleman, L.A., El-Sabeawy, F. & McAllister, A.K. (2011) MHCI negatively regulates synapse density during the establishment of cortical connections. *Nat Neurosci,* 14(4), 442-51.

Goddard, C.A., Butts, D.A. & Shatz, C.J. (2007) Regulation of CNS synapses by neuronal MHC class I. *Proc Natl Acad Sci U S A,* 104(16), 6828-33.

Gunther, E. & Walter, L. (2001) The major histocompatibility complex of the rat (Rattus norvegicus). *Immunogenetics,* 53(7), 520-42.

Heynen, A.J., Yoon, B.J., Liu, C.H., Chung, H.J., Huganir, R.L. & Bear, M.F. (2003) Molecular mechanism for loss of visual cortical responsiveness following brief monocular deprivation. *Nat Neurosci,* 6(8), 854-62.

Hong, S. & Van Kaer, L. (1999) Immune privilege: keeping an eye on natural killer T cells. *J Exp Med,* 190(9), 1197-200.

Huh, G.S., Boulanger, L.M., Du, H., Riquelme, P.A., Brotz, T.M. & Shatz, C.J. (2000) Functional requirement for class I MHC in CNS development and plasticity. *Science,* 290(5499), 2155-9.

Katz, L.C. & Crowley, J.C. (2002) Development of cortical circuits: lessons from ocular dominance columns. *Nat Rev Neurosci,* 3(1), 34-42.

Kipnis, J., Cohen, H., Cardon, M., Ziv, Y. & Schwartz, M. (2004) T cell deficiency leads to cognitive dysfunction: implications for therapeutic vaccination for schizophrenia and other psychiatric conditions. *Proc Natl Acad Sci U S A,* 101(21), 8180-5.

Kumanovics, A., Takada, T. & Lindahl, K.F. (2003) Genomic organization of the mammalian MHC. *Annu Rev Immunol,* 21, 629-57.

Li, Q., Cheung, C., Wei, R., Hui, E.S., Feldon, J., Meyer, U., Chung, S., Chua, S.E., Sham, P.C., Wu, E.X. & McAlonan, G.M. (2009) Prenatal immune challenge is an environmental risk factor for brain and behavior change relevant to schizophrenia: evidence from MRI in a mouse model. *PLoS One,* 4(7), e6354.

Loconto, J., Papes, F., Chang, E., Stowers, L., Jones, E.P., Takada, T., Kumanovics, A., Fischer Lindahl, K. & Dulac, C. (2003) Functional expression of murine V2R pheromone receptors involves selective association with the M10 and M1 families of MHC class Ib molecules. *Cell,* 112(5), 607-18.

Malenka, R.C. & Bear, M.F. (2004) LTP and LTD: an embarrassment of riches. *Neuron,* 44(1), 5-21.

McConnell, M.J., Huang, Y.H., Datwani, A. & Shatz, C.J. (2009) H2-K(b) and H2-D(b) regulate cerebellar long-term depression and limit motor learning. *Proc Natl Acad Sci U S A,* 106(16), 6784-9.

Needleman, L.A., Liu, X.B., El-Sabeawy, F., Jones, E.G. & McAllister, A.K. (2010) MHC class I molecules are present both pre- and postsynaptically in the visual cortex during postnatal development and in adulthood. *Proc Natl Acad Sci U S A,* 107(39), 16999-7004.

Neumann, H., Cavalie, A., Jenne, D.E. & Wekerle, H. (1995) Induction of MHC class I genes in neurons. *Science,* 269(5223), 549-52.

Nicoll, R.A. & Schmitz, D. (2005) Synaptic plasticity at hippocampal mossy fibre synapses. *Nat Rev Neurosci,* 6(11), 863-76.

Oliveira, A.L., Thams, S., Lidman, O., Piehl, F., Hokfelt, T., Karre, K., Linda, H. & Cullheim, S. (2004) A role for MHC class I molecules in synaptic plasticity and regeneration of neurons after axotomy. *Proc Natl Acad Sci U S A,* 101(51), 17843-8.

Olson, R., Dulac, C. & Bjorkman, P.J. (2006) MHC homologs in the nervous system--they haven't lost their groove. *Curr Opin Neurobiol,* 16(3), 351-7.

Olsson, L., Goldstein, A. & Stagsted, J. (1994) Regulation of receptor internalization by the major histocompatibility complex class I molecule. *Proc Natl Acad Sci U S A,* 91(19), 9086-90.

Parham, P. (2005) MHC class I molecules and KIRs in human history, health and survival. *Nat Rev Immunol,* 5(3), 201-14.

Parker-Athill, E.C. & Tan, J. (2010) Maternal immune activation and autism spectrum disorder: interleukin-6 signaling as a key mechanistic pathway. *Neurosignals,* 18(2), 113-28.

Patterson, P.H. (2002) Maternal infection: window on neuroimmune interactions in fetal brain development and mental illness. *Curr Opin Neurobiol,* 12(1), 115-8.

Patterson, P.H. (2009) Immune involvement in schizophrenia and autism: etiology, pathology and animal models. *Behav Brain Res,* 204(2), 313-21.

Patterson, P.H. (2011) Modeling autistic features in animals. *Pediatr Res,* 69(5 Pt 2), 34R-40R.

Ramalingam, T.S., Chakrabarti, A. & Edidin, M. (1997) Interaction of class I human leukocyte antigen (HLA-I) molecules with insulin receptors and its effect on the insulin-signaling cascade. *Mol Biol Cell,* 8(12), 2463-74.

Ribic, A., Flugge, G., Schlumbohm, C., Matz-Rensing, K., Walter, L. & Fuchs, E. (2011) Activity-dependent regulation of MHC class I expression in the developing primary visual cortex of the common marmoset monkey. *Behav Brain Funct,* 7, 1.

Ribic, A., Zhang, M., Schlumbohm, C., Matz-Rensing, K., Uchanska-Ziegler, B., Flugge, G., Zhang, W., Walter, L. & Fuchs, E. (2010) Neuronal MHC class I molecules are involved in excitatory synaptic transmission at the hippocampal mossy fiber synapses of marmoset monkeys. *Cell Mol Neurobiol,* 30(6), 827-39.

Rolleke, U., Flugge, G., Plehm, S., Schlumbohm, C., Armstrong, V.W., Dressel, R., Uchanska-Ziegler, B., Ziegler, A., Fuchs, E., Czeh, B. & Walter, L. (2006) Differential expression of major histocompatibility complex class I molecules in the brain of a New World monkey, the common marmoset (Callithrix jacchus). *J Neuroimmunol,* 176(1-2), 39-50.

Roumier, A., Bechade, C., Poncer, J.C., Smalla, K.H., Tomasello, E., Vivier, E., Gundelfinger, E.D., Triller, A. & Bessis, A. (2004) Impaired synaptic function in the microglial KARAP/DAP12-deficient mouse. *J Neurosci,* 24(50), 11421-8.

Shatz, C.J. (1996) Emergence of order in visual system development. *Proc Natl Acad Sci U S A,* 93(2), 602-8.

Smith, S.E., Li, J., Garbett, K., Mirnics, K. & Patterson, P.H. (2007) Maternal immune activation alters fetal brain development through interleukin-6. *J Neurosci,* 27(40), 10695-702.

Solheim, J.C. (1999) Class I MHC molecules: assembly and antigen presentation. *Immunol Rev,* 172, 11-9.

Soumiya, H., Fukumitsu, H. & Furukawa, S. (2011) Prenatal immune challenge compromises the normal course of neurogenesis during development of the mouse cerebral cortex. *J Neurosci Res,* 89(10), 1575-85.

Stagsted, J. (1998) Journey beyond immunology. Regulation of receptor internalization by major histocompatibility complex class I (MHC-I) and effect of peptides derived from MHC-I. *APMIS Suppl,* 85, 1-40.

Stagsted, J., Olsson, L., Holman, G.D., Cushman, S.W. & Satoh, S. (1993a) Inhibition of internalization of glucose transporters and IGF-II receptors. Mechanism of action of MHC class I-derived peptides which augment the insulin response in rat adipose cells. *J Biol Chem,* 268(30), 22809-13.

Stagsted, J., Reaven, G.M., Hansen, T., Goldstein, A. & Olsson, L. (1990) Regulation of insulin receptor functions by a peptide derived from a major histocompatibility complex class I antigen. *Cell,* 62(2), 297-307.

Stagsted, J., Ziebe, S., Satoh, S., Holman, G.D., Cushman, S.W. & Olsson, L. (1993b) Insulinomimetic effect on glucose transport by epidermal growth factor when combined with a major histocompatibility complex class I-derived peptide. *J Biol Chem,* 268(3), 1770-4.

Stubbs, E.G. & Magenis, R.E. (1980) HLA and autism. *J Autism Dev Disord,* 10(1), 15-9.

Sur, M. & Rubenstein, J.L. (2005) Patterning and plasticity of the cerebral cortex. *Science,* 310(5749), 805-10.

Syken, J., Grandpre, T., Kanold, P.O. & Shatz, C.J. (2006) PirB restricts ocular-dominance plasticity in visual cortex. *Science,* 313(5794), 1795-800.

Thams, S., Brodin, P., Plantman, S., Saxelin, R., Karre, K. & Cullheim, S. (2009) Classical major histocompatibility complex class I molecules in motoneurons: new actors at the neuromuscular junction. *J Neurosci,* 29(43), 13503-15.

Thompson, I. (2000) Cortical development: Binocular plasticity turned outside-in. *Curr Biol,* 10(9), R348-50.

Torres, A.R., Sweeten, T.L., Cutler, A., Bedke, B.J., Fillmore, M., Stubbs, E.G. & Odell, D. (2006) The association and linkage of the HLA-A2 class I allele with autism. *Hum Immunol,* 67(4-5), 346-51.

Wang, Y.T. & Linden, D.J. (2000) Expression of cerebellar long-term depression requires postsynaptic clathrin-mediated endocytosis. *Neuron,* 25(3), 635-47.

Xu, H.P., Chen, H., Ding, Q., Xie, Z.H., Chen, L., Diao, L., Wang, P., Gan, L., Crair, M.C. & Tian, N. (2010) The immune protein CD3zeta is required for normal development of neural circuits in the retina. *Neuron,* 65(4), 503-15.

4

Human Leukocyte Antigen Class II in Stimulated Polymorphnuclear Neutrophils

Bahaa K. A. Abdel-Salam
Zoology Department, Faculty of Science,
Minia University, El-Minia,
Egypt

1. Introduction

1.1 Polymorphonuclear neutrophils (PMN)

Polymorphnuclear neutrophils (PMN) possess a very short half-life in the circulation because they constitutively undergo apoptosis (Gasmi et al., 1996; Stringer et al., 1996; Moulding et al., 1998). Under certain conditions PMN play an important role in the effectors arm of host immune defense through the clearance of immune complexes, the phagocytosis of opsonized particles, and the release of inflammatory mediators (Shen et al., 1987; Petroni et al., 1988; Lloyd et al., 1992). During the recent years the image of PMN has changed considerably. Traditionally considered to be the first line defense against bacterial infection. It became increasingly clear that PMN also participate in chronic inflammatory disease and regulation of the immune response when appropriately activated (Iking-Konert et al., 2002). Persistent *Staphylococcus aureus*-mediated local infection induces the local activation and transdifferentiation of PMN to cells with dendritic-like characteristics (Wagner et al., 2006).

1.2 Interleukin (IL)

Interleukin is involved in processes of cell activation, cell differentiation, proliferation and cell to cell interactions. Each IL acts on a specific group of cells that express the correct receptor for the IL. The same IL can be produced by different cell types and an individual IL may act on different cell types, eliciting variable biological responses depending on the particular cell and its environment (Bhandari, 2002).

1.2.1 Interleukin (IL)-2

IL-2 has been considered to be a lymphocyte-activating and growth-promoting factor, and has been widely studied on T cells and NK cells (Waldmann, 1989). Monocytes have been reported to express IL-2R□ and to be activated by IL-2 for tumoricidal activity (Espinoza-Delgado et al., 1990). Thus far, PMN have not been studied for their interaction with IL-2, and their possession of IL-2R is unknown. The direct effect of IL-2 on PMN, especially the mechanisms involved in the activation of PMN, is unknown, although the ability of other immune cells to respond to IL-2 is well studied. Preliminary studies have shown that PMN have the capacity to respond to IL-2 with increased antifungal activity (Djeu et al., *1993*).

More importantly it have identified that PMN express surface receptors for IL-2, but only IL-2Rß and not IL-2Rα is present (Djeu et al., 1993).

1.2.2 Interleukin (IL)-4

IL-4 production has been found to occur in thymocytes, mature T-cells, certain malignant T-cells, mast-cells and basophiles and occasionally, in transformed B-cells (Holter, 1997). It has an effect on B-cells, T-cells, monocytes, mast-cells, endothelial cells, and fibroblasts (Paul, 1991). Directly and/or indirectly, IL-2 has a prominent role in the regulation of IL-4 producing cells (Holter, 1997). IL-4 binds to a high-affinity cell-surface receptor (IL-4R) to exert its effects (Idzerda et al., 1990). It promotes the growth and differentiation of activated human B-lymphocytes and shares many biological functions with IL-13 (Aversa et al., 1993).

1.2.3 Interleukin (IL)-15

IL-15 is a pleiotropic cytokine which shares biological activities with IL-2. IL-15 uses both β- and γ-chains of the IL-2 receptor for binding and signaling. The IL-15 receptor (IL-15R) complex also includes a specific α subunit (IL-15Rα) , distinct from the IL-2Rα chain. IL-15R is expressed on various cells of the immune response, including T- and B-cells, NK cells and more recently, peripheral blood neutrophils (Girard et al., 1999).

IL-15 plays an important role in both innate and adaptive immunity. It induces T-cell proliferation and cytokine production, stimulates the locomotion and chemotaxis of T-cells and delays its apoptosis. IL-15 has been shown to stimulate the growth and cytotoxicity of NK cells and to induce antibody-dependent cell-mediated cytotoxicity. It was also demonstrated that this cytokine induces macrophages function and B-cell proliferation (Girard et al., 1999). Recent investigation has shown that IL-15 potentiated several antimicrobial functions of normal PMN involved in the innate immune response against invading pathogens (Casatella and McDonald, 2000). IL-15 was observed to enhance phagocytosis, NF-ḱB activation, and IL-8 production and to delay apoptosis of these cells. In addition, IL-15 has been shown to prime the metabolic burst of PMN in response to N-formyl-methionyl-eucyl- phenylalanine (fMLP) (Casatella and McDonald, 2000; *Girard et al., 1996*; McDonald et al., 1998; Mastroianni et al., 2000).

The main source of IL-15 are macrophages / monocytes and lymphocytes as well as neutrophils (Casatella and McDonald, 2000; Muro and Taha, 2001; Zissel and Baumer, 2000).

1.3 Human leukocyte antigen (HLA) class II

For surface molecules, there are several reports that PMN from a variety of species can express HLA class II (Vachiery et al., 1999; Radsak et al., 2000; Iking-Konert et al., 2001a; Iking-Konert et al., 2002; Tyler et al., 2006). Under certain stimulation murine neutrophils present Class II restricted antigen (Shauna et al., 2008). Coexpression of HLA class II would potentially endow PMN with the capacity to influence the adaptive immune system through antigen presentation. Previous investigations with mouse, human, and goat PMN defined conditions whereby HLA class II expression was observed following stimulation with IFN-γ, granulocyte macrophage-colony stimulating factor (GM-CSF), or IL-3 (Gosselin et al., 1993; Smith et al., 1995; Mudzinski et al., 1995; Reinisch et al., 1996) or in human patients, with Wegener's granulomatosis (Haensch et al., 1999; Iking-Konert et al., 2001b). In some cases, PMN expression of HLA II was reported as constitutive (Okuda et al., 1979; Vachiery et al., 1999), and human PMN were also shown to function as accessory cells for primed T-cell activation with protein antigens and superantigens (Okuda et al., 1980; Fanger et al., 1997; Iking-Konert et al., 2001a; Tyler et al., 2006). Bovine PMN expressed detectable levels of HLA class II on their surface, only when cocultured with peripheral blood mononuclear cells (PBMC). This observation suggested that PMN may up-regulate endogenous HLA class II expression or passively acquire HLA class II protein from other leukocytes.

To better understand the role of IL-2 in the activation of PMN and to explore the possibility that the activation of PMN by IL-2 may reflect the interaction between T-cells and PMN. These findings provide useful insight for understanding some mechanisms of T-cell and PMN interactions and the possible role of PMN in IL-2 immunotherapy. There is evidence that HLA class II-positive PMN are able to present the superantigen staphylococcus enterotoxin E (SEE) to T-cells in an HLA class II-dependent manner (Fanger et al., 1997). Moreover, PMN pulsed with peptide was shown to activate antigen-specific memory T-cells (Reali et al., 1996). In addition, PMN stimulated with GM-CSF and IFN-γ has the capacity to present antigen to naive T-cells (Fanger et al., 1997). Those PMN with antigen-presenting capacity are thought to be a relatively mature population (Mudzinski et al., 1995). There is a large production of proinflammatory cytokines from both T-cells and monocytes following superantigen activation: T-cells produce IL-1β, IFN-γ, TNF-α, and IL-2 (Jupin et al., 1988; See et al., 1992a; Lagoo et al., 1994). While monocytes produce both IL-1β and IFN-γ (See and Chow 1992; See et al., 1992; Trede et al., 1994). It has shown that human PMN can be induced to express HLA class II molecules both *in vitro* and *in vivo*. Specifically, *in vitro* incubation of human PMN from healthy donors with either GM-CSF, IFN-γ, or IL-3 resulted in low-level expression of HLA-DR (Gosselin et al., 1993; Smith et al., 1995). In rheumatoid arthritis, there is an evidence for T-cells activation, where PMN act as dendritic-like cells at the site of inflammation (Iking-Konert et al., 2005).

1.4 Aim of the study

The aim of this study was to insure that IL-2, IL-4 or IL- 15 stimulated PMN might be involved in T-cell proliferation by acquiring HLA class II antigens.

2. Materials and methods

2.1 Immunocytochemistry

Blood was taken by venous puncture using 7·5 ml heparin-coated tubes (Sarstedt; Nümbrecht, Germany) and was analyzed within 2 hours

The IL-2R of PMN could be detected by immunofluorescence. Freshly isolated PMN by two hypotonic/hypertonic lyses steps with 0.2%/1.6% saline were fixed on slides (2 X 105 cells / slide) by a cytoSpin 4 centrifuge (Shandon; Frankfurt, Germany) and ice-cold methanol. Cells were incubated with 5% goat serum (Sigma; Saint Louis, MO, USA) in PBS followed by 2 μg anti-CD25-FITC (Becton Dickinson; San Jose, USA), 2μg anti-CD122-FITC (Serotec; Oxford, UK). Anti-mouse IgG-FITC and anti-CD66-FITC (Immunotech. Marseille, France) were used as positive and negative control respectively. The slides were examined by confocal laser microscopy (Leica, Bensheim, Germany) using Windows TC as software.

2.2 Cytofluorometry

IL-2R was detected on PMN by direct and indirect extracellular fluorescence-activated cell sorter (FACS). In direct sets of experiments cells in whole blood were stained with 2µg anti-CD122-FITC and 2µg anti-CD25 (Serotic; Oxford, UK) as a markers for IL-2Rβ chain and IL-2Rα chain. Primary an unlabeled antibody for IL-2Rβ chain was added to cells before staining with anti-CD122-FITC. Anti-mouse IgG-FITC and anti-CD66-FITC (Immunotech.; Marseille, France) were used as a negative and a positive control, respectively.

For HLA class II detection cells in whole blood were double labeled with 2µg anti-CD66b-FITC (Immunotech.; Marseille, France) as a PMN marker and 2µg PE-labeled antibodies to HLA DP-DQ-DR (Serotec; Oxford, UK), respectively, using standard procedures. They were analyzed by FACSCalibur and CellQuest software (Becton-Dickinson, Heidelberg, Germany). Results are expressed as percentage of positive cells in the respective gate or quadrant.

2.3 Cells purification and cultivation

For co-culture, cells were isolated by PolymorphPrep® (Nycomed; Oslo, Norway). PMN, Monocytes and T-cells fraction was further purified by adsorption to CD15, CD14 and CD3 beads (Miltenyi Biotech; Bergisch Gladbach, Germany), respectively, by magnetic cell separation using the devices supplied by Milteny Biotech (Bergisch-Gladbach, Germany).

Highly purified PMN (1 x 106 /ml) were cultivated in AIM V (Gibco BRL; Paisley, Scotland)) with 2.5% autologous normal human serum, NHS (inactivated at 56°C for 30 min.). T-cells and monocytes were cultured in RPMI 1640 (Gibco BRL; Paisley, Schottland) supplemented with 10% FCS (PAN Biotech GmbH; Aidenbach, Germany), 100U/ml penicillin/streptomycin (Gibco BRL; Paisley, Schottland), 2mM L-glutamine (Gibco BRL; Paisley, Schottland)), and 10mM HEPES (Gibco BRL; Paisley, Scottland). All the three types of cells were incubated at 37°C and 5 % CO_2 for the times indicated.

2.4 Stimulation of PMN

Highly purified PMN were placed into 24-well plate (Nunc™; Roskilde, Danmark)), 2ml/well, and incubated in the presence or absence of 10ng/ml IL-2 (Sigma; St Louis, MO, USA)) for about 48 hours at 37°C with 5% CO_2.

2.5 RNA isolation and reverse transcription-polymerase chain reaction (RT-PCR)

Total cellular RNA was isolated using the RNeasy kit from Qiagen (Hilden, Germany). For RT, 2 mg of RNA was incubated with 50 pmol random primer, 1 U RNase inhibitor, 10 pmol dNTP and 20 U Moloney Murine Leukemia Virus (MMuLV) reverse transcriptase (all purchased from Boehringer Mannheim, Germany) for 60 min at 37u, followed by 15 min at 94u. PCR for HLA class II was carried out in a Perkin-Elmer (UÈ berlingen, Germany) thermocycler as follows: 10 pmol dNTP was added to 5 ml of cDNA, followed by 50 pmol of the primers and 1 U Taq DNA polymerase in 2 mM MgCl2. After preheating to 94u for 10 min, 30 cycles for HLA class II were performed (30 seconds at 94u, 30 seconds at 60u, 60 seconds at 72u) followed by a final extension step at 72u for 10 min. The HLA-DR primer was used: sense: 5k-CGGATCCTTCGTGTCCCCAC-3k; antisense: 5k-

CTCCCCAACCCCGTAGTTGTGTCTGCA-3k, amplifying a 270-bp fragment (Nadler et al., 1994). This primer were synthesized by ARK Scientific Biosystems (Darmstadt, Germany). The PCR products were analyzed by gel electrophoresis (1.5% agarose) and staining with Sybr green (Molecular Probes; Leiden, the Netherlands). As a size marker, DNA molecular weight marker VI (Boehringer: Mannheim, Germany) was used. For sequencing, the PCR product was extracted by using the QIAquick gel extraction kit (Qiagen; Hilden, Germany); sequencing was performed using the ABI PRISM2 Big Dye2 Terminator Cycle Sequencing Ready Reaction Kit (PE Applied Biosystems; Warrington, UK). Data were measured and analyzed by Fluorescent Image Analyzer (FLA)-2000 (Becton Dickinson, San Jose, USA).

2.6 Coculture expreiments

Unstimulated and stimulated PMN ($1x10^3$) or monocytes (1x10) in 100μl were added per well of a 96-well concave-bottom plate (Greiner; Nuertingen, Germany). Then, $1x10^4$ T cells (100μl) were added to each well together with 25ng *Staphylococcal aueurs* Enterotoxins A (Sigma; München, Germany). The effect of IL-2 stimulation was blocked by ant-IL-2R (Serotec; Oxford, UK). After coincubation for 4 days at 37°C with 5% CO_2, proliferation was tested by adding 1 mCi of ^{3}H-thymidine (Amer-sham Life Science; Braunschweig, Germany) for 6-8 hours [^{3}H]TdR incorporation into DNA was measured and expressed as counts per minute (cpm). The values represent the mean±SD of 6-12 parallel wells.

2.7 Statistical analysis

Data were analyzed by student's t test. And a P value of 0.05 was a considered as the limit of significance.

3. Results

3.1 Visualization of the IL-2Rβ chain by immunocytochemistry

Isolated PMN by a hypotonic solution were examined by confocal laser microscopy. The IL-2Rα chain was not detectable (Fig. 1c). However the IL-2Rβ chain was seen in all cells (Fig. 2c). Mouse IgG-FITC was used as a negative control (Fig. 1a and 2a), while CD66b-FITC was used as a positive control (Fig. 1b and 2b), respectively.

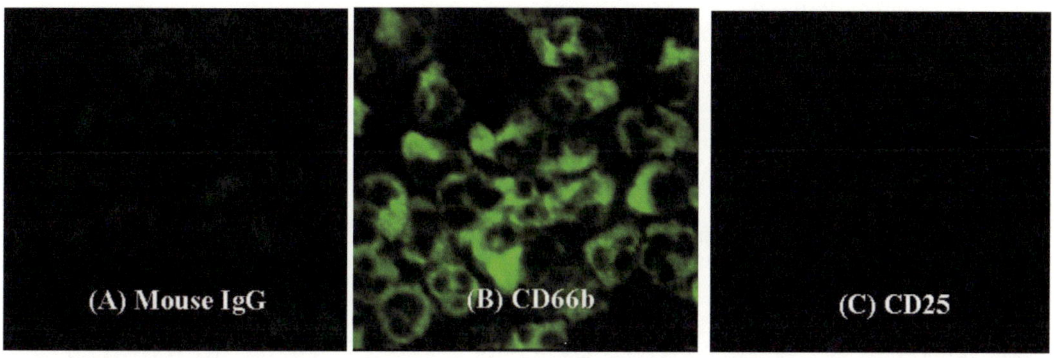

Fig. 1. Detection of IL-2Rα chain on PMN: The negative and positive controls were in panels A and B, respectively, while the panel C showed the CD25 (magnification: 1 X 400).

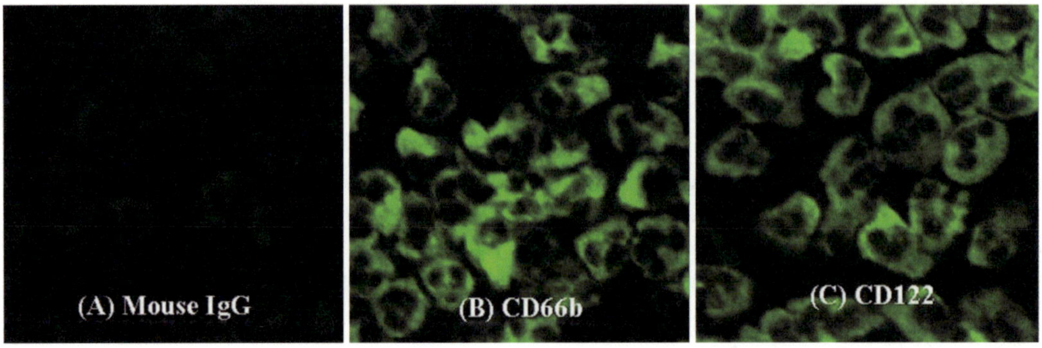

Fig. 2. Detection of IL-2Rβ chain on PMN: The negative and positive controls were in panels A and B, respectively, while the panel C showed the CD122 (magnification: 1 X400).

3.2 Direct immunofluorescence analysis of IL-2R

In order to investigate constitutive expression of IL-2R, we tested the presence of the two IL-2R chains (IL-2α and IL-2β) on the PMN cell surface by FACS. In line with previous data by others, the α chain (CD25) could not be detected (< 1 % positive cells), while PMN expressed CD122, though rather small amounts (Fig. 3).

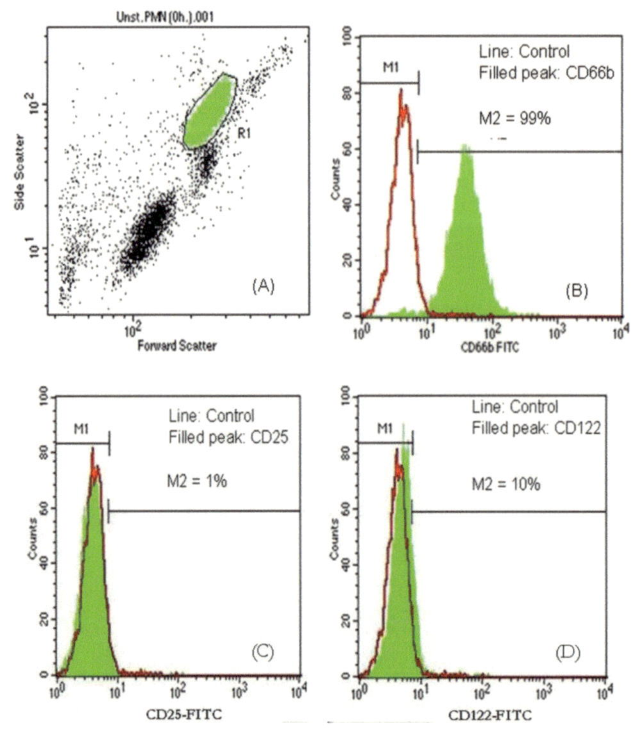

Fig. 3. Detection of IL-2R on PMN: (A) Forward-scatter (FSC) versus side-scatter (SSC) of whole blood flow cytometry showed different populations of leukocytes. R1 was set for PMN identified by expression of CD66b (B) filled peak. PMN expressed only IL-2Rβ chain (D), while IL-2Rα chain was absent (C) (filled peaks: antibody; line isotype control).

When comparing cells of different donors, the mean fluorescence intensity varied (a summary of 6 donors is shown in Table 1).

No. of tested donors	Mean fluorescence intensity
1-	10
2-	22
3-	16
4-	14
5-	32
6-	25

Table 1. Expression IL-2Rβ chain (CD122) on PMN of different donors.

3.3 Indirect immunofluorescence for the IL-2Rβ chain

By indirect labeling, using first an unlabeled antibody to IL-2Rβ, followed by a FITC-labeled antibody to mouse IgG, the signal for the IL-2Rβ chain could be amplified. Of note is that nearly all cells were positive (Fig. 4).

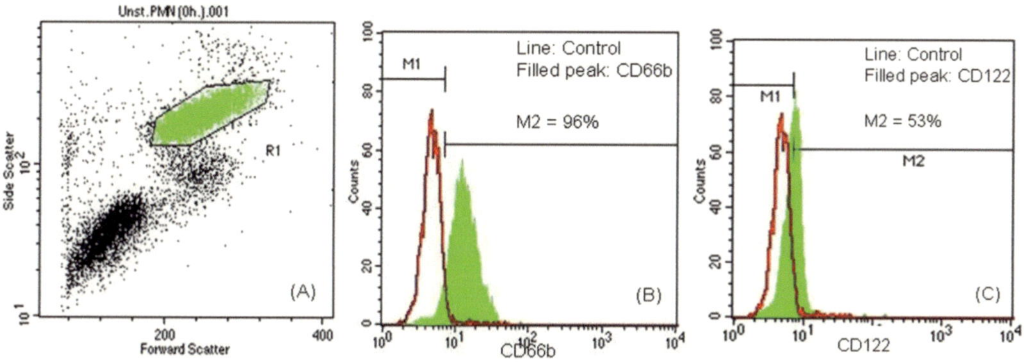

Fig. 4. Indirect extracellular detection of IL-2Rβ chain: (A) the forward-side scatter analysis of whole blood flow cytometry showed different populations of leukocytes. PMN were identified in R1. (B) M2 is the percentage of CD66b–positive cells (filled peak). (C) PMN expressed IL-2Rβ chain as detected by anti-CD122 (filled peak); the line is the negative control using mouse IgG in place of anti-CD122.

3.4 *In vitro* expression of HLA class II on PMN stimulated with IL-2

To test effects of IL-2 on HLA class II expression, the induction of HLA class II in highly purified PMN 48 hours cultured with IL-2 increased recording 20% (Fig. 5c). Freshly isolated PMN had 2% (Fig. 5a). PMN cultured with medium alone for 48 hours had also small amount (4%) of HLA class II (Fig. 5b).

3.5 Effect of IL-2 on HLA class II gene up-regulation on PMN

In another set of experiments, highly purified PMN exposed to IL-2 for various hours showed an increase in HLA class II specific RNA. This was tested by RT-PCR. When the

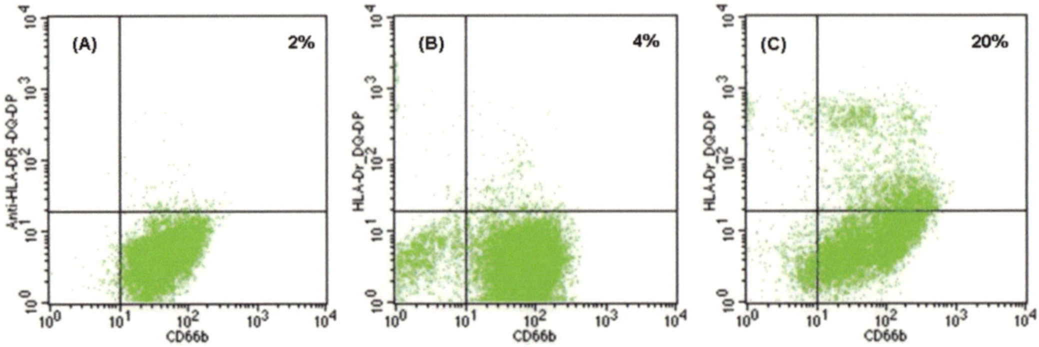

Fig. 5. Direct flow cytometry of the HLA class II induction in highly purified PMN:
A) Unstimulated PMN (0 hour). B) Unstimulated PMN (48 hours). C) Stimulated PMN with IL-2 (48 hours).

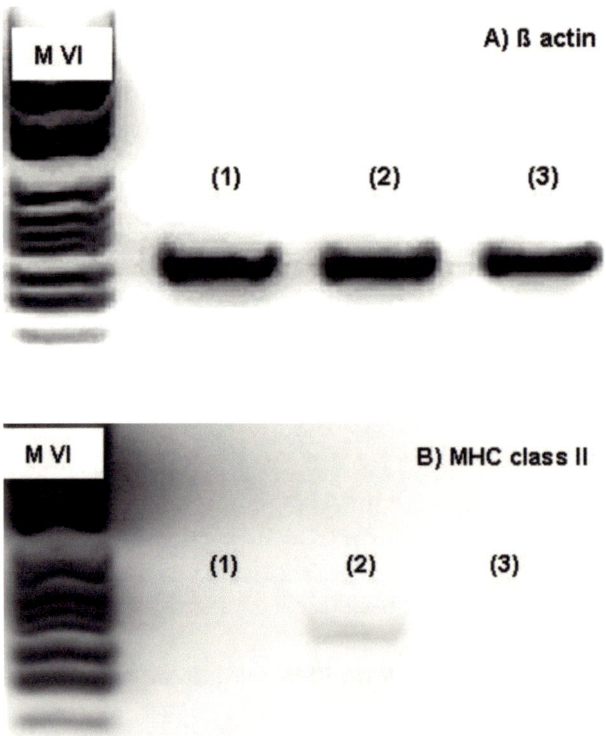

Fig. 6. RT-PCR detection of HLA class II mRNA in PMN activated with IL-2: PMN were incubated with IL-2 for 6 hours. The M VI was the used marker (154-2176 bp). Freshly isolated PMN were in Lane (1). Lane (2) showed the stimulated PMN after 6 hours, while the unstimulated PMN after 6 hours was in lane (3).

values were corrected for the input of the PCR-product by using β-actin as a housekeeping gene (Fig. 6a), it was seen that HLA class II RNA increased only when PMN were cultivated for 6 hours. The increase was more pronounced in the presence of IL-2 (Fig. 6b).

3.6 *In vitro* expression of HLA class II on PMN stimulated with IL-4

The majority of healthy donors PMN expressed CD66b (Fig. 7a, b & c). In the first set of experiments the effect of IL-4 on the expression of HLA class II was tested, where we found that PMN on whole blood showed expression of HLA class II recording 7.77% (Fig.7c) by using IL-4, as stimulators. In contrast, fresh and unstimulated cells cultured with medium only counting 1.05% (Fig.7a) and 2.71 % (Fig.7b), respectively.

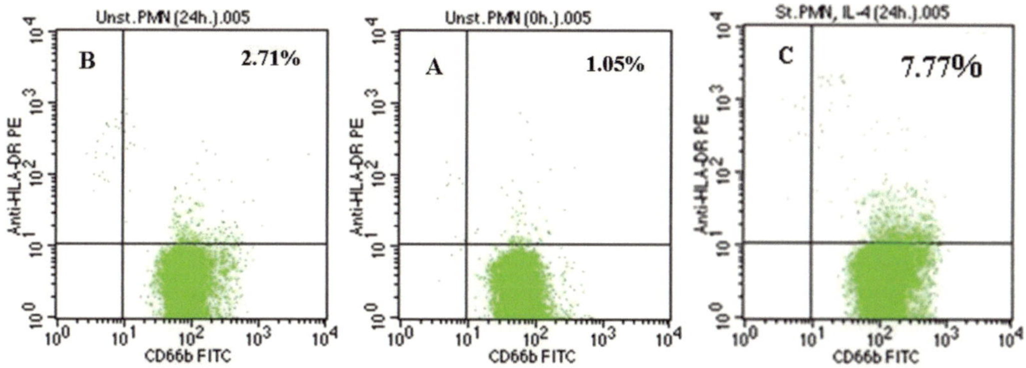

Fig. 7. Direct flow cytometry of the HLA Class II induction in whole blood PMN.
A) Unstimulated PMN (0 hour). B) Unstimulated PMN (24 hours). C) Stimulated PMN with IL-4 (24 hours).

3.7 *In vitro* expression of HLA class II on PMN stimulated with IL-15

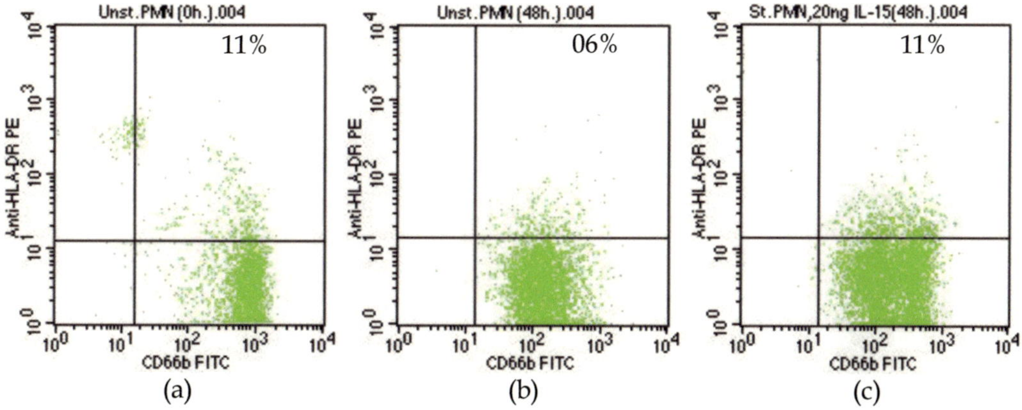

Fig. 8. Flow cytometric analysis of HLA class II expression on PMN treated with IL-15 (20ng / ml). PMN in whole blood were labeled with CD66b-FITC as a specific marker for PMN and HLA class II-PE. (A) Fresh PMN. (B) PMN cultured for 48hrs in medium.
(C) PMN cultured for 48hrs in medium with IL-15.

To test effects of IL-15 on HLA class II expression, in a first set of experiments the induction of HLA class II in PMN 24hrs co-cultured with IL-15 was very minor. Although, after 48hrs this induction increased recording 11% (Fig. 8c). Freshly PMN had 11% also (Fig. 8a). while PMN cultured with medium alone had smaller amout (06%) of HLA class II (Fig. 8b).

3.8 Interaction of HLA class II positive PMN with peripheral T-cells

The question was addressed, whether PMN stimulated to express HLA class II antigen, would be able to induce T-cell proliferation. For these experiments highly purified PMN were cultivated with IL-2 for 24 hours and then cocultivated with highly purified isolated T-cells in the absence or presence of *Staphylococcus* enterotoxin A (SEA), a well-known superantigen.

It was imperative to rule out the participation of professional antigen presenting cells, such as dendritic cell, monocytes or B-cells. Therefore great care was taken for purification of the cells, which was controlled cytofluorometry. Using this method, less than 1% contaminating cells could be detected in either the PMN or the T-cell preparation.

In a first set of experiments PMN in various numbers and for comparison monocytes were cocultivated with the T-cells and SEA and proliferation of T-cells was measured after 4 days. The experiment showed that about 10 times more PMN than monocytes were required to achieve comparable proliferation and that 100 monocytes were barely sufficient to induce T-cell proliferation above controls (T-cells alone or T-cells with SEA without PMN or monocytes, respectively) (Fig. 9).

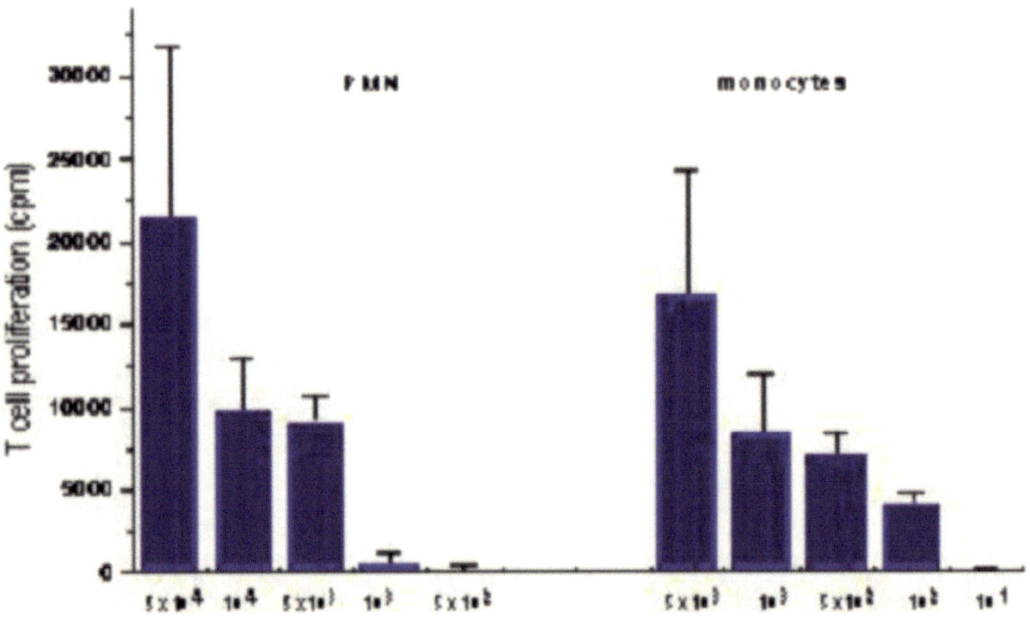

Fig. 9. Cells were cocultured with PMN or monocytes in the numbers indicated and in the presence of SEA. After 4 days proliferation of T-cells was measured by incorporation of [^{3}H] -thymidine, where proliferation was seen with at least 100 monocytes or 1000 PMN.

Based on the initial experiments, in the following 1000 PMN were used, because this would rule out participation of monocytes assuming a 1% contamination.

We could show that the T-cell proliferation was dependent not only on the number of PMN, but also on the presence or absence of SEA, and also dependent on the prestimulation of the PMN (Fig. 10).

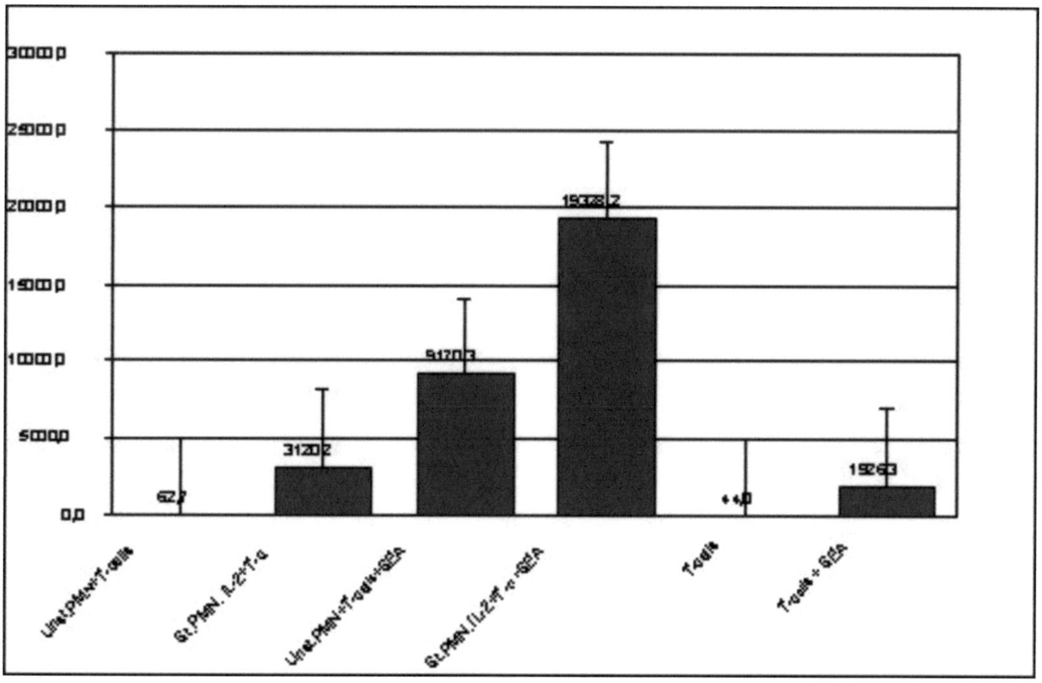

Fig. 10. Effects of bacterial Superantigens SEA on the proliferation of T-cells cocultured with 1 x 10^3 PMN stimulated with IL-2.

Moreover, the T-cell proliferation could - at least to some extent - be inhibited, when the PMN had been cultivated with IL-2 in the presence of an antibody to the IL-2 receptor (Fig. 11).

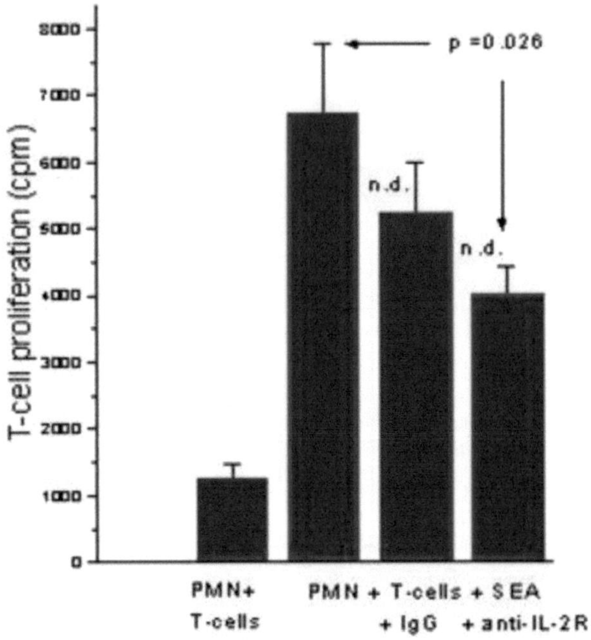

Fig. 11. Inhibition effect of anti-IL-2R on the proliferation of T-cells cocultured with 1 x 10^3 PMN stimulated with IL-2 and bacterial superantigens SEA.

The above data indicated that a high level of IL-2 in our body increases immunity by its effect on PMN to act as antigen presenting cells by the expression of HLA class II and consequently increased T-cells proliferation (cell mediated immunity).

The differences between the groups in the sets of experiments related to the interaction of HLA class II positive PMN with peripheral T-cells were calculated by t-test using $p < 0.05$ as limit.

4. Discussion

PMN are important effectors cells in host defense and inflammation. They are considered short-lived cells undergoing spontaneous apoptosis *in vivo* as well as in culture (Savill, 1997). In recent years it has become increasingly evident that culturing PMN in the presence of cytokines extends their life span (Colotta et al., 1992; Klebanoff et al., 1992; Lee et al., 1993; Biffl et al., 1996).

Previous data by others suggested that PMN express a receptor for IL-2. The present study confirms these data and provides evidence that PMN express constitutively IL-2R. As shown for monocytes and NK cells only the IL-2Rβ chain is expressed, but not IL-Rα (Espinoza-Delgado et al., 1990). This was in accordance with the present immunofluorosence results, where we detected only Il-2Rβ chain on resting PMN and confirmed my choosing of IL-2 as an activator of PMN.

Increasing evidence suggests that human PMN have an important role to play in regulating specific immune responses and in antigen presentation (Fanger et al., 1997; Radsak et al., 2000). In this study we have demonstrated that HLA Class II antigen was also detected, at the protein level by cytofowmetry, and also at the gene level by RT-PCR. These observations therefore agree well with the findings of others who have detected these antigens on the surface of activated neutrophils (Matsumoto et al., 1987; Radsak et al., 2000). The detection of these molecules therefore provides strong support for the hypothesis that human PMN can actively synthesize immunoregulatory molecules (Newburger et al., 2000) and have the potential to act as APCs (Fanger et al., 1997; Radsak et al., 2000). The observation that PMN may also express HLA class II antigens when appropriately stimulated (Gosselin et al., 1993 and Fanger et al., 1997), high lighted the possibility that PMN might function as accessory cells for T-cell activation. HLA class II expression was found on PMN of patients with active Wegener's disease (Haensch, et al., 1999). The close correlation of HLA class II expression to disease activity prompted the present study with the objective of investigating whether or not HLA class II-positive PMN might activate or support activation of T lymphocytes.

Induction of the above membrane-bound molecules was higher when PMN were stimulated in whole blood. The explanation of this phenomena may be due to the loss of some PMN IL-2R and IL-15R and other activities during their isolation procedure.

The absence or low detection of MHC class II on human PMN stimulated with IL-2, IL-4 and IL-15 could be due to: 1) The relatively long time (44 hrs) required for class II induction, which is beyond the period of PMN survival in most culture systems. 2) IL-2 and IL-15 receptor numbers may vary with the individual. 3) Synthetic capacity of the PMN may vary. 4) The capacities of cytokine receptors to signal may not be the same. 5) It may also be possible that the PMN themselves produce factors that inhibit class II induction. 6) Synthetic capacity of the PMN may vary. 7) The capacities of cytokine receptors to signal may not be the same. 8) It may also be possible that the PMN themselves produce factors that inhibit class II induction (Gosselin et al., 1993).

When comparing the number of monocytes and PMN required inducing T-cell proliferation, it was observed that 10 times more PMN than monocytes were necessary to yield the same extent of T-cell proliferation. However, the cell preparation used in this work never contained more than 1% of contaminating cells and certainly not the 10% of monocytes that would be required to affect the results. The observation that ten times more PMN than monocytes were required to induce a similar extent of T-cell proliferation has to be considered together with the observation that only a proportion of PMN acquired HLA class II. Thus, when only fully equipped PMN are considered, the ability to process and to present antigen is similar to that of monocytes. Whether HLA class II-positive PMN participate in the immune defense or play a role in pathophysiological events, is a matter of speculation. The fact that only a minor proportion of PMN acquire HLA class II might lead to the conclusion that a possible accessory function of PMN would be rather weak. One has, however, to bear in mind that PMN are numerous in the peripheral blood, and that even a low percentage of PMN expressing HLA class II would exceed both circulating monocytes and dendritic cells in number.

Because of the notion that the presence of *Staphylococcus entrotoxin* coincides with relapses of Wagner's granulomatosis (Cohn-Terveart et al., 1999), we tested whether PMN was able to also present *Staphylococcus enterotoxin A* is a superantigen, so-called because it binds outside of the peptide-binding groove of the HLA class II and the antigen-specific domain of the T-cell receptor, and consequently activates a large portion of T-cells, preferentially those with a V beta 2 domain (Simpson et al., 1995). In accordance with previous studies (Fanger et al., 1997; Radsak et al., 2000), co-culture of PMN with T-cells and SE resulted in T-cell proliferation. Taken together, our data demonstrate that by synthesizing and expressing of HLA class II antigens, PMN acquire the capacity to present superantigens to T-cells.

5. Conclusion

In conclusion, PMN possession of IL-2R β and γ chains that have the ability to bind with IL-2, IL-4 and IL-15 prompted us to use IL-2, IL-4 and IL-15 as stimuli for PMN. They stimulated PMN to express HLA class II which is the main antigen presenting molecules. PMN expressed HLA class II present SEA to T-cells causing their proliferation. T-cells proliferations lead to antigen destruction, B-cells activation and consequently immunoglobulin production, and activation of phagocytic cells.

6. Acknowledgement

I thank Prof. Dr. G. M. Haensch (Immunology Institute, Heidelberg, Germany) for using her laboratory in this study. I also thank her advice and encouragement throughout the work.

7. References

[1] Aversa, G., Punnonen, J., Cocks, B.G., de Waal Malefyt, R., Vega, F. Jr , Zurawski, S. M. , et al. (1993). An interleukin 4 (IL-4) mutant protein inhibits both IL-4 and IL-13-induced human immunoglobulin G4 (IgG4) and IgE synthesis and B cell proliferation: support for a common component shared by IL-4 and IL-13 receptors. *J Exp Med.,* 178:2213-2218.

[2] Bhandari, V. (2002). Developmental differences in the role of interleukins in hyperoxic lung injury in animal models. *Frontiers in Bioscience,* 7: 1624-1633.

[3] Biffl, W. L., Moore, E. E., Moore, F. A., Barnett, C. C., Carl, V. S., Peterson V. M. (1996). Interleukin-6 delays neutrophil apoptosis. *Arch. Surg.,* 131:24-30.

[4] Casatella, M.A., McDonald, P.P. (2000). Interleukin-15 its impact on neutrophil function. *Curr. Opin. Hematol.,* 4:174-177.

[5] Cohn-Terveart, J. W., Popa, E. R., Bos, N. A. (1999). The role of superantigen in vasculitis. *Curr. Opin. Rheumatol.,* 11:24-33.

[6] Colotta, F., Re, F., Polentarutti, N., Sozzani, S., Mantovani, A. (1992). Modulation of granulocyte survival and programmed cell death by cytokines and bacterial products. *Blood,* 80:2012-2020.

[7] Djeu, J. Y., Liu, J. H., Wei, S., Rui, H., Pearson, C. A., Leonard, W. J., Blanchard, D. K. (1993). Function associated with IL-2 receptor β on human neutrophils: Mechanism of activation of antifungal activity against Candida alhicuns by IL-2. *J. Immunol.,* 150:960-970.

[8] Espinoza-Delgado, I., Ortaldo, J. R., Winkler-Pickett, R., Sugamura, K., Varesio, L., Longo, D. L. (1990). Expression and role of p75 interleukin-2 receptor on human monocytes. *J. Exp. Med.*, 171:1821-1826.

[9] Fanger, N. A., Liu, C., Guyre, P. M., Wardwell, G. K., Neil, J. O., Guo, T. L., Christian, T. P., Mudzinski, S. P., Gosselin, E. J. (1997). Activation of human T cells by major histocompatibility complex class II-expressing neutrophils: proliferation in the presence of superantigen, but not tetanus toxoid. *Blood*, 89:4128-4135.

[10] Gasmi, L., McLennan, A. G., Edwards, S. W. (1996). The diadenosine polyphosphates Ap3 A and Ap4 A and adenosine triphosphate interact with granulocyte-macrophage colony-stimulating factor to delay neutrophil apoptosis: implications for neutrophil-platelet interactions during inflammation. *Blood*, 87:3442-3449.

[11] Girard, D, Boiani, N, Beaulieu, AD. (1999). Human neutrophils express the interleukin-15 receptor alpha chain (IL-15R alpha) but not the IL-9R alpha component. *Clin. Immunol. Immunophatol.*, 88: 232-240.

[12] Girard, D, Paquet, ME, Paquin, R, Beaulieu, AD. (1996). Differential effects of interleukin-15 (IL-15) and IL-2 on human neutrophils: modulation of phagocytosis, cytoskeleton rearrangement, gene expression, and apoptosis by IL-15. *Blood*, 88: 3176-3184.

[13] Gosselin, E. J., Wardwell, K., Rigby, W. F., Guyre, P. M. (1993). Induction of HLA class II on human polymorphonuclear neutrophils by granulocyte/macrophage colony-stimulating factor, IFN-gamma, and IL-3. *J. Immunol.*, 151:1482-1490.

[14] Haensch, G. M., Radsak, M., Wagner, C., Reis, B., Koch, A., Breitbart, A., Andrassy, K. (1999). Expression of major histocompatibility class II antigens on polymorphonuclear neutrophils in patients with Wegener's granulomatosis. *Kidney Int.*, 55: 1811-1818.

[15] Holter, W. (1997). Interleukin-4: structure and function. In: Remick DG, Friedland JS, editors. Cytokines in health and disease. New York, NY: Marcel Dekker;. p. 53.

[16] Idzerda, R. L., March, C. J., Mosley, B., Lyman, S D., Vanden Bo, s T., Gimpel, S. D. et al. (1990). Human interleukin-4 receptor confers biological responsiveness and defines a novel receptor superfamily. *J Exp Med.*, 171:861-873.

[17] Iking-Konert, C., Ostendorf, B., Sander, O., Jost, M., Wagner, C., Joosten, L., Schneider, M., Haensch, G. M. (2005). Transdifferentiation of polymorphonuclear neutrophils to dendritic-like cells at the site of inflammation in rheumatoid arthritis: evidence for activation by T cells. *Ann. Rheum. Dis.* 64:1436-1442.

[18] Iking-Konert, C., Cseko, C., Wagner, C., Stegmaier, S., Andrassy, K., Hansch, G. M. (2001a). Transdifferentiation of polymorphonuclear neutrophils: acquisition of CD83 and other functional characteristics of dendritic cells. *J. Mol. Med.* 79:464-474.

[19] Iking-Konert, C., Vogt, S., Radsak, M., Wagner, C., Hansch, G. M., Andrassy, K. (2001b). Polymorphonuclear neutrophils in Wegener's granulomatosis acquire characteristics of antigen presenting cells. *Kidney Int.*, 60:2247-2262.

[20] Iking-Konert, C., Wagner, C., Denefleh, B., Hug, F., Schneider, M., Andrassy, K., Hansch, G. M. (2002). Up-regulation of the dendritic cell marker CD83 on polymorphonuclear neutrophils (PMN): divergent expression in acute bacterial infections and chronic inflammatory disease. *Clin. Exp. Immunol.* 130:501-508.

[21] Jupin, C., Anderson, S. Damais, C. Alouf, J. E. and Parant. M. (1988). Toxic shock syndrome toxin-1 as an inducer of human tumour necrosis factors and γ interferon. *J. Exp. Med.* 167:752-761.

[22] Klebanoff, S. J., Olszowski, S., van Voorhis, W. C., Ledbetter, J. A., Waltersdorph, A. M., Schlechte, K. G. (1992). Effects of gamma interferon on human neutrophils, protection from deterioration on storage. *Blood,* 80:225-234.

[23] Lagoo, A. S., Lagoo-Deenadayalan, S., Lorenz, H. M., Byrne, J., Barber, W. H., Hardy, K. J. (1994). IL-2, IL-4, and IFN-γ gene expression versus secretion in superantigen-activated T-cells. *J. Immunol.* 152: 1641-1652.

[24] Lee, A., Whyte, M. B. K., Haslett, C. (1993). Inhibition of apoptosis and prolongation of neutrophil functional longevity by inflammatory mediators. *J. Leukoc. Biol.* 54:283-289.

[25] Lloyd, A. R., Oppenheim, J. J. (1992). Poly's lament: The neglected role of the polymorphonuclear neutrophil in the afferent limb of the immune response. *Immunol. Today,* 13:169-172.

[26] Matsumoto, S., Takei, M., Moriyama, M., Imanishi, H. (1987). Enhancement of Ia like antigen expression by interferon gamma in polymorphonuclear leukocytes. *Chem. Pharm. Bull.,* 35:436-439.

[27] Mastroianni, C. M., D 'Ettore, G., Forcina, G., Lichtner, M., Mengoni, F. D., Agostino, C., Corpolongo, A., Massetti, A., Vullo, V. (2000). Interleukin-15 enhances neutrophil functional activity in patients with human immunodeficiency virus infection. *Blood,* 96: 1979-1984.

[28] Moulding, D. A., Quayle, J. A., Hart, C. A., Edwards, S. W. (1998). Mcl-1 expression in human neutrophils: regulation by cytokines and correlation with cell survival. *Blood,* 92:2495-2502.

[29] McDonald, P. P., Russo, M. P., Cassatella, M.A. (1998). Interleukin-15 (IL-15) induces NF-ќ B activation and IL-8 production in human neutrophils. *Blood,* 4828-4835.

[30] Mudzinski, S. P., Christian, T. P., Guo, T. L., Cirenza, E., Hazlett, K. R., Gosselin, E. J. (1995). Expression of HLA-DR (major histocompatibility complex class II) on neutrophils from patients treated with granulocyte macrophage colony-stimulating factor for mobilization of stem cells. *Blood,* 86:2452-2453.

[31] Muro, S, Taha, R. (2001). Expression of IL-15 in inflammatory pulmonary disease. *J. Allergy Clin. Immunol.,* 108: 970-975.

[32] Nadler, S. G., Rankin, B. M., Moran-Davis, P., Cleaveland, J. S., Kiener, P. A. (1994). Effect of interferon-c on antigen processing in human monocytes. *Eur. J. Immunol.,* 24:3124-2130.

[33] Newburger, P. E., Subrahmanyam, Y. V. B. K., Weissman, S. M. (2000). Global analysis of neutrophil gene expression. *Curr. Opin. Hematol.,* 7:16-20.

[34] Okuda, K., Neely, B. C., David, C. S. (1979). Expression of H-2 and Ia antigens on mouse peritoneal neutrophils. *Transplantation,* 28:354-356.

[35] Okuda, K., Tani, K., Ishigatsubo, Y., Yokota, S., David, C. S. (1980). Antigen-pulsed neutrophils bearing Ia antigens can induce T lymphocyte proliferate response to the syngeneic or semisyngeneic antigen-primed T lymphocytes. *Transplantation,* 30:368-372.

[36] Petroni, K.C., Shen, L., Guyre, P. M. (1988). Modulation of human polymorphonuclear leukocyte IgG Fc receptors and Fc receptor-mediated functions by IFN-g and glucocorticoids. *J. Immunol.*, 140:3467-3472.

[37] Radsak, M., Iking-Konert, C., Stegmaier, S., Andrassy, K., Hänsch, G. M. (2000). Polymorphonuclear neutrophils as accessory cells for T-cell activation: major histocompatibility complex Class II restricted antigen-dependent induction of T-cell proliferation. *Immunology*, 101:521-530.

[38] Reali, E., Guerrini, R., Moretti, S., Spisani, S., Lanza, F., Tomatis, R., Traniello, S., Gavioli, R. (1996). Polymorphonuclear neutrophils pulsed with synthetic peptides efficiently activate memory cytotoxic T lymphocytes. *J. Leukoc. Biol.*, 60:207-213.

[39] Reinisch, W., Tillinger, W., Lichtenberger, C., Gangl, A., Willheim, M., Scheiner, O., Steger, G. (1996). *In vivo* induction of HLA-DR on human neutrophils in patients treated with interferon-γ. *Blood*, 87:3068.

[40] Savill, J. (1997). Apoptosis in resolution of inflammation. *J. Leukoc. Biol.*, 61:375-380.

[41] See, R. H., Chow, A. W. (1992). Role of the adhesion molecule lymphocyte function associated antigen 1 in toxic shock syndrome toxin 1-induced tumor necrosis factor alpha and interleukin-1β secretion by human monocytes. *Infect. Immunol.*, 60:4957-4960.

[42] See, R. H., Kum, W. W. S., Chang, A. H., Goh, S. H., Chow, A. W. (1992). Induction of tumor necrosis factor and interleukin-1 by purified staphylo-coccal toxic shock syndrome toxin 1 requires the presence of both monocytes and T lymphocytes. *Infect. Immunol.*, 60:2612-2618.

[43] Shauna, C., Owain, R. M., James, M. B., Iain, B. M. (2008). Murine neutrophils present Class II restricted antigen. *Immunol. Lett.*, 15: 49-54.

[44] Shen, L., Guyre, P. M., Fanger, M. W. (1987). Polymorphonuclear leukocyte function triggered through the high affinity Fc receptor for monomeric IgG. *J. Immunol.*, 139:534-538.

[45] Simpson, I. J., Skinner, M. A., Geursen, A. (1995). Peripheral blood T-lymphocytes in systemic vasculitis: Increased T-cell receptor V beta 2 gene usage in microscopic polyarteritis. *Clin. Exp. Immunol.*, 101: 220-236.

[46] Smith, W. B., Guida, L., Sun, Q., Korpelainen, E. I., van den Heuvel, C., Gillis, D., Hawrylowicz, C. M., Vadas, M. A., Lopez, A. F. (1995). Neutrophils activated by granulocyte-macrophage colony-stimulating factor express receptors for interleukin-3 which mediate class II expression. *Blood*, 86;3938-3944.

[47] Stringer, R. E., Hart, C. A., Edwards, S. W. (1996). Sodium butyrate delays neutrophil apoptosis: role of protein biosynthesis in neutrophil survival. *Br. J. Hematol.*, 92:169-175.

[48] Trede, N. S., Moris, T., Scholl, P. R., Geha, R. S., Chatila, T. (1994). Early activation events induced by the staphylococcal superantigen toxic shock syndrome toxin-1 in human peripheral blood monocytes. *Clin. Immunol. Immunopathol.*, 70:137-144.

[49] Tyler, A. W., Terry, K. B., Lorne, A. B., Philip, J. G. (2006). Bovine polymorphonuclear cells passively acquire membrane lipids and integral membrane proteins from apoptotic and necrotic cells. *J. Leukoc. Biol.*, 79:1226-1233.

[50] Vachiery, N., Totte, P., Balcer, V., Martinez, D., Bensaid, A. (1999). Effect of isolation techniques, *in vitro* culture and IFN-γ treatment on the constitutive expression of HLA class I and class II molecules on goat neutrophils. *Vet. Immunol. Immunopathol.,* 70:19-32.

[51] Wagner, C., Iking-Konert, C., Hug, F., Stegmaier, S., Heppert, V., Wentzensen, A., Haensch G. M. (2006). Cellular inflammatory response to persistent localized Staphylococcus aureus infection: phenotypical and functional characterization of polymorphonuclear neutrophils (PMN). *Clin. Exp. Immunol.,* 143:70-77.

[52] Waldmann, T. A. (1989). The multi-subunit interleukin-2 receptor. *Ann. Rev. Biochem,* 58:875-911.

[53] Zissel, G, Baumer, I. (2000). In vitro release of interleukin- 15 by bronchoalveolar lavage cells and peripheral blood mononuclear cells from patients with different lung disease. *Eur. Cytokine Netw.,* 11: 105-112.

5

Dicer Regulates the Expression of Major Histocompatibility Complex (MHC) Class I Chain-Related Genes A and B

Kai-Fu Tang
Wenzhou Medical College
China

1. Introduction

RNAi constitutes a key component of the innate immune response to viral infection in both plants and invertebrate animals, and has been postulated to function as the genome or intracellular immune system (Fire A., 2005; Plasterk RH., 2002; Umbach JL. & Cullen BR., 2009). Knockdown of Dicer, the key component of the RNAi pathway, elicits DNA damage and induces the expression of MHC class I chain-related gene A and B (MICA and MICB), two ligands of the NKG2D receptor expressed by natural killer cells and activated $CD8^+$ T cells (Tang KF. et al, 2008b). In this chapter, I discuss the possible molecular mechanisms by which decreased Dicer expression elicits DNA damage and induces the expression of MICA and MICB. MICA and MICB are frequently up-regulated in epithelial tumors of diverse tissue origins (Gasser S. & Raulet DH., 2006). Dicer is down-regulated in most tumor tissues (Merritt WM. et al, 2008; Wu JF. et al, 2011), and DNA damage response is activated in human tumors and precancerous lesions (Bartkova J. et al, 2005, 2006; DiTullio RA Jr. et al, 2002; Gorgoulis VG. et al, 2005). Therefore, the possible roles of Dicer, DNA damage, and MICA and MICB in tumorigenesis are also discussed.

2. RNA interference and the intracellular immune system

Experimental introduction of antisense RNA into cells was once used to interfere with the function of endogenous genes (Izant JG. & Weintraub H., 1984; Nellen W. & Lichtenstein C., 1993). However, Fire and colleagues found in 1991 that plasmid-encoded sense RNA is sufficient to cause interference (Fire A. et al, 1991); Guo and Kemphues reported in 1993 that, in addition to antisense RNA, sense RNA and double-stranded RNA (dsRNA) interfere with the function of endogenous genes (Guo S. & Kemphues KJ., 1995). In 1998, Fire and colleagues found that double-stranded RNA is substantially more effective at producing interference than either strand individually (Fire A. et al, 1998). After injection into adult animals, purified single strands had at most a modest effect, whereas double-stranded mixtures caused potent and specific interference (Fire A. et al, 1998). This phenomenon is now termed RNA interference (RNAi). Historically, RNAi was also known as other names, including posttranscriptional gene silencing (PTGS) and co-suppression in plants (Napoli C. et al, 1990; van der Krol AR. et al, 1990), RNA-mediated virus resistance in plants (Lindbo JA. & Dougherty WG., 1992), and"quelling" in Neurospora (Cogoni C., 1996) and algae (Wu-Scharf D. et al, 2000). It was postulated that the main functions of the RNAi pathway include antiviral defense, heterochromatic silencing, and transposon regulation (Martienssen RA. et al, 2008; Umbach JL. & Cullen BR., 2009). Therefore, Plasterk and Fire proposed that RNAi is the genome or intracellular immune system (Fire A., 2005; Plasterk RH., 2002).

3. Dicer is the key component of the RNAi pathway

RNAi is characterized by the presence of RNAs of about 22 nucleotides in length that are homologous to the gene being suppressed (Hamilton AJ. & Baulcombe DC., 1999; Hammond SM. et al, 2000; Zamore PD. et al, 2000). These 22-nucleotide sequences, called short interfering RNAs (siRNAs), serve as guide sequences that instruct a multicomponent nuclease, RNA-Induced Silencing Complex (RISC), to destroy the homologous messenger RNAs (Hammond SM. et al, 2000). Dicer, the key component of the RNAi pathway, was identified by Bernstein and colleagues (Bernstein E. et al, 2001). They demonstrated that immunoprecipitated Dicer can generate 22-nucleotide RNAs from dsRNA substrates, and that inhibition of Dicer expression significantly reduces processing of long dsRNA in whole-cell lysates or in Dicer immunoprecipitates (Bernstein E.et al, 2001). In addition to the extrogenous siRNAs, Dicer is also responsible for the biogenesis of endogenous siRNAs. In Schizosaccharomyces pombe, Dicer processes endogenous dsRNA derived from centromeric repeats. The small RNAs are then associated with Ago1, Chp1, and Tas3 to form the RNA-induced initiation of transcriptional gene silencing (RITS) complex that is required for heterochromatin assembly in fission yeast (Verdel A. et al, 2004). Deletion of Dicer results in the aberrant accumulation of complementary transcripts from centromeric heterochromatic repeats. This is accompanied by transcriptional de-repression of transgenes integrated at the centromere, loss of histone H3 lysine-9 methylation, and impaired centromere function (Volpe TA. et al, 2002). The Drosophila endogenous siRNAs are derived from transposons, heterochromatic sequences, and stem-loop structures containing RNAs. Normal accumulation of these endogenous siRNAs requires the siRNA-generating ribonuclease, Dicer, and the RNA interference effector protein, Ago2; mutations in Dicer causes an increase in these transcripts (Czech B. et al, 2008; Ghildiyal M. et al, 2008; Kawamura Y. et al, 2008; Okamura K. et al, 2008). SiRNAs are target-dependent amplified in some organisms. DsRNA is cut into siRNAs, the double-stranded siRNAs are converted into single-stranded siRNAs by the slicer activity of Ago2, the sense strands are degraded, and the antisense strands anneal to their targets and induce target degradation. Alternatively, the antisense RNAs may serve as primers, inducing dsRNA synthesis by the RNA-dependent RNA polymerase (RdRP); Dicer then cuts the dsRNAs to generate secondary siRNAs (Plasterk RH., 2002). Whether there are endogenous siRNAs in organisms lacking RdRP activity was investigated by means of deep sequencing. Two groups found that endogenous siRNAs derived from pseudogenes, natural antisense transcripts, and transposable elements exist in mouse oocytes (Tam OH. et al, 2008; Watanabe T. et al, 2008).

In addition to producing siRNA, Dicer is also required for the biogenesis of other types of small RNAs. Hutvagner and colleagues presented evidence that in Drosophila, a developmentally regulated microRNA (miRNA) precursor, pre-let-7, is cleaved by an RNA interference-like mechanism to produce mature let-7 miRNA (Hutvágner G. et al, 2001). In cultured human cells, knockdown of Dicer leads to accumulation of the let-7 precursor. This is the first evidence that the RNA interference and miRNA pathways intersect (Hutvágner G. et al, 2001). In addition to the biogenesis of siRNAs and miRNAs, Dicer is also required for the degradation of unstable RNAs containing AU-rich elements (AREs) in 3-prime untranslated regions (UTRs) (Jing Q. et al, 2005). Morever, Dicer also functions in fragmenting chromosomal DNA during apoptosis. Nakagawa and colleagues reported that inactivation of the Caenorhabditis elegans Dicer gene compromises apoptosis and blocks apoptotic chromosome fragmentation (Nakagawa A. et al, 2010). Dicer is cleaved by the Ced3 caspase to generate a C-terminal fragment with deoxyribonuclease activity, which produces 3-prime hydroxyl DNA breaks on chromosomes and promotes apoptosis (Nakagawa A. et al, 2010).

4. Dicer is essential for heterochromatin formation

Depletion of Dicer disrupts heterochromatin formation in Schizosaccharomyces pombe, Arabidopsis thaliana, Caenorhabditis elegans, Tetrahymena thermophila, and Drosophila melanogaster (Grewal SI., 2010; Lejeune E. & Allshire RC., 2011; Martienssen RA. et al, 2008; Riddle NC. & Elgin SC., 2008). However, whether Dicer is involved in heterochromatin formation in mammalian cells is still controversial. Kanellopoulou and colleagues reported that knockout of Dicer in mouse ES cells disrupts centromeric heterochromatin formation, with reduced histone H3K9 di-methylation and tri-methylation, reduced DNA methylation, and increased levels of centromeric repeat RNAs. The decondensation of heterochromatin is accompanied by markedly reduced levels of the 25-30 nt centromeric small dsRNAs, suggesting that Dicer-dependant small RNAs are required for the formation of centromeric heterochromatin (Kanellopoulou C. et al, 2005). Two groups found that the retinoblastoma-like 2 protein (Rbl2) is the target of miR-290 family miRNAs, and that Rbl2 can inhibit the expression of DNA methyltransferases (Dnmts), including Dnmt1, Dnmt3a and Dnmt3b (Benetti R. et al, 2008; Sinkkonen L. et al, 2008). Dicer deficiency in mice leads to decreased DNA methylation. DNA-methylation defects correlate with decreased expression of Dnmts and miR-290 family miRNAs, and can be reversed by transfection with miR-290 family miRNAs. These results indicate that the DNA hypomethylation in Dicer knockout cells is the consequence of low levels of miR-290 family miRNAs (Benetti R. et al, 2008; Sinkkonen L. et al, 2008). However, Benetti and colleagues found that Dicer is not required for histone tri-methylation. They observed that Dicer-null cells have a normal density of H3K9me3 and H4K20me3 marks and of HP1-binding at pericentric repeats, and that these heterochromatic histone marks are significantly increased at telomeric chromatin in Dicer-null cells compared to wild-type controls. They also found that the active chromatin mark, AcH3K9, is decreased at Dicer-null telomeres compared to wild-type telomeres, and that the density of this mark was not significantly decreased at pericentric chromatin. These results suggest that Dicer knockout cells have a higher degree of chromatin compaction and silencing at telomeric chromatin (Benetti R. et al, 2008). Hannon's group reported that although loss of Dicer affects the abundance of transcripts from centromeres in mouse ES cells, the histone modification status at pericentric repeats and methylation of centromeric DNA are not affected in Dicer knockout ES cells (Murchison EP. et al, 2005). Cobb and colleagues reported that the maintenance of constitutive and facultative heterochromatin seemed to be unperturbed in Dicer knockout thymocytes (Cobb BS. et al, 2005).

5. Decreased Dicer expression elicits DNA damage

The timing of DNA replication is tightly regulated and correlates with chromatin state. Highly condensed heterochromatin replicates late in S phase, while less condensed euchromatin tends to replicate early (Donaldson AD., 2005). Although the replication times of many single copy loci, including a 5 Mb contiguous region surrounding the Rex1 gene, are unchanged in Dicer mutant ES cells, the temporal control of satellite DNA replication is sensitive to loss of Dicer (Jørgensen HF. et al, 2007). Misregulation of the timing of DNA replication may cause stalled and collapsed replication forks, which in turn elicit a DNA damage response (Sancar A. et al, 2004). Loss of Dicer in Drosophila cells not only results in decondensation of heterochromatin but also leads to accumulation of extrachromosomal circular (ecc) repeated DNAs. Ligase IV, an essential regulator of nonhomologous end-joining and perhaps other DNA damage-repair machinery, participates in eccDNA formation (Peng JC. & Karpen GH., 2007). This suggests that, while heterochromatin decondensation increases the access of DNA repair and recombination proteins to repeated DNA, activation of DNA damage response may also contribute to the formation of eccDNA in Dicer mutant cells. RNAi is postulated to function as the genome's immune system, defending against molecular parasites such as transposons and viruses, and loss of Dicer may activate transposition (Fire A., 2005; Plasterk RH., 2002). Transposition generates double strand DNA breaks and elicits a DNA damage response (Gasior SL. et al, 2006). Chromatin structure is essential for maintaining genome integrity (Peng JC. & Karpen GH., 2008). For example, Drosophila cells that lack the Su(var)3-9 H3K9 methyltransferase have significantly elevated frequencies of spontaneous DNA damage in heterochromatin. Accumulated DNA damage in these mutants correlates with chromosomal defects, such as translocations and loss of heterozygosity. Based on the observation that S-phase in Su(var)3-9 mutants is significantly shorter than that in wild type cells, the authors proposed that accumulation of DNA damage in Su(var)3-9 mutants is the consequence of defective DNA replication (Peng JC. & Karpen GH., 2009). The regions of repetitive DNA may be incompletely replicated or defective in chromatin reassembly because of a shortened S phase. Alternatively, repeated DNA in heterochromatin may undergo faster replication, resulting in more replication errors. However, the demonstration that DNA damage is detected in G1, S, and G2 stages in Su(var)3-9 mutants suggests that defective DNA replication is not the only cause of the increased DNA damage. HP1β, whose localization requires H3K9me, is needed for efficient DNA damage detection in mammalian cells (Ayoub et al, 2008). Therefore, another explanation for the increased frequencies of DNA damage in Su(var)3-9 mutant cells may be that proper DNA damage detection and subsequent DNA repair response are impaired (Peng JC. & Karpen GH., 2009). We also demonstrated that 5-Aza-2'-deoxycytidine (5-aza-dC), a DNA methyltransferase inhibitor, induces DNA damage in human cells (Tang KF. et al, 2008a).

To test whether loss of Dicer can induce DNA damage, we knocked down Dicer in HEK293T cells and human hepatoma HepG2 cells and measured markers for DNA damage. Immunostaining assays for the phosphorylated form of histone H2AX (γ-H2AX), a widely used marker for double-strand DNA breaks (Foster ER. & Downs JA., 2005), and for the replication protein A 70 (RPA70), a protein that becomes phosphorylated and forms intranuclear foci upon exposure of cells to DNA damage (Zou Y. et al, 2006), revealed that a much higher percentage of Dicer knockdown cells display intense γ-H2AX foci and RPA foci compared to control cells (Tang KF. et al, 2008b). Using a comet assay to directly assess DNA damage, we confirmed that knockdown of Dicer resulted in accumulation of DNA breaks (Tang KF. et al, 2008b). Consistent with our results, Peng and Karpen reported a significant increase in spontaneous DNA damage in heterochromatic DNAs of Dicer mutant Drosophila cells (Peng JC. & Karpen GH., 2009). Mudhasani and colleagues reported that loss of Dicer activates a DNA damage checkpoint, up-regulates p19(Arf)-p53 signaling, and induces senescence in primary cells (Mudhasani R. et al, 2008).

In Figure 1, I summarize the possible mechanisms on how loss of Dicer leads to DNA damage. First, loss of Dicer reduces the level of endogenous siRNAs, resulting in heterochromatin decondensation. Heterochromatin decondensation may induce DNA damage via the following mechanisms: (i) loss of H3K9 methylation compromises DNA damage detection and subsequent DNA repair response, leading to DNA damage accumulation; (ii) disruption of DNA replication timing induces DNA damage; and (iii) mobilization of transposon and retrotransposon creates DNA double-strand breaks. Second, loss of Dicer stabilizes dsRNA derived from transposons and retrotransposons, causing a high level of transposition and generating DNA double-strand breaks. Third, loss of Dicer compromises miRNA biogenesis. Some miRNAs, such as the miR290 family, can suppress the expression of DNA methyltransferases or histone modifiers; loss of such miRNAs may cause heterochromatin decondensation, which in turn results in DNA damage. Loss of miRNAs that target to components of the DNA damage repair pathway may cause insufficient DNA damage repair, leading to DNA damage accumulation. These molecular events may act synergically or additively in Dicer mutant cells to induce DNA damage.

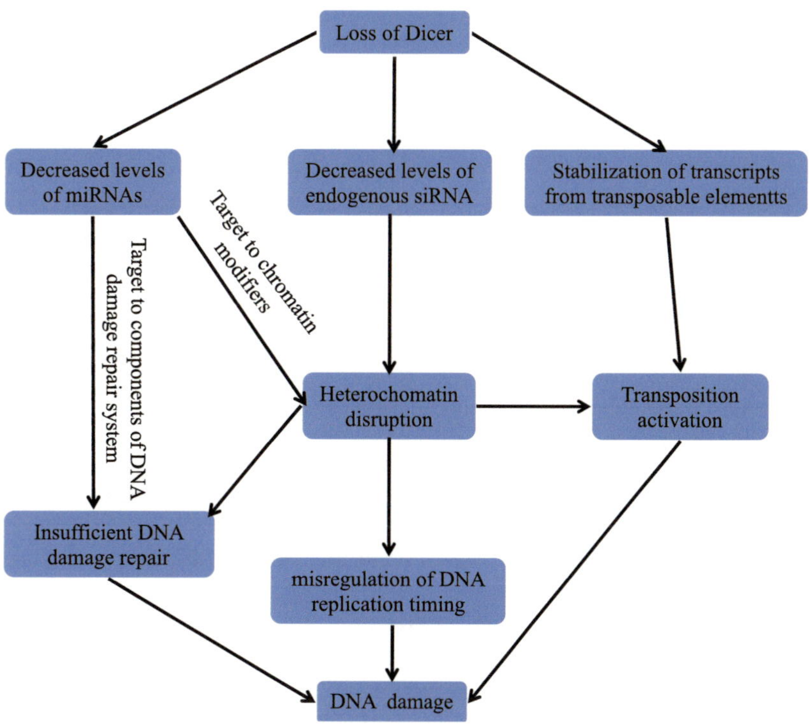

Fig. 1. Molecular mechanisms of DNA damage arising from decreased Dicer expression.

6. DNA damage response induces the expression of ligands for the NKG2D receptor

Natural killer (NK) cells, components of the innate immune system, can kill certain transformed or virus-infected cells lacking MHC class I, yet spare the cells expressing MHC class I. The ability to attack cells missing 'self' markers predicted the existence of both inhibitory and activating receptors on NK cells (Lanier LL., 2008). Unlike T and B cells, which possess a single antigen receptor that dominates cellular development and activation, NK cells do not possess one dominant receptor, but instead have a vast array of receptors to initiate effector functions. None of the receptors alone, with the exception of CD16, is able to elicit cytolytic activity or cytokine secretion (Lanier LL., 2008). The NKG2D receptor complex is one of the activating NK receptors. It is a hexamer, with one NKG2D homodimer associated with two DAP10 homodimers. A single gene encodes NKG2D, which is a C-type lectin-like superfamily member, and a type II transmembrane-anchored glycoprotein expressed as a disulfide-bonded homodimer on the surface of NK cells, γδ T cells, and $CD8^+$ T cells (Lanier LL., 2008). Engagement of NKG2D by its ligands leads either to the direct activation of killing and cytokine secretion by NK cells or to a costimulation of cytotoxic T-lymphocyte cytotoxicity (Lanier LL., 2008; Stern-Ginossar N. & Mandelboim O., 2009). In humans, NKG2D ligands are divided into two families: the MHC class I polypeptide-related chain (MIC) protein family, which contains MICA and MICB; and the cytomegalovirus UL16-binding proteins (ULBP) family, which consists of five members (ULBP1, ULBP2, ULBP3, ULBP4, and REAT1G) (Stern-Ginossar N. & Mandelboim O., 2009).

Gasser and colleagues found that NKG2D ligands are up-regulated in non-tumor cell lines by genotoxic stress and stalled DNA replication, conditions known to activate a major DNA damage checkpoint pathway (Gasser S. et al, 2005). The DNA damage checkpoints employ damage sensor proteins, such as ATM, ATR, the Rad17-RFC complex, and the 9-1-1 complex, to detect DNA damage and to initiate signal transduction cascades that employ Chk1 and Chk2 Ser/Thr kinases and Cdc25 phosphatases. The signal transducers activate p53 and inactivate cyclin-dependent kinases to inhibit cell cycle progression from G1 to S (the G1/S checkpoint), DNA replication (the intra-S checkpoint), or G2 to mitosis (the G2/M checkpoint) (Sancar A. et al, 2004). The up-regulation of NKG2D ligand induced by genotoxic stress was prevented by pharmacological or genetic inhibition of ATR, ATM, or Chk1, indicating that up-regulation of NKG2D ligands is a consequence of DNA damage response (Gasser S. et al, 2005). Induction of DNA damage leads to p53 activation. The role of p53 in the up-regulation of NKG2D ligands was addressed by Textor and colleagues. They found that induction of wild-type p53, but not mutant p53, strongly up-regulated mRNA and cell surface expression of ULBP1 and ULBP2, and that the intronic p53 responsive elements in these two novel p53 target genes are responsible for the up-regulation of ULBP1 and ULBP2 (Textor S. et al, 2011). The biological and medical implications of these findings have been addressed by several groups. Soriani and colleagues demonstrated that treatment with low doses of therapeutic agents such as doxorubicin, melphalan, and bortezomib commonly used in the management of patients with multiple myeloma leads to up-regulation of NKG2D ligands, and that the drug-induced expression of NKG2D ligands was abolished after treatment with the ATM and ATR pharmacologic inhibitors (Soriani A. et al, 2009). We showed that treatment with 5-Aza-2'-deoxycytidine (5-aza-dC), a DNA methyltransferase inhibitor, induces DNA damage-dependant up-regulation of NKG2D ligands (Tang KF. et al, 2008a). Cerboni and colleagues demonstrated that in response to superantigen, alloantigen, or a specific antigenic peptide, the expression of NKG2D ligands on the surface of T lymphocytes is induced, and that the induction of NKG2D ligand expression is the consequence of DNA damage (Cerboni C. et al, 2007). In addition, they demonstrated that activated T cells became susceptible to autologous NK lysis via NKG2D/NKG2DLs interaction and granule exocytosis, suggesting that NK lysis of T lymphocytes via NKG2D may be one of the mechanisms limiting T-cell responses (Cerboni C. et al, 2007). HIV up-regulates cell-surface expression of NKG2D ligands, including ULBP1, ULBP2, and ULBP3, but not MICA or MICB, in infected cells both in vitro and in vivo. HIV-1-induced up-regulation of NKG2D ligands contributes to HIV-1-induced $CD4^+$ T-lymphocyte depletion. Recently, two groups demonstrated that the HIV-1 Vpr protein activates the DNA damage response, which specifically induces surface expression of ULBP1 and ULBP2 (Richard J. et al, 2010; Ward J. et al, 2009).

7. Decreased Dicer expression elicits up-regulation of MICA and MICB

The DNA damage pathway regulates expression of innate immune system ligands for the NKG2D receptor. Human NKG2D ligands are up-regulated by genotoxic stress and stalled DNA replication. Dicer knockdown elicits DNA damage in human cells. These observations prompted us to test whether NKG2D ligands were up-regulated in Dicer knockdown cells. Quantitative RT-PCR and flow cytometry revealed markedly increased levels of MICA and MICB mRNAs and proteins in Dicer knockdown cells compared with mock-transfected or control siRNA-transfected cells. In contrast, inhibiting the expression of Dicer did not significantly alter the levels of ULBP1, ULBP2, and ULBP3 mRNAs. Up-regulation of MICA and MICB by Dicer knockdown is prevented by pharmacologic or genetic inhibition of DNA damage pathway components, including ATM, ATR, or Chk1. This finding suggests that up-regulation of MICA and MICB is the result of DNA damage response activated by Dicer knockdown. Dicer knockdown cells also exhibited greater sensitivity to lysis by NKL, a cell line derived from an aggressive form of human natural killer cell leukemia. Lysis was partially inhibited by anti-NKG2D antibody, which indicated that up-regulated NKG2D ligands make the cells more susceptible to lysis by NK cells. This result suggests that Dicer-deficient cells may be cleared by NK or other immune cells (Tang KF. et al, 2008b).

Although we have shown that up-regulation of MICA and MICB in Dicer knockdown cells is the result of DNA damage response activation, further studies are necessary to determine whether other mechanisms are also involved in the regulation of MICA and MICB in Dicer knockdown cells. Stern-Ginossar and colleagues reported that one of the human cytomegalovirus encoded miRNAs, hcmv-miR-UL112, specifically down-regulates MICB expression during viral infection, leading to decreased binding of NKG2D and reduced killing by NK cells (Stern-Ginossar N. et al, 2007). The hcmv-miR-UL112 binding site in the MICB 3′-untranslated region is conserved among different MICB alleles and a similar site exists in the MICA 3′-untranslated region, suggesting that these sites are targeted by cellular microRNAs (Stern-Ginossar N. et al, 2007). To test this hypothesis, Stern-Ginossar and colleagues expressed MICB with or without its 3′-UTR in primary human foreskin fibroblast (HFF) cells. MICB expression was much higher when it was expressed without its 3′-UTR. Fusion of the 3′-UTR of MICA to green fluorescent protein (GFP) also inhibited GFP expression. These results indicated that the 3′-UTRs of MICA and MICB inhibit expression of the corresponding proteins. Knockdown of Drosha, an enzyme essential for miRNA biogenesis (Lee Y. et al, 2003), relieved the inhibitory effects, suggesting that cellular microRNAs do indeed regulate MICA and MICB expression. Further studies demonstrated that miR-20a, miR-93, miR106b, miR-372, miR-373, and miR-520d are involved in the regulation of MICA and MICB expression (Stern-Ginossar N. et al, 2008). Yadav and colleagues reported that miR-520b acted on both the MICA 3′-UTR and the promoter region, causing a decrease in the levels of the MICA transcript and protein. However, an antisense oligonucleotide inhibitor of miR-520b increased the expression of a reporter construct containing the MICA 3′-UTR (Yadav D. et al, 2009). Dicer is the key enzyme involved in miRNA biogenesis, and knockdown of Dicer reduces levels of miRNAs. Therefore, it is conceivable that reduced levels of miRNAs may contribute to the up-regulation of MICA and MICB in Dicer knockdown cells.

Interferon-alpha promotes expression of MICA in tumor cells (Zhang C. et al, 2008). Some siRNAs are found to activate protein kinase R (PKR) and induce global up-regulation of interferon-stimulated genes (Marques JT. & Williams BR., 2005; Sledz CA. et al, 2003). Because dsRNAs are natural substrates of Dicer, knockdown of Dicer may stabilize endogenous dsRNAs. Elevated levels of endogenous dsRNAs may activate the interferon pathway. Therefore, it seems possible that up-regulation of MICA and MICB is the consequence of nonspecific activation of the interferon pathway in Dicer knockdown cells. Our results indicated that the phosphorylation status of PKR and the expression of interferon-stimulated genes are not changed in Dicer knockdown cells compared to control cells (Tang KF. et al, 2008b). However, we cannot exclude the possibility that complete depletion of Dicer may yield levels of endogenous dsRNAs high enough to activate the interferon pathway, and eventually up-regulate the expression of MICA and MICB.

The expression of MICA and MICB is tightly correlated with cell proliferation status. Highly confluent HCT116 cells grown to quiescence contain small amounts of MICA and MICB mRNAs and display low MIC surface protein expression. In rapidly proliferating cells, MICA and MICB mRNAs and surface proteins are strongly induced (Venkataraman GM. et al, 2007). Knockout of Dicer in hepatocytes leads to increased cell proliferation (Sekine S. et al, 2009), and Dicer knockdown lung adenocarcinoma (LKR13) cells grow faster than control cells (Kumar MS. et al, 2007). Therefore, it is possible that up-regulation of MICA and MICB is the consequence of increased cell proliferation induced by down-regulation of Dicer.

Further studies are necessary to elucidate why loss of Dicer leads to up-regulation of MICA and MICB. Some possible mechanisms, summarized in Figure 2, are as follows: (i) decreased Dicer expression elicits DNA damage , which in turn induces up-regulation of MICA and MICB; (ii) loss of Dicer impairs biogenesis of miRNAs, some miRNAs, such as miR-20a, miR-93, miR106b, miR-372, miR-373, miR-520 and miR-520d, can repress the expression of MICA and MICB transcriptionally and posttranscriptionally; (iii) loss of Dicer may result in increased cell proliferation, and increased proliferation induces the transcription of MICA and MICB; and (iv) loss of Dicer stabilizes endogenous dsRNAs, and increased levels of the dsRNAs activate the interferon pathway, which in turn induces the expression of MICA and MICB.

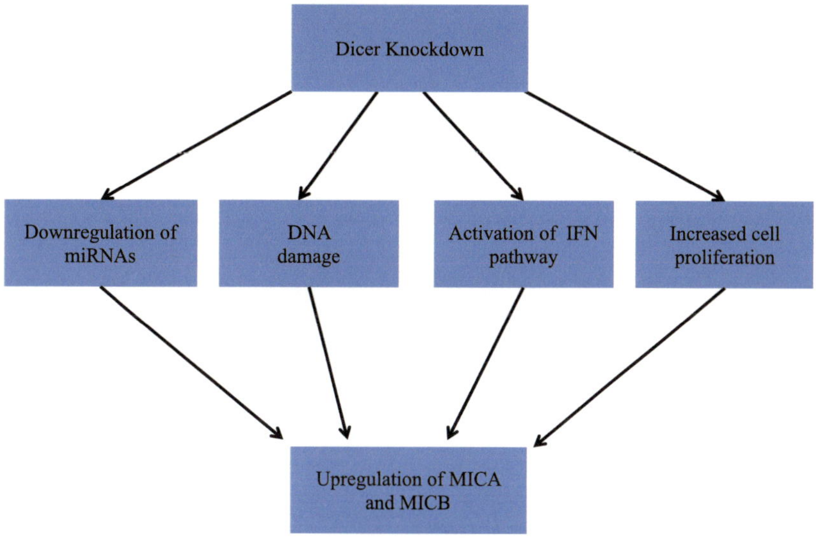

Fig. 2. Molecular mechanisms linking decreased Dicer expression to increased MICA and MICB expression

8. Dicer, DNA damage, and tumorigenesis

Compared with normal tissue, miRNAs are generally down-regulated in tumor tissue (Lu J. et al, 2005). Levels of Dicer mRNA and protein are decreased in 60% of ovarian-cancer specimens. Low Dicer expression is significantly associated with advanced tumor stage and poor prediagnosis (Merritt WM. et al, 2008). We found that compared to the adjacent non-cancerous liver tissues, Dicer mRNA and protein are reduced in hepatocellular carcinoma tissues in 34 of 36 patients (Wu JF. et al, 2011). Signs of a DNA damage response, including histone H2AX and Chk2 phosphorylation, p53 accumulation, focal staining of p53 binding protein 1, are widely found in clinical specimens from different stages of human tumors and precancerous lesions, but not in normal tissues (Bartkova J. et al, 2005, 2006; DiTullio RA Jr. et al, 2002; Gorgoulis VG. et al, 2005). Decreased Dicer expression elicits DNA damage (Mudhasani R. et al, 2008; Peng JC. & Karpen GH., 2009; Tang KF. et al, 2008b). Therefore, the following questions are intriguing: Is there an association between DNA damage and Dicer down-regulation in cancer tissues? If the answer is yes, what is the causal relationship between DNA damage and Dicer down-regulation in the process of carcinogenesis? What is the role of Dicer in carcinogenesis?

Kumar and colleagues found that loss of Dicer promotes tumorigenesis (Kumar MS. et al, 2007). They showed that Dicer knockdown cancer cells had a more pronounced transformed phenotype. In animals, Dicer knockdown cells formed tumors with accelerated growth; the tumors were also more invasive than control tumors. Furthermore, conditional deletion of Dicer enhanced tumor development in a K-Ras-induced mouse model of lung cancer (Kumar MS. et al, 2007). Sekine and colleagues disrupted Dicer in hepatocytes using a conditional knockout mouse model and found that Dicer elimination induces hepatocyte proliferation and overwhelming apoptosis. Unexpectedly, they found that two-thirds of the mutant mice spontaneously developed hepatocellular carcinomas (HCCs) at 1 year of age. The fact that the majority of Dicer deficient hepatocytes undergo apoptosis and that only a minor subset of Dicer-deficient hepatocytes gives rise to HCCs suggests the requirement of a "second hit" that promotes hepatocarcinogenesis in Dicer-deficient hepatocytes (Sekine S. et al, 2009). Based on these observations, I propose a simple model to explain how Dicer knockout leads to hepatocarinogenesis (Figure 3). Dicer depletion induces DNA damage via the mechanisms described in Figure 1, and DNA damage response leads to cell apoptosis or senescence. DNA damage may also result in DNA mutation such that cells containing oncogenic mutations may escape from apoptosis and senescence, eventually forming cancer.

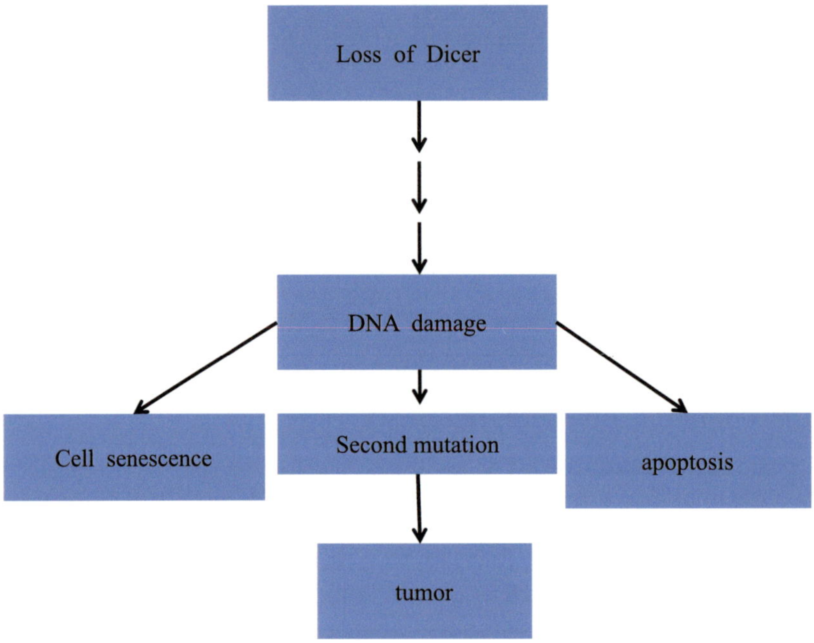

Fig. 3. Molecular mechanisms of Dicer knockout-induced tumorigenesis

Oncogene activation leads to augmented numbers of active DNA replicons and to alterations in DNA replication fork progression. These alterations activate DNA damage response, and eventually cell senescence or apoptosis. Genetic analyses indicate that early in tumorigenesis (before genomic instability and malignant conversion), human cells activate an ATR/ATM-regulated DNA damage response network that delays or prevents cancer. Mutations compromising this DNA damage response network might allow cell proliferation, survival, increased genomic instability and tumor progression (Bartkova J. et al, 2005, 2006; Di Micco R. et al, 2006).

Comparison of the mechanisms of oncogene-induced carcinogenesis (Figure 4) and Dicer depletion induced carcinogenesis suggests that Dicer is a tumor suppressor gene. However, Kumar and colleagues demonstrated that Dicer functions as a haploinsufficient tumor suppressor gene (Kumar MS. et al, 2009). Deletion of a single copy of Dicer in tumors from Dicerfl/+ animals reduced survival compared with controls. Moreover, tumors from Dicerfl/fl animals always maintained one functional Dicer allele; forced deletion of Dicer inhibited tumorigenesis. Analysis of human cancer genome copy number data reveals frequent deletion of Dicer. However, the gene has not been reported to undergo homozygous deletion (Kumar MS. et al, 2009).

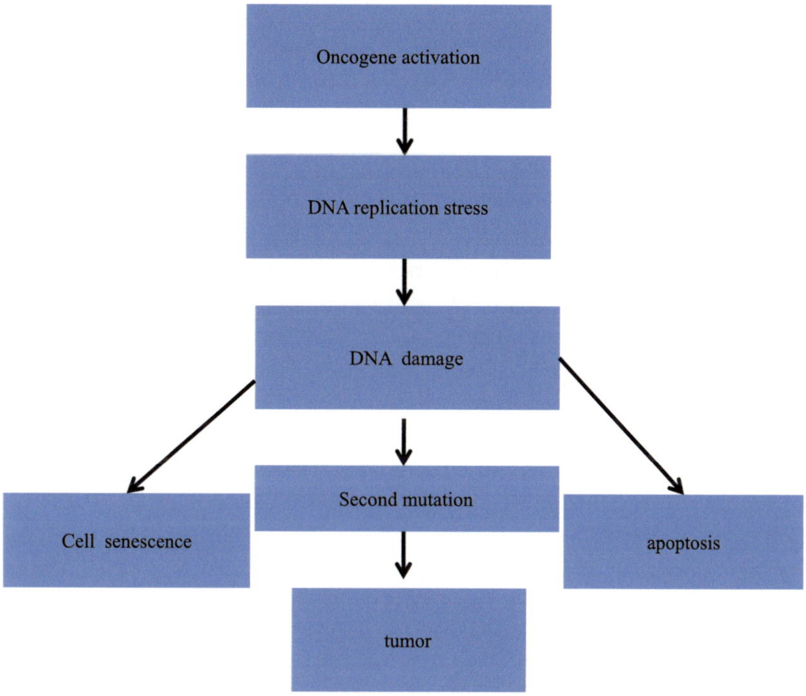

Fig. 4. Molecular mechanisms of oncogene-induced tumorigenesis

9. MIC molecules, DNA damage and tumorigenesis

Although evolved in parallel with the human MHC class I genes, MIC molecules (MICA and MICB) are quite different from MHC class I molecules. The characteristics of MIC molecules include the lack of association with beta-2-microglobulin, stable expression without conventional class I peptide ligands, and the absence of a CD8 binding site. The MIC genes are highly polymorphic. Around 60 alleles of MICA and 25 alleles of MICB have so far been identified (Bahram S. et al, 1994; Eagle RA. & Trowsdale J., 2007;). T cells with variable region V-delta-1 gamma/delta T-cell receptors are distributed throughout the human intestinal epithelium and may function as sentinels that respond to self-antigens. MIC molecules are expressed on the surface of the intestinal epithelium cells, and are recognized by intestinal epithelial T cells expressing diverse V-delta-1 gamma/delta TCRs. These data suggest that MIC molecules may regulate the protective responses by the V-delta-1 gamma/delta T cells in the epithelium of the intestinal tract (Groh V. et al, 1998). Cytomegalovirus (CMV) infection induces MIC expression and a concurrent down-regulation of MHC class I molecules on fibroblasts and endothelial cells (Groh V. et al, 2001). Functional analysis of T-cell cytotoxicity against CMV-infected fibroblasts showed that early after infection when MIC expression was low, antibodies to MHC class I, but not to MIC or NKG2D, could block T cell-mediated cytolysis (Groh V. et al, 2001). As MIC expression increased, antibody masking of MIC or NKG2D reduced target-cell lysis; anti-MHC class I antibodies further reduced cytolysis. This study suggests that MIC molecules are involved in the immune clearance of virus-infected cells (Groh V. et al, 2001). MICA binds NKG2D on gamma/delta T cells, $CD8^+$ alpha/beta T cells, and natural killer cells. Engagement of NKG2D activates cytolytic responses of gamma/delta T cells and NK cells against transfectants and epithelial tumor cells expressing MICA (Bauer S. et al, 1999). These results indicate that MICA and MICB play important roles in anti-viral and anti-tumor immune response.

DNA damage response is activated in clinical specimens from different stages of human tumors and precancerous lesions, but not in normal tissues (Bartkova J. et al, 2005, 2006; DiTullio RA Jr. et al, 2002; Gorgoulis VG. et al, 2005). Activation of the DNA damage response results in cell cycle arrest, senescence, and apoptosis. It was proposed that tumor progression requires the appearance of mutations that misregulate the DNA damage response pathway, such as p53 mutations, which allay the cell cycle block and allow tumor outgrowth (Gasser S. & Raulet DH., 2006; Halazonetis TD., 2004). DNA damage induces up-regulation of NKG2D ligands (including MICA and MICB). Some components of the DNA damage checkpoints, including ATM and ATR (two proteins involved in DNA damage detection), and Chk1 (a protein that transduces the DNA damage signal to effector proteins), are essential for the up-regulation of NKG2D ligands (Gasser S. et al, 2005; Tang KF. et al, 2008b). p53 is one of the effector proteins of the DNA damage checkpoints, but is not required for up-regulation of NKG2D ligands, as indicated by DNA damage-induced expression of the ligands in p53-deficient cell lines (Gasser S. et al, 2005). The fact that other components of the DNA damage response, such as ATR and Chk1, are rarely mutated in tumors might explain why NKG2D ligands are frequently up-regulated in cancer cells (Gasser S. & Raulet DH., 2006; Halazonetis TD., 2004). These findings suggest a possible role of the immune system, via the DNA damage response and NKG2D, in the elimination of precancerous cells and cancer cells.

In addition to promoting anti-tumor immune response, MICA and MICB can also suppress tumor immune surveillance. MICA associates with endoplasmic reticulum protein-5 (ERP5) on the surface of tumor cells, and the association is required for MICA shedding. Detailed analysis indicated that ERP5 and membrane-anchored MICA form transitory, mixed disulfide complexes, from which soluble MICA is released after proteolytic cleavage near the cell membrane. The secreted form of MIC molecules may bind to NKG2D receptor and inhibit the killing activity of effector cells (Kaiser BK. et al, 2007). NKG2D binding of MIC can induce endocytosis and degradation of NKG2D. In cancer patients, NKG2D expression was markedly reduced in both $CD8^+$ tumor-infiltrating T cells and in peripheral blood T cells, and the reduction of NKG2D expression is associated with increased level of circulating tumor-derived soluble MICA. Down-regulation of NKG2D severely impairs the function of tumor antigen-specific effector T cells (Groh V. et al, 2002). MICA can also mediate strong suppressive effects on T cell proliferation. Responsiveness to MICA-mediated suppression involves a receptor other than NKG2D. This finding might explain the observation that strong in vivo NKG2D ligand expression, such as in tumor cells, sometimes fails to support effective immune responses (Kriegeskorte AK. et al, 2005).

10. Conclusion

Dicer is misregulated in tumor tissues, and decreased Dicer expression induces the expression of MICA and MICB. MICA and MICB play important roles in anti-tumor immune response, and are frequently up-regulated in epithelial tumors of diverse tissue origins. These observations suggest that the intracellular immune system and the innate immune system have a good synergistic or additive effect in tumor immune surveillance. In addition, decreased Dicer expression elicits DNA damage, which in turn induces cell apoptosis and senescence. However, disruption of Dicer in hepatocytes promotes hepatocarcinogenesis. Therefore, the role and mechanism of Dicer in tumorigenesis need further investigation.

11. Acknowledgment

The author is supported by National Natural Science Foundation of China (grant Nos. 30700708, 30971621 & 81171967), Zhejiang Provincial Natural Science Foundation of China (grant No. R2110503), Wenzhou Science and Technology Foundation of China (grant Nos. Y20100203), and the key project of Chongqing Medical Science Foundation (grant No. 09-1-17). The author wish to thank Dr. Gui-Ling Li for proof reading, Lu Lv and Yu-Xiao Fang for editing the reference.

12. References

Ayoub N, Jeyasekharan AD, Bernal JA, & Venkitaraman AR.(2008). HP1-beta mobilization promotes chromatin changes that initiate the DNA damage response. Nature. （May 2008）, pp. 682-6, ISSN 0028-0836

Bahram S., Bresnahan M., Geraghty DE., & Spies T. (1994). A second lineage of mammalian major histocompatibility complex class I genes.*Proc Natl Acad Sci U S A*, Vol. 91, No. 14,(Jul 1994), pp.6259-63,ISSN 0027-8424

Bartkova J., Horejsí Z., Koed K., Krämer A., Tort F., Zieger K., Guldberg P., Sehested M., Nesland JM., Lukas C., Ørntoft T., Lukas J., & Bartek J. (2005).DNA damage response as a candidate anti-cancer barrier in early human tumorigenesis. *Nature*, Vol. 434, No. 7035,(Apr 2005), pp.864-70,ISSN 0028-0836

Bartkova J., Rezaei N., Liontos M., Karakaidos P., Kletsas D., Issaeva N., Vassiliou LV., Kolettas E., Niforou K., Zoumpourlis VC., Takaoka M., Nakagawa H., Tort F., Fugger K.,Johansson F., Sehested M., Andersen CL., Dyrskjot L., Ørntoft T., Lukas J., Kittas C., Helleday T., Halazonetis TD., Bartek J., & Gorgoulis VG. (2006).Oncogene-induced senescence is part of the tumorigenesis barrier imposed by DNA damage checkpoints. *Nature*, Vol. 444, No. 7119,(Nov 2006), pp.633-7,ISSN 0028-0836

Bauer S., Groh V., Wu J., Steinle A., Phillips JH., Lanier LL., & Spies T. (1999). Activation of NK cells and T cells by NKG2D, a receptor for stress-inducible MICA. *Science*, Vol. 285, No. 5428,(Jul 1999), pp.727-9,ISSN 0036-8075

Benetti R., Gonzalo S., Jaco I., Muñoz P., Gonzalez S., Schoeftner S., Murchison E., Andl T., Chen T., Klatt P., Li E., Serrano M., Millar S., Hannon G., & Blasco MA. (2008).A mammalian microRNA cluster controls DNA methylation and telomere recombination via Rbl2-dependent regulation ofDNA methyltransferases. *Nat Struct Mol Biol.* Vol. 15, No. 9,(Sep 2008), pp.998,ISSN 1545-9985

Bernstein E., Caudy AA., Hammond SM., & Hannon GJ. (2001).Role for a bidentate ribonuclease in the initiation step of RNA interference. *Nature.* Vol. 409, No. 6818,(Jan 2001), pp.363-6,ISSN 0028-0836

Cerboni C., Zingoni A., Cippitelli M., Piccoli M., Frati L., & Santoni A. (2007).Antigen-activated human T lymphocytes express cell-surface NKG2D ligands via an ATM/ATR-dependent mechanism and become susceptible to autologous NK- cell lysis. *Blood.* Vol. 110, No. 2,(July 2007), pp.606-15, ISSN 0006-4971

Cobb BS., Nesterova TB., Thompson E., Hertweck A., O'Connor E., Godwin J., Wilson CB., Brockdorff N., Fisher AG., Smale ST., & Merkenschlager M. (2005).T cell lineage choice and differentiation in the absence of the RNase III enzyme Dicer. *J Exp Med.* Vol. 201, No. 9,(May 2005), pp.1367-73,ISSN 0022-1007

Cogoni C., Irelan JT., Schumacher M., Schmidhauser TJ., Selker EU., & Macino G. (1996).Transgene silencing of the al-1 gene in vegetative cells of Neurospora is mediated by a cytoplasmic effector and does not depend on DNA-DNA interactions or DNA methylation. *EMBO J.* (Jun 1996), Vol. 15, No. 12,pp. 3153-63, ISSN 0261-4189

Czech B., Malone CD., Zhou R., Stark A., Schlingeheyde C., Dus M., Perrimon N., Kellis M., Wohlschlegel JA., Sachidanandam R., Hannon GJ., & Brennecke J. (2008).An endogenous small interfering RNA pathway in Drosophila. *Nature,* Vol. 453, No. 7196,2008 Jun 5, pp.798-802. 22, ISSN 0028-0836

Kawamura Y, Saito K, Kin T, Ono Y, Asai K, Sunohara T, Okada TN, Siomi MC, & Siomi H. (2008).Drosophila endogenous small RNAs bind to Argonaute 2 in somatic cells. *Nature,* Vol. 453, No. 7196,(Jun 2008), pp.793-7,ISSN 0028-0836

Di Micco R., Fumagalli M., Cicalese A., Piccinin S., Gasparini P., Luise C., Schurra C., Garre' M., Nuciforo PG., Bensimon A., Maestro R., Pelicci PG., & d'Adda di Fagagna F. (2006). Oncogene-induced senescence is a DNA damage response triggered by DNA hyper-replication. *Nature,* Vol. 444, No. 7119,(Nov 2006), pp.638-42, ISSN 0028-0836

DiTullio RA Jr., Mochan TA., Venere M., Bartkova J., Sehested M., Bartek J., & Halazonetis TD. (2002). 53BP1 functions in an ATM-dependent checkpoint pathway that is constitutively activated in human cancer. *Nat Cell Biol,* Vol.4, No.12, (Dec 2002), pp.998-1002, ISSN 1465-7392

Donaldson AD. (2005).Shaping time, chromatin structure and the DNA replication programme. Trends Genet, Vol.21, No.8, (Aug 2005), pp.444-9, ISSN 0168-9525

Eagle RA., & Trowsdale J. (2007).Promiscuity and the single receptor, NKG2D. *Nat Rev Immunol,* Vol.7, No.9,(Sep 2007), pp.737-44, ISSN 1474-1733

Fire A., Albertson D., Harrison SW., & Moerman DG. (1991).Production of antisense RNA leads to effective and specific inhibition of gene expression in C. elegans muscle. *Development,* Vol.113, No.2,(Oct 1991), pp.503-14, ISSN 0950-1991

Fire A., Xu S., Montgomery MK., Kostas SA., Driver SE., & Mello CC. (1998). Potent and specific genetic interference by double-stranded RNA in Caenorhabditis elegans. *Nature,* Vol. 391, No. 6669,(Feb 1998), pp.806-11, ISSN 0028-0836

Fire A. (2005).Nucleic acid structure and intracellular immunity, some recent ideas from the world of RNAi. *Q Rev Biophys,* Vol. 38, No. 4,(Nov 2005), pp.303-9,ISSN 0033-5835

Foster ER., & Downs JA. (2005).Histone H2A phosphorylation in DNA double-strand break repair. *FEBS J,* Vol. 272, No. 13,(Jul 2005), pp.3231-40,ISSN 1742-464X

Gasior SL., Wakeman TP., Xu B., & Deininger PL. (2006).The human LINE-1 retrotransposon creates DNA double-strand breaks. *J Mol Biol,* Vol. 357, No. 5,(Apr 2006), pp.1383-93,ISSN 0022-2836

Gasser S., Orsulic S., Brown EJ., & Raulet DH. (2005).The DNA damage pathway regulates innate immune system ligands of the NKG2D receptor. *Nature,* Vol. 436, No. 7054,(Aug 2005), pp.1186-90,ISSN 0028-0836

Gasser S., & Raulet DH. (2006).The DNA damage response arouses the immune system. *Cancer Res,* Vol. 66, No. 8,(Apr 2006), pp.3959-62, ISSN 0008-5472

Ghildiyal M., Seitz H., Horwich MD., Li C., Du T., Lee S., Xu J., Kittler EL., Zapp ML., Weng Z., & Zamore PD. (2008).Endogenous siRNAs derived from transposons and mRNAs in Drosophila somatic cells. *Science,* Vol. 320, No. 5879,(May 2008), pp.1077-81,ISSN 0036-8075

Gorgoulis VG., Vassiliou LV., Karakaidos P., Zacharatos P., Kotsinas A., Liloglou T., Venere M., Ditullio RA Jr., Kastrinakis NG., Levy B., Kletsas D., Yoneta A., Herlyn M., Kittas C., & Halazonetis TD. (2005).Activation of the DNA damage checkpoint and genomic instability in human precancerous lesions. *Nature,* Vol. 434, No. 7035,(Apr 2005), pp.907-13,ISSN 0028-0836

Grewal SI. (2010).RNAi-dependent formation of heterochromatin and its diverse functions. *Curr Opin Genet Dev,* Vol. 20, No. 2,(Apr 2010), pp.134-41,ISSN 0959-437X

Groh V., Rhinehart R., Randolph-Habecker J., Topp MS., Riddell SR., & Spies T. (2001).Costimulation of CD8alphabeta T cells by NKG2D via engagement by MIC induced on virus-infected cells. *Nat Immunol,* Vol. 2, No. 3,(Mar 2001), pp.255-60,ISSN 1529-2908

Groh V., Steinle A., Bauer S., & Spies T. (1998). Recognition of stress-induced MHC molecules by intestinal epithelial gammadelta T cells. *Science,* Vol. 279, No. 5357,(Mar 1998), pp.1737-40, ISSN 0036-8075

Groh V., Wu J., Yee C., & Spies T. (2002).Tumour-derived soluble MIC ligands impair expression of NKG2D and T-cell activation. *Nature,* Vol. 419, No. 6908,(Oct 2002), pp.734-8, ISSN 0028-0836

Guo S., & Kemphues KJ. (1995).par-1, a gene required for establishing polarity in C. elegans embryos, encodes a putative Ser/Thr kinase that is asymmetrically distributed. *Cell,* Vol. 81, No. 4,(May 1995), pp.611-20, ISSN 0092-8674

Halazonetis TD. (2004). Constitutively active DNA damage checkpoint pathways as the driving force for the high frequency of p53 mutations in human cancer. *DNA Repair (Amst),* Vol. 3, No. 8-9,(Aug-Sep 2004), pp.1057-62,ISSN 1568-7864

Hamilton AJ., & Baulcombe DC. (1999). A species of small antisense RNA in posttranscriptional gene silencing in plants. *Science,* Vol. 286, No. 5441,(Oct 1999), pp.950-2,ISSN 0036-8075

Hammond SM., Bernstein E., Beach D., & Hannon GJ. (2000).An RNA-directed nuclease mediates post-transcriptional gene silencing in Drosophila cells. *Nature*, Vol. 404, No. 6775,(Mar 2000), pp.293-6, ISSN 0028-0836

Hutvágner G, McLachlan J, Pasquinelli AE, Bálint E, Tuschl T, & Zamore PD. (2001). A cellular function for the RNA-interference enzyme Dicer in the maturation of the let-7 small temporal RNA. *Science*, Vol. 293, No. 5531,(Aug 2001), pp.834-8, ISSN 0036-8075

Izant JG., & Weintraub H. (1984).Inhibition of thymidine kinase gene expression by anti-sense RNA, molecular approach to genetic analysis. *Cell*, Vol. 36, No. 4,(Apr 1984), pp.1007-15,ISSN 0092-8674

Jing Q., Huang S., Guth S., Zarubin T., Motoyama A., Chen J., Di Padova F., Lin SC., Gram H., & Han J. (2005).Involvement of microRNA in AU-rich element-mediated mRNA instability. *Cell*, Vol. 120, No. 5,(Mar 2005), pp.623-34,ISSN 0092-8674

Jørgensen HF., Azuara V., Amoils S., Spivakov M., Terry A., Nesterova T., Cobb BS., Ramsahoye B., Merkenschlager M., & Fisher AG. (2007).The impact of chromatin modifiers on the timing of locus replication in mouse embryonic stem cells. *Genome Biol*, Vol.8, No.8,(2007), pp.R169,ISSN 1474-7596

Kaiser BK., Yim D., Chow IT., Gonzalez S., Dai Z., Mann HH., Strong RK., Groh V., & Spies T. (2007). Disulphide-isomerase-enabled shedding of tumour-associated NKG2D ligands. *Nature*, Vol. 447, No. 7143,(May 2007), pp.482-6,ISSN 0028-0836

Kanellopoulou C., Muljo SA., Kung AL., Ganesan S., Drapkin R., Jenuwein T., Livingston DM., & Rajewsky K. (2005).Dicer-deficient mouse embryonic stem cells are defective in differentiation and centromeric silencing. *Genes Dev*, Vol. 19, No. 4, (Feb 2005), pp.489-501,ISSN 0890-9369

Kriegeskorte AK., Gebhardt FE., Porcellini S., Schiemann M., Stemberger C., Franz TJ., Huster KM., Carayannopoulos LN., Yokoyama WM., Colonna M., Siccardi AG., Bauer S., & Busch DH. (2005).NKG2D-independent suppression of T cell proliferation by H60 and MICA. *Proc Natl Acad Sci U S A*, Vol. 102, No. 33,(Aug 2005), pp.11805-10,ISSN 0027-8424

Kumar MS., Lu J., Mercer KL., Golub TR., & Jacks T. (2007).Impaired microRNA processing enhances cellular transformation and tumorigenesis. *Nat Genet*, Vol. 39, No. 5,(May 2007), pp.673-7,ISSN 1061-4036

Kumar MS., Pester RE., Chen CY., Lane K., Chin C., Lu J., Kirsch DG., Golub TR., & Jacks T. (2009). Dicer1 functions as a haploinsufficient tumor suppressor. *Genes Dev*, Vol. 23, No. 23,(Dec 2009), pp.2700-4,ISSN 0890-9369

Lanier LL. (2008). Up on the tightrope, natural killer cell activation and inhibition. *Nat Immunol*, Vol. 9, No. 5,(May 2008), pp.495-502,ISSN 1529-2908

Lee Y., Ahn C., Han J., Choi H., Kim J., Yim J., Lee J., Provost P., Rådmark O., Kim S., & Kim VN. (2003).The nuclear RNase III Drosha initiates microRNA processing. *Nature*, Vol. 425, No. 6956,(Sep 2003), pp.415-9, ISSN 0028-0836

Lejeune E., & Allshire RC. (2011).Common ground, small RNA programming and chromatin modifications. *Curr Opin Cell Biol*, Vol. 23, No. 3,(Jun 2011), pp.258-65, ISSN 0955-0674

Lindbo JA., & Dougherty WG. (1992).Untranslatable transcripts of the tobacco etch virus coat protein gene sequence can interfere with tobacco etch virus replication in transgenic plants and protoplasts. *Virology*, Vol. 189, No. 2,(Aug 1992), pp.725-33, ISSN 0042-6822

Lu J., Getz G., Miska EA., Alvarez-Saavedra E., Lamb J., Peck D., Sweet-Cordero A., Ebert BL., Mak RH., Ferrando AA., Downing JR., Jacks T., Horvitz HR., & Golub TR. (2005).MicroRNA expression profiles classify human cancers. *Nature*, Vol. 435, No. 7043,(Jun 2005), pp.834-8,ISSN 0028-0836

Marques JT., & Williams BR. (2005).Activation of the mammalian immune system by siRNAs. *Nat Biotechnol*, Vol. 23, No. 11,(Nov 2005), pp.1399-405,ISSN 1087-0156

Martienssen RA., Kloc A., Slotkin RK., & Tanurdzić M. (2008).Epigenetic inheritance and reprogramming in plants and fission yeast. *Cold Spring Harb Symp Quant Biol*, (2008), pp.265-71,ISSN 0091-7451

Merritt WM., Lin YG., Han LY., Kamat AA., Spannuth WA., Schmandt R., Urbauer D., Pennacchio LA., Cheng JF., Nick AM., Deavers MT., Mourad-Zeidan A., Wang H., Mueller P,Lenburg ME., Gray JW., Mok S., Birrer MJ., Lopez-Berestein G., Coleman RL., Bar-Eli M., & Sood AK. (2008).Dicer, Drosha, and outcomes in patients with ovarian cancer. *N Engl J Med*, Vol. 359, No. 25,(Dec 2008), pp.2641-50,ISSN 0028-4793

Mudhasani R., Zhu Z., Hutvagner G., Eischen CM., Lyle S., Hall LL., Lawrence JB., Imbalzano AN., & Jones SN. (2008).Loss of miRNA biogenesis induces p19Arf-p53 signaling and senescence in primary cells. *J Cell Biol*, Vol. 181, No. 7,(2008 Jun), pp.1055-63,ISSN 0021-9525

Murchison EP., Partridge JF., Tam OH., Cheloufi S., & Hannon GJ. (2005).Characterization of Dicer-deficient murine embryonic stem cells. *Proc Natl Acad Sci U S A*, Vol. 102, No. 34,(Aug 2005), pp.12135-40,ISSN 0036-8075

Nakagawa A., Shi Y., Kage-Nakadai E., Mitani S., & Xue D. (2010).Caspase-dependent conversion of Dicer ribonuclease into a death-promoting deoxyribonuclease. *Science*, Vol. 328, No.5976,(Apr 2010), pp.327-34,ISSN 0036-8075

Napoli C., Lemieux C., & Jorgensen R. (2007).Introduction of a Chimeric Chalcone Synthase Gene into Petunia Results in Reversible Co-Suppression of Homologous Genes in trans. *Plant Cell*, Vol.2, No.4,(Apr 1990) ,pp. 279-289, ISSN 1040-4651

Nellen W., & Lichtenstein C. (1993).What makes an mRNA anti-sense-itive? *Trends Biochem Sci*, Vol. 18, No. 11,(Nov 1993), pp.419-23,ISSN 0036-8075

Okamura K., Chung WJ., Ruby JG., Guo H., Bartel DP., & Lai EC. (2008).The Drosophila hairpin RNA pathway generates endogenous short interfering RNAs. *Nature*, Vol. 453, No. 7196,(Jun 2008), pp.803-6,ISSN 0028-0836

Peng JC., & Karpen GH. (2007).H3K9 methylation and RNA interference regulate nucleolar organization and repeated DNA stability. *Nat Cell Biol.* Vol. 9, No.1,(Jan 2007), pp.25-35,ISSN 1465-7392

Peng JC., & Karpen GH. (2008).Epigenetic regulation of heterochromatic DNA stability. *Curr Opin Genet Dev*, Vol. 18, No. 2,(Apr 2008), pp.204-11,ISSN 0959-437X

Peng JC., & Karpen GH. (2009).Heterochromatic genome stability requires regulators of histone H3 K9 methylation.*PLoS Genet*, Vol. 5, No. 3, (Mar 2009), pp.e1000435,ISSN 1553-7390

Plasterk RH. (2002).RNA silencing, the genome's immune system. *Science*, Vol. 296, No. 5571,(May 2002), pp.1263-5,ISSN 0036-8075

Richard J., Sindhu S., Pham TN., Belzile JP., & Cohen EA. (2010). HIV-1 Vpr up-regulates expression of ligands for the activating NKG2D receptor and promotes NK cell-mediated killing. *Blood*, Vol. 115, No. 7,(Feb 2010), pp.1354-63,ISSN 0006-4971

Riddle NC., & Elgin SC. (2008).A role for RNAi in heterochromatin formation in Drosophila. *Curr Top Microbiol Immunol*, Vol. 320,(2008) , pp.185-209,ISSN 0070-217X

Sancar A, Lindsey-Boltz LA, Unsal-Kaçmaz K., & Linn S. (2004).Molecular mechanisms of mammalian DNA repair and the DNA damage checkpoints. *Annu Rev Biochem*, Vol. 73 (Volume publication date July 2004), (July 2004), pp.39-85,ISSN 0066-4154

Sekine S., Ogawa R., Ito R., Hiraoka N., McManus MT., Kanai Y., & Hebrok M. (2009).Disruption of Dicer1 induces dysregulated fetal gene expression and promotes hepatocarcinogenesis. *Gastroenterology*, Vol. 136, No. 7,(Jun 2009), pp.2304-2315.e1-4,ISSN 0016-5085

Sinkkonen L., Hugenschmidt T., Berninger P., Gaidatzis D., Mohn F., Artus-Revel CG., Zavolan M., Svoboda P., & Filipowicz W. (2008).MicroRNAs control de novo DNA methylation through regulation of transcriptional repressors in mouse embryonic stemcells. *Nat Struct Mol Biol*, Vol. 15, No. 3,(Mar 2008), pp.259-67, ISSN 1545-9985

Sledz CA., Holko M., de Veer MJ., Silverman RH., & Williams BR. (2003). Activation of the interferon system by short-interfering RNAs. *Nat Cell Biol*, Vol. 5, No. 9,(Sep 2003), pp.834-9,ISSN 1465-7392

Soriani A., Zingoni A., Cerboni C., Iannitto ML., Ricciardi MR., Di Gialleonardo V., Cippitelli M., Fionda C., Petrucci MT., Guarini A., Foà R., & Santoni A. (2009). ATM-ATR-dependent up-regulation of DNAM-1 and NKG2D ligands on multiple myeloma cells by therapeutic agents resultsin enhanced NK-cell susceptibility and is associated with a senescent phenotype. *Blood*, Vol. 113, No. 15,(Apr 2009), pp.3503-11,ISSN 0006-4971

Stern-Ginossar N., Elefant N., Zimmermann A., Wolf DG., Saleh N., Biton M., Horwitz E., Prokocimer Z., Prichard M., Hahn G., Goldman-Wohl D., Greenfield C., Yagel S., Hengel H., Altuvia Y., Margalit H., & Mandelboim O. (2007).Host immune system gene targeting by a viral miRNA. *Science*, Vol. 317, No. 5836,(Jul 2007), pp.376-81,ISSN 0036-8075

Stern-Ginossar N., Gur C., Biton M., Horwitz E., Elboim M., Stanietsky N., Mandelboim M., & Mandelboim O. (2008). Human microRNAs regulate stress-induced immune responses mediated by the receptor NKG2D. *Nat Immunol*, Vol.9, No.9,(Sep 2008), pp.1065-73,ISSN 1529-2908

Stern-Ginossar N., & Mandelboim O. (2009).An integrated view of the regulation of NKG2D ligands. *Immunology*, Vol. 128, No.1,(Sep 2009), pp.1-6,ISSN 0019-2805

Tam OH., Aravin AA., Stein P., Girard A., Murchison EP., Cheloufi S., Hodges E., Anger M., Sachidanandam R., Schultz RM., & Hannon GJ. (2008).Pseudogene-derived small interfering RNAs regulate gene expression in mouse oocytes. *Nature*, Vol. 453, No. 7194, (May 2008), pp.534-8,ISSN 0028-0836

Tang KF., He CX., Zeng GL., Wu J., Song GB., Shi YS., Zhang WG., Huang AL., Steinle A., & Ren H. (2008a). Induction of MHC class I-related chain B (MICB) by 5-aza-2'-deoxycytidine. *Biochem Biophys Res Commun*, Vol. 370, No. 4,(Jun 2008), pp.578-83,ISSN 0006-291X

Tang KF., Ren H., Cao J., Zeng GL., Xie J., Chen M., Wang L., & He CX. (2008b).Decreased Dicer expression elicits DNA damage and up-regulation of MICA and MICB. *J Cell Biol*, Vol. 182, No. 2,(Jul 2008), pp.233-9,ISSN 0021-9525

Textor S., Fiegler N., Arnold A., Porgador A., Hofmann TG., & Cerwenka A. (2011).Human NK cells are alerted to induction of p53 in cancer cells by upregulation of the NKG2D ligands ULBP1 and ULBP2. *Cancer Res*, [Epub ahead of print] (Sep 2011). ISSN 0008-5472

Umbach JL., & Cullen BR. (2009).The role of RNAi and microRNAs in animal virus replication and antiviral immunity. *Genes Dev*, Vol. 23, No. 10,(May 2009), pp.1151-64,ISSN 0890-9369

van der Krol AR., Mur LA., Beld M., Mol JN., & Stuitje AR. (1990). Flavonoid genes in petunia, addition of a limited number of gene copies may lead to a suppression of gene expression. *Plant Cell*, Vol.2, No.4,(Apr 1990), pp.291-9,ISSN 1040-4651

Venkataraman GM., Suciu D., Groh V., Boss JM., & Spies T. (2007).Promoter region architecture and transcriptional regulation of the genes for the MHC class I-related chain A and B ligands of NKG2D. *J Immunol*, Vol. 178, No. 2,(Jan 2007), pp.961-9,ISSN 0022-1767

Verdel A., Jia S., Gerber S., Sugiyama T., Gygi S., Grewal SI., & Moazed D. (2004).RNAi-mediated targeting of heterochromatin by the RITS complex. *Science*, Vol. 303, No. 5658,(Jan 2004), pp.672-6,ISSN 0036-8075

Volpe TA., Kidner C., Hall IM., Teng G., Grewal SI , & Martienssen RA. (2002). Regulation of heterochromatic silencing and histone H3 lysine-9 methylation by RNAi. *Science*, Vol. 297, No. 5588,(Sep 2002), pp.1833-7,ISSN 0036-8075

Ward J., Davis Z., DeHart J., Zimmerman E., Bosque A., Brunetta E., Mavilio D., Planelles V., & Barker E. (2009).HIV-1 Vpr triggers natural killer cell-mediated lysis of infected cells through activation of the ATR-mediated DNA damageresponse. *PLoS Pathog*, Vol. 5, No. 10,(Oct 2009), pp.e1000613,ISSN 1553-7366

Watanabe T, Totoki Y, Toyoda A, Kaneda M, Kuramochi-Miyagawa S, Obata Y, Chiba H, Kohara Y, Kono T., Nakano T., Surani MA., Sakaki Y., & Sasaki H. (2008).Endogenous siRNAs from naturally formed dsRNAs regulate transcripts in mouse oocytes. *Nature*, Vol. 453, No. 7194, (May 2008), 539-43, ISSN 0028-0836

Wu JF., Shen W., Liu NZ., Zeng GL., Yang M., Zuo GQ., Gan XN., Ren H., & Tang KF. (2011).Down-regulation of Dicer in hepatocellular carcinoma. *Med Oncol*, Vol. 28, No. 3,(Sep 2011), pp.804-9,ISSN 1357-0560

Wu-Scharf D., Jeong B., Zhang C., & Cerutti H. (2000).Transgene and transposon silencing in Chlamydomonas reinhardtii by a DEAH-box RNA helicase. *Science*, Vol. 290, No. 5494,(Nov 2000), pp.1159-62,ISSN 0036-8075

Yadav D., Ngolab J., Lim RS., Krishnamurthy S., & Bui JD. (2009).Cutting edge, down-regulation of MHC class I-related chain A on tumor cells by IFN-gamma-induced microRNA. *J Immunol*, Vol. 182, No. 1,(Jan 2009), pp.39-43,ISSN 0022-1767

Zamore PD., Tuschl T., Sharp PA., & Bartel DP. (2000).RNAi, double-stranded RNA directs the ATP-dependent cleavage of mRNA at 21 to 23 nucleotide intervals. *Cell*, Vol. 101, No. 1, (Mar 2000), pp.25-33,ISSN 0092-8674

Zhang C., Niu J., Zhang J., Wang Y., Zhou Z., Zhang J., & Tian Z. (2008). Opposing effects of interferon-alpha and interferon-gamma on the expression of major histocompatibility complex class I chain-related A in tumors. *Cancer Sci*, Vol. 99, No. 6,(Jun 2008), pp.1279-86,ISSN 1347-9032

Zou Y., Liu Y., Wu X., & Shell SM. (2006). Functions of human replication protein A (RPA), from DNA replication to DNA damage and stress responses. *J Cell Physiol*, Vol. 208, No. 2,(Aug 2006), pp.267-73,ISSN 0021-9541

6

Killer Immunoglobulin-Like Receptors and Their Ligands

Roberto Biassoni, Irene Vanni and Elisabetta Ugolotti
Molecular Medicine, Istituto Giannina Gaslini
Italy

1. Introduction

In immunology, the concept of alloreactivity is universally linked to the mechanism of T-cell recognition, where the T cell receptors (TCR) may interact with peptides mounted on major histocompatibility complex (MHC) molecules. The mechanisms responsible for the generation of TCR specificity and thus for the T cell activation depend on the repertoire of the genes coding for T cell receptor following the gene rearrangements of their variable regions and on the development and maturation of T-cells (Felix & Allen, 2007). Alloreactivity is not only important in the regulation of the adaptive immune responses, but it is also involved in the function of a major component of the *innate immune system* represented by the Natural killer (NK) cells (Ciccone et al., 1988, 1992; Kärre et al., 1986), and the rationale of this phenomena has been shown useful in some leukemia treatments (Ruggeri et al., 2005). NK cells are known to play a major role in the rejection of viral-infected or tumour-transformed cells (Herberman et al., 1975; Kiessling et al., 1975) following the "missing self" mechanism (Ljunggren & Kärre, 1990). Their function is controlled by a multifaceted collection of receptors able to deliver either inhibitory or activating signals. Differently than T lymphocytes, NK cells display receptors encoded by germline loci, and some of them are able to interact specifically with particular alleles of the MHC class I.

In humans and in primates these molecules are the killer immunoglobulin-like receptors (KIR) that display a clonal and stochastic distribution on the cell surface and are encoded by a multigene family. In particular, NK cells are known to express at least a one dominant self class I inhibitory receptor responsible for the self-tolerance (Moretta et al., 1996, Biassoni et al., 2009a). The activation of NK cells is based on continuous surveillance for MHC class I expression on autologous cells by inhibitory KIR cell surface receptors and by a balance of functions depending by integration of activating and inhibitory receptors responses (Biassoni, 2009b). All conditions that alter the surface expression level of the MHC class I on target cell, such as virus infection or tumour-transformation, are sufficient to trigger NK-mediated cytolysis.

In humans, higher primates and cattle, the inhibition of NK cell function depends by the expression of KIR encoded by a multigene family evolved in the last 135 million years from the two *KIR3DL* and *KIR3Dx* ancestral gene loci (Parham et al., 2011). Humans and higher primates have generated the KIR repertoire from the ancestral *KIR3DL* gene, while in cattle NK receptors have evolved from the other ancestral gene locus *KIR3Dx*, that is still conserved in primates genomes as remnant of genes evolution during speciation. The human KIR genes map on chromosome 19q13.42, in the telomeric region of Leukocyte Receptor complex (LRC). Rodents and other species conversely evolved a completely different set of MHC class I-specific NK receptors, the Ly49 multigene family, which encode for type II transmembrane proteins belonging to the C-type lectin molecules.

Also the CD94/NKG2A receptor, conserved during speciation, is involved in the negative-control of NK cell function. In humans and in mice, it is specific for the HLA-E or Qa-1 molecules able to bind conserved peptides derived from the processing of different MHC class I leader sequences. Thus, CD94/NKG2A receptors sense the expression of different HLA class I molecules at once, indirectly monitoring the overall presence and level of expression of MHC class I alleles, making it particularly sensitive to any modification induced in transformed cells (Borrego et al., 2006).

KIR and HLA loci are both highly polymorphic and within this review we discuss the vast polymorphism of the KIR gene complex, which rivals that of the HLA complex. Indeed, one of the purposes of this chapter is to summarize our current knowledge of how KIR and their ligand diversities may influence the outcome of a number of key human diseases. For this reason, it is imperative for the accurate and reliable typing to determine the presence/absence of specific KIR genes, since the interactions of specific KIR and specific ligands have important roles in several diseases.

2. Killer immunoglobulin-like receptors (KIR)

KIR receptors vary in length from 306 to 456 amino acid residues and are characterized by immunoglobulin-like (Ig-like) domains on their extracellular regions, by a transmembrane and cytoplasmic region that are functionally relevant as they define the type of signal which is transduced by a defined NK cell (Colonna & Samaridis, 1995; D'Andrea et al., 1995; Wagtmann et al., 1995).

KIR proteins are classified by the number of extracellular Ig-like C2-type domains (2D or 3D) by the presence of a long (L) or short (S) cytoplasmic tail represented as KIR2DL and KIR2DS, respectively (Anfre' et al., 2001). *Inhibitory* KIR have a transmembrane region containing only hydrophobic amino acids and a long cytoplasmic tail (KIR2DL and KIR3DL) containing Immune Tyrosine-based Inhibitory Motifs (ITIM) involved in negative signalling. Upon ligand recognition ITIM are phosphorylated and lead to the association with the intracellular Src homology-2 (SH2) domain-containing phosphatases 1 or 2 (SHP1 or SHP2), which are responsible for turning off locally all triggering signalling pathways induced by activating NK cell receptors.

In contrast, some KIR are known to induce triggering of NK cell functions displaying a transmembrane region characterized by a positively charged amino acid (lysine) involved in the association with ITAM-bearing subunits and by a short cytoplasmic tail (KIR2DS, KIR3DS). Intracytoplasmic signalling and activation induced by these receptors are linked to the DAP12 receptor-associated signalling molecules that form a multichain immune recognition receptor (Sigalov, 2010). Different from all the other members of the KIR family, KIR2DL4 exhibits low polymorphism and high conservation, being one of the KIR framework genes. Although, it is characterized by a long cytoplasmic tail containing a single N-terminal ITIM, a feature shared with KIR3DL2 and KIR3DL3, KIR2DL4 transduces weak triggering signals mainly associated with cytokine releases rather than cytolysis (Cantoni et al., 1998; Faure & Long, 2002; Kikuchi-Maki et al., 2003; Rajagopalan et al., 2001; Selvakumar et al., 1996). The activating function depends by the association with FcεRIγ-chain, as signalling adapter molecule, instead of the DAP12, due to the positively charged arginine residue present in the transmembrane region (Kikuchi-Maki et al., 2005).

2.1 Organization of Killer immunoglobulin-like gene loci

The KIR genes are polymorphic, although highly homologous and are found in a region of 150 kb on chromosome 19q13.4 within the 1 Mb leukocyte receptor complex (LRC). The KIR loci and the genes coding for the Human Leukocyte Antigens (HLA) class I molecules reside on different chromosomes so they segregate independently and probably constitute the most diverse loci in the human genome. Indeed, the polygenic region coding for KIR has underwent rapid evolution and selection through mechanisms of homologous recombination, domain shuffling, and point mutations (Rajalingam et al., 2004); finally its diversity is achieved from the polymorphism of KIR genes and by the numbers of genes present in a haplotype. In detail, there are at least fifteen KIR genes and 2 pseudogenes (*KIR3DP1, KIR2DP1*) exhibiting substantial allelic diversity (Figure 1). Among them we may find 4 frameworks KIR genes/pseudogene present in nearly all individuals (*KIR2DL3, KIR3DP1, KIR2DL4, KIR3DL2*). Overall, KIR genes encode eight inhibitory receptors (*KIR2DL1, KIR2DL2, KIR2DL3, KIR2DL4, KIR2DL5A, KIR2DL5B, KIR3DL1, KIR3DL2*), six activating molecules (*KIR2DS2, KIR2DS3, KIR2DS5, KIR3DS1, KIR2DS1, KIR2DS4*), and two pseudogenes (*KIR2DP1, KIR3DP1*). Genes coding for KIR molecules, vary in length from 4 to 16 kb and may contain from four to nine exons, and with signal peptides encoded by sequences present in the first two exons. KIR genes are classified as belonging into either Type I (Cw Group I, 80 Asn) (KIR2D), Type II (Cw Group II, 80 Lys) (KIR2D), or KIR3D grouping. These depend on the presence of pseudoexon-3, partial or complete deletion of coding regions, and by the homology of the sequences encoding the immunoglobulin like (Ig-C2) domains. In detail, KIR3D genes encode proteins with three extra-cellular Ig-like domains (termed D0, D1 and D2), while KIR2D receptors are encoded by either

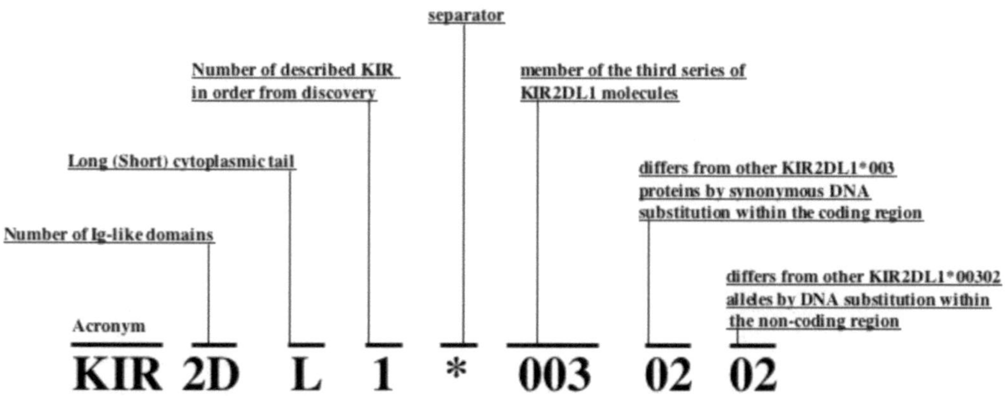

EMBL-EBI/IPD-KIR database at the following address, http://www.ebi.ac.uk/ipd/kir/

Fig. 1. Nomenclature Killer cell Immunoglobulin-like Receptors (KIR) genes and alleles.

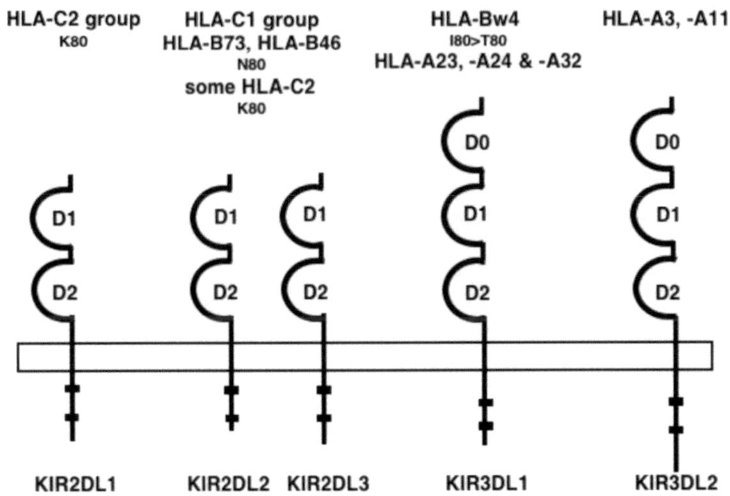

a)

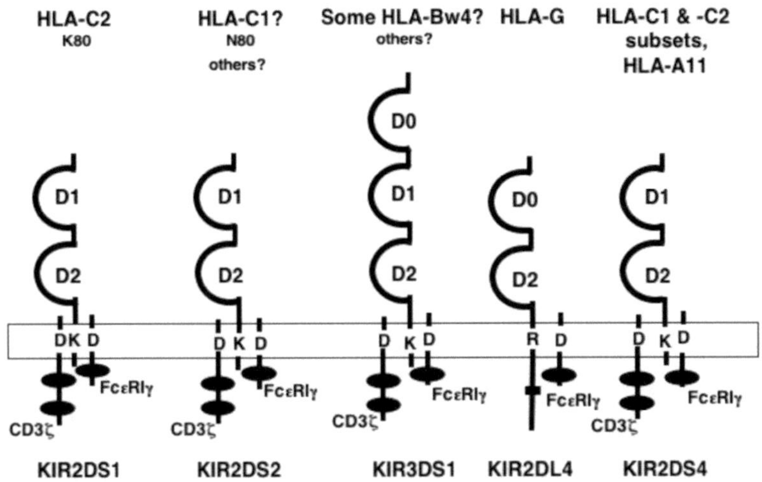

b)

Panel A: Inhibitory KIR named on the bottom and the relative HLA-ligand recognized by the same receptors (shown on the top). D0, D1 and D2 Ig-like domain structures are shown. Cell membrane is shown as an open rectangle. Small black-filled parallelograms represent ITIM in the cytoplasmic tail of the receptors.
Panel B: Activating KIR named on the bottom and the relative HLA-ligand recognized by the same receptors (shown on the top). D0, D1 and D2 Ig-like domain structures are shown. Cell membrane is shown as an open rectangle. Small black-filled parallelogram represent ITIM in the cytoplasmic tail of the KIR2DL4. Small black-filled ovals represent ITAM in the cytoplasmic tail of the associated chains. These signal transducing molecules are associated with the receptors through a polar interaction, inside the hydrophobic tranmembrane environment, involving either lysine (K) or arginine (R) present in the cytoplasmic tail of triggering KIR with an aspartic acid residue (D) in the cytoplasmic tail of the signalling transducing molecules.
I80>T80: indicates the affinity of interaction with KIR3DL1

Fig. 2. Structural representation of either inhibitory (A) or activating (B) KIR.

Type I KIR2D genes characterized by the presence of pseudoexon 3 and displaying two extra-cellular domains with a D1 and D2 conformation or Type II KIR2D genes, which encode two extra-cellular domain proteins with a D0 and D2 conformation having deleted the corresponding region of exon 4 (Figure 2). Type I KIR2D genes (*KIR2DP1, KIR2DL1-3* and *KIR2DS1-5* genes) are all characterized by eight exons and by the presence of pseudoexon 3, that it is inactivated due to a nucleotide substitution located on the intron 2-exon 3 splice-site. The nucleotide sequences of pseudoexon 3 share a high-degree of nucleotide identity with to KIR3D exon 3 corresponding sequences. Within the Type I KIR2D group of genes, *KIR2DL1* and *KIR2DL2* have an additional identical partial deletion in exon 7, a characteristic of these genes, only. *KIR2DS1-5* differ from the other type I KIR2D genes only in the length of the coding sequences for the cytoplasmic tail in exon 9. Finally, the *KIR2DP1* pseudogene structure shows a shorter exon 4 sequence due to a single base pair deletion. Type II KIR2D genes (*KIR2DL4, KIR2DL5A* and *KIR2DL5B*) have a translated exon 3 and a deletion of exon 4 sequence. Within the Type II KIR2D genes, *KIR2DL4* is further differentiated from *KIR2DL5A/B* and from all other KIR genes, on the base of the length of its exon 1 sequence. In *KIR2DL4*, exon 1 was found to be longer by six nucleotides displaying a different initiation codon, interestingly in better agreement with the 'Kozak transcription initiation consensus sequence' than those present in the other KIR genes. KIR3D genes are characterized by nine exons and include the structurally related *KIR3DL1, KIR3DS1, KIR3DL2* and *KIR3DL3* genes, where the *KIR3DL2* locus has the longest genomic nucleotide sequence among all KIR genes (16,256 bp). Within the KIR3D group the genes differ in the length of exon 9, so that the cytoplasmic tail encoded sequences vary in length from 23 to 116 amino acid residues in *KIR3DS1* or in *KIR2DL4*, respectively. Moreover, *KIR3DS1* differs from *KIR3DL1* or *KIR3DL2* loci for the presence of a short exon 8 sequence, while *KIR3DL3* is lacking exon 6. Finally, *KIR3DP1* shares a high degree of sequence identity to *KIR3DL3* sequences, but it lacks sequences from exon 6 to exon 9, and occasionally also exon 2.

2.1.1 KIR haplotypes

The assortment of KIR genotypes may vary significantly in different subjects due to duplication or deletion of gene loci that have occurred during evolution. This has lead to two major groups of haplotypes, "A" or "B", based on the relative KIR gene content. Members of haplotype B are characterized by a higher number of genes coding for activating receptors than members of the haplotype A group. Immunogenetic analyses of different ethnic populations show significant differences in terms of the distribution of group A and B haplotypes. The linkage disequilibrium analyses of the centromeric and telomeric regions clearly indicate the evolutionary histories of these regions, which may have undergone different gene assortment and may also have been inherited separately during evolution. Thus, the complexity of haplotypes is such that the genomic region belonging to the KIR complex is structurally organized having as centromeric boundaries the gene *KIR3DL3* and at the telomeric ends the *KIR3DL2* locus (Figure 3). In addition it is possible to define separate partial haplotypes since a centromeric portion distinct from the telomeric one is structurally separated by the two framework genes *KIR3DP1* and *KIR2DL4* (Figure 3). Based on this classification, members of the haplotype "A" group needs to display both centromeric (CenA) and telomeric (TelA) genotype organization A/A (Uhrberg et al., 1997). We have also to consider that KIR gene inheritance is the result of distinct diploid combinations of genotypes so that haplotype A is only the result of Cen A/A and

Tel A/A combinations, i.e., both parents having CenA and TelA, and both parents passing both sets to their offspring who then has CenAA/TelAA (Cooley et al., 2010). Thus in this situation *KIR2DL3, KIR2DP1, KIR2DL1* loci are typically present in the centromeric portion while a single activating gene (*KIR2DS4*) could be present in its telomeric region together with *KIR3DL1* (Figure 3). All other haplotypes are described as members of the B haplotype, which is the more variable in terms of genotype, having at least one of the following genes: KIR2DL5A/B, KIR2DL2, KIR2DS1, KIR2DS2, KIR2DS3, KIR2DS5 and KIR3DS1. Interestingly, KIR3DL1 and KIR3DS1 segregate as alleles of the same gene locus, the former associated with TelA haplotype, while the latter with TelB group of genes; in addition, the unexpressed KIR2DL5B variant is usually present together with KIR2DS3 or more rarely with KIR2DS5 that conversely is frequently present with KIR2DL5A. It is of note that in

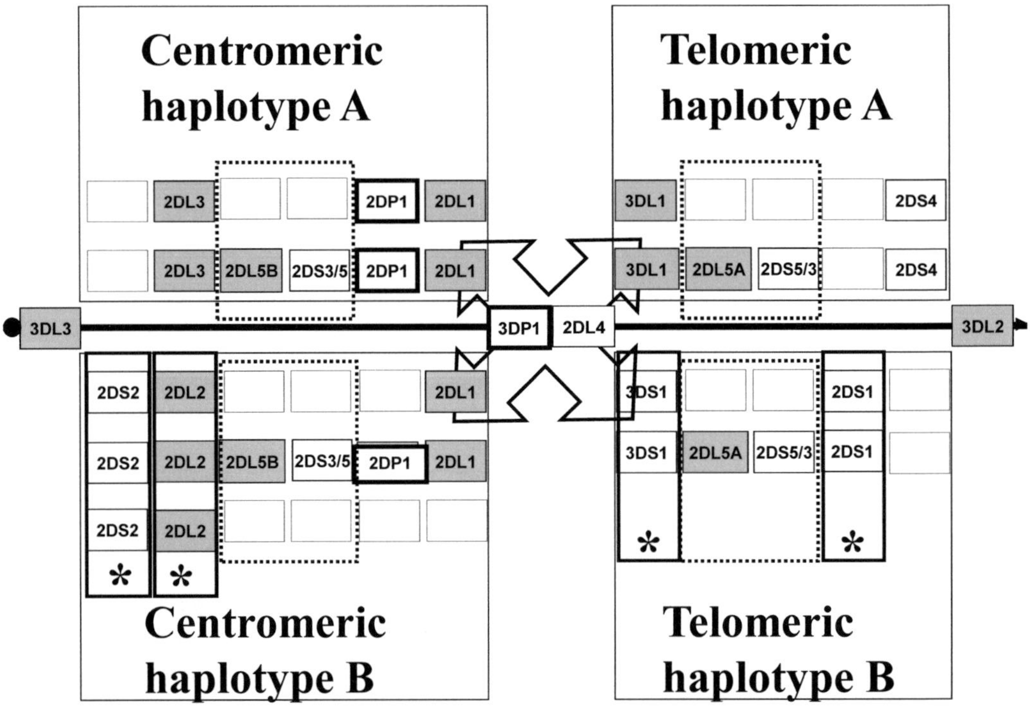

The framework 3DL3, 3DP1, 2DL4 and 3DL2 gene loci are drawn on the line representing chromosome19q13.42 region oriented from centromer (left) to telomer (right). Inhibitory receptors (shown gray boxes), activating ones (unfilled boxes) and pseudogenes (boxed with thicker line) are indicated. The genomic organizations of centromeric and telomeric regions are boxed with continuous line trait. The genes defining A haplotype are drawn on top, while the ones typical for B haplotype on the bottom. Boxes represented with dotted lines indicate gene regions frequently deleted, in detail KIR2DL5B is more frequently, but no exclusively associated with KIR2DS3 and on the opposite the gene telomeric to KIR2DL5A is KIR2DS5 and rarely KIR2DS3. The KIR3DP1 may be also present as KIR3DP1 Δex2. Centromeric and/or telomeric haplotye B need to have at least one of the genes indiacted with *. The four ways arrow indicate possible combination of centromeric and telomeric regions to determine CenAA-TelAA, CenAA-TelAB, CenAA-TelBB, CenAB-TelAA, CenAB-TelAB, CenAB-TelBB, CenBB-TelAA, CenBB-TelAB, CenBB-TelBB.

Fig. 3. Simplified genomic organization defining the KIR haplotypes

KIR	Aliases	Ligand	Function
2DL1	CD158a, cl-42, 47.11,nkat1, p58.1	HLA-C2^{Lys80} (Biassoni et al., 1995; Colonna et al., 1995; Wagtmann et al., 1995 ; Winter & Long, 1997)	Inhibition
2DS1	CD158h, EB6Actl, EB6Actll	HLA-C2^{Lys80} (weak) (Biassoni et al., 1997)	Activation
2DL2	CD158b1, cl-43, nkat6	HLA-C1^{Asn80}, HLA-B*73, -B*46, some HLA-C2 (Biassoni et al., 1995; Moesta et al., 2008)	Inhibition
2DL3	CD158b2, cl-6, nkat2, nkat2a, nkat2b, p58	HLA-C1^{Asn80}, HLA-B*73, -B*46 (Moesta et al.,2008; Winter et al., 1998)	Inhibition
2DS2	CD158j, 183Actl, cl-49, nkat5	HLA-C1^{Asn80} (weak) (Stewart et al., 2005)	Activation
2DL4	CD158d, 15.212, 103AS,	HLA-G	Activation Inhibition ?
2DL5A/B	CD158f, KIR2DL5.1/KIR2DL5.2,KIR2DL5.3, KIR2DL5.4	Unknown	Inhibition
2DS3	nkat7	Unknown	Activation
2DS4	CD158i, cl-39, KKA3, nkat8	Various HLA-C1 and HLA-C2 alleles, HLA-A*11(Graef et al., 2009)	Activation
2DS5	CD158g, nkat9	Unknown	Activation
3DL1	CD158e1, cl-2, cl-11, AMB11, nkat3, NKB1, NKB1B	HLA-Bw4 $^{(I80>T80)}$ except HLA-B*13:01/02 (Foley et al., 2008) HLA-A*23,-*24,-*32 (Stern et al., 2008; Thananchai et al., 2007) HLA-A*25 (Foley et al., 2008 : but not by Stern et al., 2008)	Inhibition
3DS1	CD158e2, nkat10	HLA-Bw4 ?	Activation
3DL2	CD158k, cl-5, nkat4, nkat4a, nkat4b	HLA-A*3,-*11 (weak) (Pende et al., 1996; Hansasuta et al., 2004)	Inhibition
3DL3	CD158z, KIR3DL7, KIR44, KIRC1	Unknown	Inhibition

I80>T80: indicates the affinity of interaction with KIR3DL1

Definition of KIR-mismatch in the case of HSCT

- **ligand-ligand model**: incompatibility between the donor KIR ligand and recipient KIR ligand is based on the "missing-self" hypothesis. Thus a ligand-ligand mismatch is possible if the donor has a ligand that is absent in the recipient (Ruggeri et al., 2002).
- **missing ligand model**: the above ligands-ligand paradigm is complicated by the fact that not all the individual genomes contain the complete set of KIR genes. Thus, you have to take in consideration that incompatibility between the donor KIR and recipient KIR ligand (receptor-ligand mismatch) is true if the donor has an inhibitory receptor for which the cognate ligand is absent in the recipient (Leung et al., 2004; Hsu et al., 2005). Thus to avoid this problem a KIR genotypic and phenotypic analysis is required.
- **receptor-receptor model:** it is known as KIR-haplotype incompatibility between the donor KIR and recipient KIR and it is valid if the donor has a receptor that is absent in the recipient (Gagne et al., 2002; McQueen et al., 2007)

Table 1. KIR ligand specificity

group A the haplotype diversity is primarily associated at the allelic polymorphism, while the group B haplotypes have greater diversity in gene content exhibiting only a moderate allelic polymorphism. In particular an analysis based on the genotype of only the four KIR2DL1, 2DL3, 3DL1 and 3DL2 loci showed at least 22 different haplotype A members with only 0.24% of unrelated individuals sharing an identical genotype (Shilling et al., 2002).The different B haplotypes may have mixed "B/x" genotypes (CenAA/TelAB, CenAB/TelAA, CenAA/TelBB, CenAB/TelAB, CenBB/TelAA, CenAB/TelBB, or CenBB/TelAB), which display all genes typical of group B plus at least an additional KIR group A gene, or may have a pure B/B genotype, without any A genes, CenBB/TelBB (Figure 3) (Cooley et al., 2010; Gourraud et al., 2010; Hsu et al., 2002; Middleton & Gonzelez, 2010; Pyo et al., 2010).

2.2 Ligand(s) of the Killer immunoglobulin-like receptors

On human NK cells, the KIR family of receptors participates in the complex regulation of NK cell responses through recognition of specific human leukocyte antigen (HLA) class I molecules on target cells. Both the KIR receptor and its cognate HLA ligand must be expressed in order to regulate NK cell activity. In fact each KIR interacts directly with distinct groups of expressed HLA alleles and the NK-mediated responses are governed by the avidity of interaction with HLA class I α1-helix around amino acid residue-80 (Figure 2). Thus, this α1-helix region is directly responsible for defining the different NK alloreactivities. In particular, inhibitory KIR2DL1, KIR2DL2 and KIR2DL3 receptors, and to a lesser extent the activating KIR2DS1 and probably KIR2DS2 are able to discriminate between two essentially non-overlapping groups of HLA-C alleles (Table 1). KIR2DL1 and KIR2DS1 (weaker) are specific for HLA-C alleles belonging to C2-group sharing V^{76}, N^{77} and K^{80} residues (essentially the majority of HLA-Cw2, 4, 5, 6 and some other alleles) (Figure 2A) (Table 1). In contrast, KIR2DL2 and to a lesser extent KIR2DL3 recognize HLA-C alleles (C1-group) characterized by V^{76}, S^{77} and N^{80} amino acids (mainly defined by HLA-Cw1, 3, 7, 8 and some other alleles). Additionally, some rare or geographically localized HLA-B allotypes (B73 and B46, respectively) containing a functional C1 epitope, originated by recombination events and sharing amino acids 66–77 with HLA-Cw3 alleles, and therefore interact with KIR2DL2 and KIR2DL3 (Biassoni et al., 1995; Abi-Rached et al., 2010) (Figure 2A). In addition, both KIR2DL2 and KIR2DL3 have also been described in having weak alloreactivity against some C2 allotypes (Moesta et al, 2008; Pende et al, 2009), probably due to allelic differences within the C2 subgroup (Figure 2A) (Table 1) (Moesta et al., 2008). Intriguingly, NK cell biology evolution drove to dominance in the recognition of HLA-C loci, where in humans at least 3 inhibitory and 2 activating receptors are able to sense the dimorphisms covering all known HLA-C alleles. It is known that MHC-C evolved only recently in humans and great apes (at least in orangutans), and not before. Apparently, the KIR and C1 loci evolved before the KIR-C2 since in Orangutans neither MHC-C2 alleles nor C2-specific KIRs could be detected (Older Aguilar et al., 2010). KIR3DL1 loci encode specific receptors for HLA-B alleles that share the public epitope Bw4 corresponding to amino acids 77-83 on the HLA class I α1-helix with the exception of HLA-B*13:01 and HLA-B*13:02 (Foley et al., 2008), and for some HLA-A alleles characterized by Bw4-supertypic specificity like A23, A24, , and A32 (Stern et al., 2008; Thananchai et al., 2007). An additional paper suggested that also HLA-A*25 alleles may be recognized by KIR3DL1 (Foley et al., 2008) although these data have not been confirmed by others (Stern et al., 2008).

KIR3DL1 has been described to strongly interact with target cells expressing homozygous Bw4 alleles sharing Isoleucine-80, and weakly with homozygous Bw4 Threonine 80 (Figure 2A) (Table 1). KIR3DL2 has been reported to be specific for HLA-A3 and -A11 allotypes, but with a limited ability to inhibit NK-mediated lysis (Döhhring et al., 1996; Pende et al., 1996) (Figure 2A) (Table 1).

Among activating KIR receptors, the direct HLA binding was demonstrated only for KIR2DS1, where the weaker avidity of interaction was been found to be dependent on the dimorphism of amino acid residue 70 (Biassoni et al., 1997) (Figure 2B). In contrast, evidence that KIR3DS1 may be associated with HLA-B recognition has been hypothesized, since it was found to be responsible for the delay of AIDS progression, but direct binding could not be demonstrated (Martin et al., 2002a; Gillespie et al., 2007). Recently a single KIR3DS1 allele (KIR3DS1*014), selected on the basis of critical D1-domain residues associated with Bw4-specificity (Figure 2B) (Norman et al., 2007), and carrying glycine-138 instead than tryptophan, was found to have direct HLA-Bw4 binding capability (O'Connor et al., 2011). The non-synonymous mutations in the extracytoplasmic domain linked with HLA-specific interaction are typical on activating KIR molecules (Biassoni et al., 1997; O'Connor et al, 2011), and also experimental shuffling of 2DS2 residue 45 from tyrosine to phenylalanine typical of 2DL2 receptor were found to enhance the affinity of the KIR2DS2 for HLA-C1 ligand (Winter et al., 1998). These observations may be the results of evolution followed by selection pressure, since activating KIR may have evolved from ancestral inhibitory receptors (Abi-Rached & Parham, 2005). Further, it is likely that the triggering ones have evolved to decrease the affinity of HLA-recognition probably to avoid autoimmune phenomena, but with time, they acquired the potential to recognize HLA class I molecules presenting peptides of viral origin (Khakoo et al., 2000; Vilches & Parham, 2002; Abi-Rached & Parham, 2005). Class I MHC tend to present peptides of ~9 amino acids in length in their binding groove bounded by the α1- and α2-helices. The amino acid residue at position 8 of the peptide in the MHC class I binding groove may be governing KIR/HLA class I-interactions. Interestingly, this amino acid in position 8 is localized near the residue 80 amino acid of the α1-helix. In particular, the KIR2DL/HLA-C and KIR3DL1/HLA-Bw4 interactions are affected by the presence of P8-residues either bearing strong negative or positive charges (Malnati et al., 1995; Peruzzi et al., 1996; Rajagopalan & Long, 1997). The relevance of pathogen derived-peptide is known to be associated with the positive association of both KIR3DS1 and Bw4 gene loci in HIV-infected subjects thus suggesting a possible role for HIV-associated peptides and by the fact that EBV infection is able to influence the KIR2DS1 HLA-C2 group interaction (Figure 2B) (Stewart et al., 2005). Pathogens present in the environment may have participated in the shaping of genetic loci of activating KIR thus explaining the hypothesis of recurrent acquisition and loss of activating KIR loci during evolution. In addition, the role of peptide in the KIR-mediated HLA class I recognition is known, since KIR3DL2 have a strong dependence from EBV-derived peptides presented by HLA-A3 and A11 alleles, and by that the presentation of particular self-peptide via HLA-Bw4 alleles were found to be protective from NK cell mediated lysis (Hansasuta et al., 1997; Malnati et al., 1995). Finally, KIR2DL4 binds to the non classical MHC class I HLA-G molecules (Ponte et al., 1999; Rajagopalan & Long EO, 1999), while KIR2DS4, probably originated from a gene conversion event with KIR3DL2 sequences, binds specifically to subsets of HLA-C1 and HLA-C2 group of alleles, and to HLA-A11 (Figure 2B) (Table 1) (Graef et al., 2009). Different analyses have demonstrated that KIR and their ligands may influence the outcome of a number of key human diseases. It is therefore obvious that accurate and reliable molecular typing, to determine the assortment of KIR genes together with HLA class I genes, is imperative. This is necessary to define the KIR-ligand associations in order to determine possible interactions associated either in the positive or negative responses to several diseases and pathologic states.

3. Molecular typing techniques

Accurate typing methods to discriminate HLA class I alleles and KIR genotypes is of great interest to establish the associations of KIR/HLA, and their activation or inhibition potentials. Due to the extraordinary polymorphism of the Human Leukocyte Antigen complex, it is recognized that serological HLA typing techniques are inadequate for this task. The correct assignment of HLA class I alleles relies on molecular typing techniques (Harville, 2009). The introduction of Polymerase chain reaction (PCR) has allowed the development of more advanced techniques for molecular typing of HLA alleles. Additional methods dedicated in the HLA typing of group of alleles relevant in the NK-mediated function have been published using either RT-PCR or pyrosequencing on genomic DNA (Shilling et al., 2002; Ugolotti et al., 2011). At present for the identification of KIR genotype there is a tendency to use methods familiar to laboratories, such as the sequence-specific primers (SSP-PCR) and sequence-specific oligonucleotide probes (SSOP). In fact, traditional KIR genotyping methods utilize SSP-PCR and requires that genomic DNA must be amplified using a collection of primers in separate reactions in order to define the various loci or alleles and to be detected by fragment lengths using gel electrophoresis. However, there are drawbacks to utilizing the SSP method for higher-throughput analysis of KIR loci in populations. Furthermore, the SSP method includes the problem of sample amplification failure, which could be due to either general PCR failure, or an as of yet undefined variant sequence. The first problem could be partially overcome using different primer combinations to amplify the same KIR locus, and if the same primer set is able to amplify different KIR loci (Martin & Carrington, 2008; Kulkarni et al., 2010). Unfortunately, the inability to detect variant KIR alleles due to primer mismatch is without a practical solution. Accordingly, amplification failure could result in erroneous KIR genotyping results. An alternative KIR genotyping assay uses sequence-specific oligonucleotide probes (SSOP) developed for locus-specific resolution of 14 KIR gene loci. The SSOP assay requires a smaller quantity of genomic DNA than SSP techniques. Although generally more efficient than SSP methods, genotyping analysis by SSOP assays is still cumbersome and may have similar pitfalls in the detection of previously unreported variants (Middleton & Gonzeles, 2010). Some groups use sequencing for the KIR allele determination, whereas others have used mass spectrometry, or real-time reverse transcription-polymerase chain reaction, which not only could prove useful for allele determination but also for determining copy number of either gene or allele (Cooley et al., 2009; Du et al., 2008; Norman et al., 2007). Recently, the possibility to discriminate the KIR alleles by the technique of high-resolution melting (HRM) has been reported (Gonzales et al., 2009).

More recently, KIR haplotypes have been completely sequenced using Next Generation Sequencer (NGS), different patents using NGS have been filed (De Re et al., 2011), and some of sequenced haplotypes are present on the EBI database (http://www.ebi.ac.uk/ipd/kir/sequenced_haplotypes.html). Further, commercial kits are available for KIR typing in the clinical setting.

4. KIR/HLA class I genotypes and their implication in disease progression

As noted, an accurate typing system to discriminate groups of HLA class I alleles of a subject together with the analysis of KIR genotypes is of great interest to establish the association KIR/HLA, and their possible involvement in different pathologic or disease states. Another issue is to accurately define the sub-population of effector cells responsible for the immune responses. In this regard, an important issue is that KIR receptors are not only expressed by NK cells, but also by a subpopulation of CD8+ T lymphocytes. In this context, the role of this latter subpopulation may mask, or may actually be, the principal subject in any association between pathologic states and KIR/HLA interactions.

4.1 Human immunodeficiency virus (HIV)

HIV was the first viral infection for which an association between specific KIR and HLA class I ligands was observed. In detail, it has been reported that specific combinations between the activating receptor KIR3DS1 and HLA-Bw4 alleles, characterized by isoleucine at position 80 (HLA-Bw4^{I80}), have a protective effect against AIDS progression (Martin et al., 2002a). In fact, the interaction between HLA-Bw4^{I80} alleles and the activating receptor KIR3DS1 could be associated with enhanced NK cell reactivity that improves antiviral immune responsiveness. Moreover, this combination was found to confer protection against the onset of opportunistic infection during AIDS (Qi et al., 2006). Additionally, others found that KIR3DL1 alleles are correlated with the outcome of HIV infection in combination with HLA-B57, also an HLA-Bw4^{I80} allele. It has been found to be more protective than the KIR3DS1/HLA-Bw4^{I80} interaction (Martin et al., 2002a). It has to be stressed that the most protective KIR allele was KIR3DL1*004, which is not expressed on the cell surface, thus suggesting that absence of inhibition, or the better the enhanced KIR/HLA triggering potential, play roles in the immune-response against HIV (Rajagopalan et al., 2006). These data may not be in contrast though, since KIR3DS1 and KIR3DL1 are allelic form of the same gene present in haplotype B or A, respectively, thus representing different aspects of a complex system of interactions.

As expected, since the KIR complex has a multiloci ligand system, in some subject not only HLA-B alleles, but also HLA-C ligands appear to play roles in the control of HIV infection. A higher expression of HLA-C has also been associated with a slower AIDS progression (Fellay et al., 2007; Jennes et al., 2006; Thomas et al., 2009). While the HLA-C*07 alleles (C1-group), which are generally less expressed probably due to a mutation in the -35 residue (C>T), are associated with the most rapid progression of disease. Whereas alleles expressed at high levels (characterized by the -35 "C" allele), are associated with slower progression (Fellay et al., 2007; Thomas et al., 2009). These data may suggest the existence in these subjects of activating KIR(s) with C1-group specificity. Recently, a correlation of NK cell responses against HIV1-derived peptides has been associated with the presence of activating KIR(s) characterized by such C1-group specificity (Tiemessen et al., 2011).

4.2 Hepatitis C virus (HCV)

KIR/HLA combinations, suggesting a weak inhibitory potential, or better suggesting a triggering interaction, are been also found to be relevant in the viral clearance in hepatitis C virus (HCV) infection. This pathogen is common worldwide and is the direct cause of chronic diseases such as cirrhosis and hepatocellular carcinoma in 85% of infected subjects due to non-efficient immune-responsiveness. Among the high number of patients with chronic infection, 17% develop complications such as cirrhosis, and 2% due the most serious progression of disease like hepatocellular carcinoma. The factor leading to these different outcomes are not clear yet, although the route of infection, size of inoculums, and the viral genotype may play major roles. Interestingly, it is known that a particular MHC polymorphism is associated with the spontaneous clearance, or a self-limited HCV infection. Thus, subjects characterized by weaker KIR-mediated inhibitory interaction (KIR2DL3/HLA-C1 group) would be protective. Probably, it is because this inhibition could be more easily overridden by activating receptors, which generate a more efficient viral clearance than a stronger inhibitory interaction such as that triggered from KIR2DL2/HLA-C1 group or KIR2DL1/HLA-C2 group. In detail, analyses on more than 1000 subjects revealed that 350 recovered spontaneously without treatment for HCV infection. The more common characteristics among them were the homozygous inheritance of the KIR2DL3 locus and of its relative HLA-C1 group ligand (Khakoo et al., 2004). When a KIR does not efficiently suppress immune cells, the cells can be more easily activated to eliminate infected cells. Another retrospective study was performed in 151 donor-recipient pairs, evaluating the KIR/HLA genotypes and the relapse of HCV disease, and its progression after liver transplantation. Liver biopsies were obtained from the recipients 1, 3, 5, 7 and 10 years post-transplant to determine when hepatitis relapsed, the degree of fibrosis, and the progression to cirrhosis (Espadas de Arias et al., 2009). They found that hepatitis was more at risk to recur when the KIR/HLA-C interacting ligands are "staggered" between donor and recipient. In addition, the presence of KIR2DL3 in the recipient was related to the progression of liver fibrosis. In general, a simple model of genetic protection has not been found in all patient populations. KIR2DL3 is found in the "A" group of haplotypes, as it is true for KIR2DS4. Consistent with this, KIR2DS4 has also been associated with protection against chronic HCV infection. Similarly, the B group of haplotypes marked with KIR2DL5, but without the presence of both KIR2DL3 and KIR2DS4, have been found to be associated with a poor response to treatment for HCV (Carneiro et al., 2010). Finally, the KIR2DL3/HLA-C1 group interaction was not found to be protective in a cohort of HIV/HCV co-infected individuals, implying that the HIV viral infection might modulate the protective effect of KIR3DL3.

4.3 Hepatitis B virus (HBV)

The same rationale of weak inhibition by the homozygous KIR2DL3 and HLA-C1/C1 group genotype has been also indicated in the protection from hepatitis B (HBV) viral infection, while the presence of KIR2DL1 in combination with HLA-C2 group ligand (stronger interaction), conferred the susceptibility to chronic hepatitis B (Gao et al., 2010). Chronic hepatitis B (CHB) is an inflammatory disease of the liver caused in 10% of people who become infected with hepatitis B virus (HBV). Many of those with chronic infection may be asymptomatic, thus increasing the risk of viral transmission. Chronic infection with hepatitis B may increase the chance of permanent damage to the liver, including cirrhosis and liver cancer. Chronic hepatitis B (CHB) affects more than 350 million persons in the world. Another study, has also investigated on the KIR gene polymorphisms in a large cohort of 150 chronic hepatitis B patients, 251 subjects with resolution of infection, and 412 healthy controls. These authors found a correlation between KIR2DS2 and

KIR2DS3 as HBV susceptible genes able to induce a persistent weak inflammatory reaction that results in continuous injury of live tissues, and thus to chronic hepatitis; whereas, KIR2DS1, KIR3DS1, and KIR2DL5 may act as protective genes that facilitate the clearance of HBV (Zhi-ming et al., 2007).

4.4 Human Cytomegalovirus (HCMV)

Human Cytomegalovirus (HCMV) is the cause of latent infections in the majority of infected individuals. In infected immuno-compromised subjects, this virus may reactivate causing life-threatening infection. Again, activating KIR genes are thought to be important for the control of CMV reactivation after haematopoietic stem cell transplantation (HSCT), and KIR2DS2 together with KIR2DS4, or a total of at least 5 loci coding for activating KIR present, could be associated with reduced CMV infection after transplantation (Zaia et al., 2009).

4.5 Human papilloma virus (HPV)

Activating KIR genes are associated with recurrent respiratory papillomatosis (RRP), a rare disease caused by human papilloma virus (HPV). In this context, activating KIR3DS1 and KIR2DS1 receptors have been found to be involved in the triggering of an effective early immune response against HPV-infected targets to establish resistance to RRP development (Bonagura et al., 2010).

4.6 Herpes simplex virus (HSV)

In the case of infections sustained by herpes simplex virus (HSV) it has been found that both KIR2DL2 and KIR2DS2 genes could be associated in all asymptomatic cases (Estefania et al., 2007). However, at present it was impossible to determine whether the inefficient responses to HSV could be associated to one of the gene loci coding for the activating or the inhibitory receptor. The uncertainty is because these genes are in tight linkage disequilibrium since they are expressed as different adjacent loci of the B-haplotypes.

4.7 Psoriasis

There is a strong genetic basis associated with the development of the chronic inflammatory condition of the skin known as psoriasis. The MHC class I region that includes HLA-A, -B, -C, and -E genes has been found associated with psoriasis (Bowcock & Krueger, 2005; Nair et al., 2000). Among them, HLA-Cw6 appears to be one of the loci most associated with psoriasis (Nair et al., 2006; Tiilikainen et al., 1980). At least 3 additional loci, an allele with a HLA-Bw4 epitope (Feng et al. 2009), HLA-E alleles representing the ligand for type II heterodimeric receptors (NKG2A/CD94, and NKG2C/CD94), and stress-induced MICA molecules, representing the ligand for the NKG2D triggering receptor (Cerwenka & Lanier, 2003; Cheng et al., 2000) may be involved in disease. Data about which KIR may be involved in psoriasis are still unresolved, since some researchers have found KIR2DS1 associated in the development of disease (Holm et al., 2005; Luszczek et al., 2005; Suzuki et al., 2004), while others could not find any association (Chang et al., 2006; Williams et al., 2005). The findings about a possible association between KIR2DS1 and psoriasis is intriguing, since this receptor may recognize the HLA-Cw6 alleles (C2-group) as ligands, making these data very attractive, although a consensus on the biological significance of this association is still without an unanimous consensus. Another study pointed out the KIR2DL5 locus as the locus associated with the development of psoriasis (Suzuki et al., 2004). KIR2DS1 and KIR2DS2 have been found to be associated with psoriatic arthritis (PsA) (Williams et al., 2005), but without the expression of their associated HLA-C ligands (Martin et al., 2002b), or conversely, in presence of their ligands (Nelson et al., 2004). Altogether, the variability of the data published on psoriasis and PsA, indicate the absence of consensus, either because the numbers of patients analyzed were too low, or because the data on KIR/HLA association could be epiphenomenon and not the real cause of disease.

4.8 Inflammatory bowel disease (IBD)

In chronic inflammatory diseases of the gastrointestinal tract (IBD), Crohn's disease (CD) and ulcerative colitis (UC), the frequency of KIR2DL1 and KIR2DL3 is lower in patients than in healthy donors. It is of note that, the KIR2DL1/HLA-C2 group interaction is less frequent in IBD patients than with controls (Zhang et al., 2008). Therefore, the data suggest that poor inhibition through the KIR/HLA interaction contribute to the genetic susceptibility of IBD, and may be the direct cause of the chronic inflammation.

4.9 Use of NK cell activity in hematopoietic stem cell transplantion (HSCT)

NK cells have been used in adoptive immunotherapy as alloreactive natural killer (NK) cells for treatment of hematologic malignancies, in particular the myeloid leukemias. The knowledge acquired have made possible the use of NK cell alloreactivity (donor-versus-recipient) for eradication of leukemia cells using KIR/HLA haplotype-mismatched transplants ('haploidentical') or haploidentical hematopoietic stem cell transplantation (haplo-HSCT) (Pende et al., 2009; Velardi, 2008). This immunotherapy is based on the selection of donor NK cell expressing appropriate KIR repertoire (Table 1). The selection of KIR mismatches in HLA-matched donors by KIR genotyping is fundamental in the clinical treatment approach to define a donor selection strategy for improving transplant outcomes (Table 1) (Leung, 2011; van der Meer et al., 2008).

4.10 Reproduction

The interaction between NK cells and uterine trophoblasts is an active process for blood vessel enlargement, and in remodelling during placentation, in order to have a more efficient blood supply to the fetus during pregnancy. Defective invasion of uterine trophoblasts is one cause of abnormal placental development, which may occur in disorders such as pre-eclampsia. In this pathological condition there is incomplete enlargement of blood vessels, which is often associated with high blood pressure, ending up in poor fetal growth, or in recurrent miscarriages. Much evidence indicates that interactions between fetal trophoblasts and maternal uterine NK cells are important in human placentation, with abnormal interaction resutling in increased risk for developing pre-eclampsia. This situation arises in a mother displaying homozygosity for KIR haplotype A (essentially absence of activating KIRs) and presence of HLA-C2 group alleles in the fetal tissues (Hiby et al., 2004). These data suggest that strong KIR inhibitory signals may be associated with a reduction of vessel enlargement, resulting in poor implantation, and increasing the risk of recurrent spontaneous abortions. More interestingly, also the HLA-C typing of the father was found to be crucial in miscarriages, where an increased frequency of HLA-C2 group alleles in both the mother and the father, associated with the lack of KIR2DS1 in the mother, seems to increase the risk of abortion. These data are the first evidence of a male factor that increases the risk in spontaneous abortions (Hiby et al., 2008). Others have found that mothers with recurrent miscarriages showed an increase of KIR2DS1 frequency, together with a decrease of HLA-C2 group alleles, in comparison with mothers without recurrent spontaneous abortions, while the expression of KIR2DL1, the inhibitory receptor for HLA-C2 group, was unchanged (Wang et al., 2007). In addition, trophoblast cells express on their cell surface the non-classical MHC class I, HLA-G, while decidual NK cells express the HLA-G-specific KIR2DL4 receptor. Thus, the HLA-G-specific KIR2DL4 receptors could play an important role in pregnancy outcome though the interaction between decidual NK cells and trophoblasts. Indeed several studies showed that higher cell surface expression of KIR2DL4 is associated with successful pregnancy (Yan et al., 2007). These data are not in conflict with the idea that activating KIR likely support placentation, since KIR2DL4 is known to have triggering potential. While KIR/HLA interactions, including maternal and paternal HLA and KIR alleles, between NK cells and trophoblasts are involved in preservation or loss of prenancies, they do not represent the only set of factors. For example, women who are missing KIR2DL4 have had successful pregnancy outcomes (Nowak et al., 2011).

5. Conclusion

Killer Ig-like receptors (KIR) expressed by NK cells and by some CD8+ T lymphocytes are known to have important roles in normal immune protection, and certain pathological conditions, such as cancer, infectious diseases, loss of pregnancy, and autoimmunity. NK cells and some CD8+ T lymphocytes, which express KIR, also express multiple other receptors on their cell surface able to modulate/regulate their function and thus influence host immune-responses through a complex matrix of intra-cytoplasmic signals. All the knowledges gathered in the last 15 years about the structure of KIR, their function, as well as defining their ligand specificity, although still not completed, have made some clinical applications possible. It is currently possible via specific HLA matching and KIR mismatching to use NK cells to kill tumor cells. It can be envisioned that via knowledge of KIR associations with specific pathogen-infected cells, directed NK cell therapy, activation and inhibition, can be utilized to result in erradication of the virus, rather than chronic infection. All of these approaches are based on the correct KIR genotyping, performed together with the determination of the HLA class I allele. And, is ultimately based on the specific residues determining the KIR specificity, and interaction with HLA. Since NK cells and a subpopulation of CD8+ T lymphocytes express KIR, efforts continue to require addressing which is the correct cell population associated with the process under investigation. In addition, due to differential KIR levels of expression and haplotypic expression, studies must consider the presence, an increase, or a decrease of expression of certain KIR locus in the analyzed population versus the control population for valid assessment of the obtained results. At the current time, published information is lacking on the relative expression levels of KIR in different populations of people. In conclusion, an accurate evaluation of KIR/HLA interaction, taking in consideration the complexity of the KIR and HLA gene systems, together with a sufficient number of subjects analyzed is needed to define the KIR involvement in natural immunity and in different disease states.

6. References

Abi-Rached, L., & Parham, P. (2005). Natural selection drives recurrent formation of activating killer cell immunoglobulin-like receptor and Ly49 from inhibitory homologues. *J. Exp. Med.*, Vol.201, No.8, (April 2005), pp. 1319-1332

Abi-Rached, L., Moesta, AK, Rajalingam, R., Guethlein, LA, & Parham, P. (2010). Human-specific evolution and adaptation led to major qualitative differences in the variable receptors of human and chimpanzee natural killer cells. *PLoS Genet*, Vol.6, No.11, (November 2010), e1001192

André, P., Biassoni, R., Colonna, M., Cosman, D., Lanier, L.L., Long, E.O., Lopez-Botet, M., Moretta, A., Moretta, L., Parham, P., Trowsdale, J., Vivier E., Wagtmann, N., & Wilson, M.J. (2001). New nomenclature for MHC receptors. *Nature Immuno*, Vol.2, No.8, (August 2001), pp. 661

Biassoni, R., Falco, M., Cambiaggi, A., Costa, P., Verdiani, S., Pende, D., Conte, R., Di Donato, C., Parham, P., & Moretta, L.(1995). Amino acidic substitutions can influence the NK-mediated recognition of HLA-C molecules. Role of serine-77 and lysine-80 in the target cell protection from lysis mediated by "group 2" or "group 1" NK clones. *J Exp Med*, Vol.182, No.2, (August 1995), pp. 605–9

Biassoni, R., Pessino, A., Malaspina, A., Cantoni, C., Bottino, C., Sivori, S., Moretta, L., & Moretta, A.(1997). Role of amino acid position 70 in the binding affinity of p50.1 and p58.1 receptors for HLA-Cw4 molecules. *Eur J Immunol*, Vol.27, No.12, (December 1997), pp. 3095–3099

Biassoni, R., Ugolotti, E. & DeMaria, A. (2009a). NK cell receptors and their interactions with MHC. *Current Pharmaceutical Design*, Vol.15, No.28, (2009), pp. 3301-3310, ISSN: 1381-6128

Biassoni, R. (2009b). Human natural killer receptors and their ligands. Current Protocols in Immunology. 14.10.1–14.10.23

Bonagura, V.R., Du, Z., Ashouri, E., Luo, L., Hatam, L.J., DeVoti, J.A., Rosenthal, D.W., Steinberg, B.M.,Abramson, A.L., Gjertson, D.W., Reed, E.F., & Rajalingam, R.(2010). Activating killer cell immunoglobulinlike receptors 3DS1 and 2DS1 protect against developing the severe form of recurrent respiratory papillomatosis. *Hum Immunol*, Vol.71, No.2, (February 2010), pp. 212-9

Borrego, F., Masilamani, M., Marusina, A.I., Tang, X., & Coligan, J.E. (2006). The CD94/NKG2 family of receptors: from molecules and cells to clinical relevance. *Immunol Res*, Vol.35, No.3, (2006), pp.263-78

Bowcock, A.M., & Krueger, J.G. (2005). Getting under the skin: the immunogenetics of psoriasis. *Nat Rev Immunol*, Vol.5, No.9, (September 2005), pp. 699-711

Cantoni, C., Verdiani, S., Falco, M., Pessino, A., Cilli, R., Conte, R., Pende, D., Ponte, M., Mikaelsson, M.S., Moretta, L., & Biassoni, R. (1998). p49, a putative HLA class I-specific inhibitory NK receptor belonging to the immunoglobulin superfamily. *Eur J Immunol*, Vol.28, No.10, (October 1998), pp.1980-1990

Cerwenka, A. & Lanier, L.L. (2003). NKG2D ligands: unconventional MHC class I-like molecules exploited by viruses and cancer. *Tissue Antigens*, Vol.61, No.5, (May 2003), pp. 335-43

Chang, Y.T., Chou, C.T., Shiao, Y.M., Lin, M.W., Yu, C.W., Chen, C.C., Huang, C.H., Lee, D.D., Liu, H.N., Wang, W.J., & Tsai, S.F.(2006).The killer cell immunoglobulin-like receptor genes do not confer susceptibility to psoriasis vulgaris independently in Chinese. *J Invest Dermatol*, Vol.126, No.10, (October 2006), pp. 2335-8

Cheng, L., T., Zhang, S.Z., Xiao, C.Y., Hou, Y.P., Li, L., Luo, H.C.,Jiang, H.Y, & Zuo, W.Q. (2000). The A5.1 allele of the major histocompatibility complex class I chain-related gene A is associated with psoriasis vulgaris in Chinese. *Br J Dermatol*, Vol.143, No.2, (August 2000), pp. 324-9

Ciccone, E., Viale, O., Pende, D., Malnati, M., Biassoni, R., Melioli, G., Moretta, A., Long, EO & Moretta, L. (1988). Specific lysis of allogeneic cells after activation of CD3- lymphocytes in mixed lymphocyte culture. *J Exp Med*, Vol.168, No.6, (December 1998), pp. 2403-8

Ciccone, E., Pende, D., Viale, O., Than, A., Di Donato, C., Orengo, AM, Biassoni, R., Verdiani, S., Amoroso, A., Moretta, A., & Moretta, L. (1992). Involvement of HLA class I alleles in natural killer (NK) cell-specific functions: expression of HLA-Cw3 confers selective protection from lysis by alloreactive NK clones displaying a defined specificity (specificity 2). *J Exp Med*, Vol.176, No.4, (October 1992), pp. 963-71

Colonna, M. & Samaridis, J. (1995). Cloning of immunoglobulin-superfamily members associated with HLA-C and HLA-B recognition by human natural killer cells. *Science*, Vol.268, No.5209, (April 1995), pp. 405-8

Cooley, S., Trachtenberg, E., Bergmann, T.L., Saeterum, K., Klein, J., Le, CT, Marsh, S.G., Guethlein, L.A., Parham, P., Miller, J.S., & Weisdorf, D.J. (2009). Donors with group B KIR haplotypes improve relapse-free survival after unrelated hematopoietic cell transplantation for acute myelogenous leukemia. *Blood*, Vol.113, No.3, (January 2009), pp. 726–32

Cooley, S., Weisdorf, DJ, Guethlein, LA, Klein, JP, Wang, T., Le, CT, Marsh, SG, Geraghty, D., Spellman, S., Haagenson, MD, Ladner, M., Trachtenberg, E., Parham, P., & Miller, JS. (2010). Donor selection for natural killer cell receptor genes leads to superior survival after unrelated transplantation for acute myelogenous leukemia. *Blood*, Vol.116, No.14, (October 2010), pp. 2411-9

D'Andrea, A., Chang, C., Franz-Bacon, K., McClanahan, T., Phillips, JH, & Lanier, LL. (1995). Molecular cloning of NKB1. A natural killer cell receptor for HLA-B allotypes. *J Immunol*, Vol.155, No.5, (Sep tember 1995), pp. 2306-10

De Re, V., Caggiari, L., De Zorzi, M., & Toffoli, G. (2011). Kir Molecules: Recent Patents of Interest for the Diagnosis and Treatment of Several Autoimmune Diseases, Chronic Inflammation, and B-Cell Malignancies. *Recent Pat DNA Gene Seq*, (June 2011)

Döhhring, C., Scheidegger, D., Samaridis, J., Cella, M., & Colonna, M. (1996). A human killer inhibitory receptor specific for HLA-A1,2. *J Immunol, Vol.*156, No.9, (May 1996), pp. 3098–3101

Du, Z., Sharm, SK, Spellman, S., Reed, E.F., & Rajalingham, R.(2008). KIR2DL5 alleles mark certain combination of activating *KIR* genes. *Genes Immun*, Vol.9, No.5, (July 2008), pp. 1–11

Espadas de Arias, A., Haworth, S., Belli, L., Burra, P., Pinzello, G., Minola, E., Boccagni, P., Torelli, R., Scalamogna, M., & Poli, F. (2009). Killer Cell Immunoglobulin-Like Receptor Genotype and Killer Cell Immunoglobulin-Like Receptor–Human Leukocyte Antigen C Ligand Compatibility Affect the Severity of Hepatitis C Virus Recurrence After Liver Transplantation. *Liver Transpl*, Vol.15, No.4,(April 2009),pp.390-399

Estefanía, E., Gómez-Lozano, N., Portero, F., de Pablo, R., Solís, R., Sepúlveda, S., Vaquero, M., González, M.A., Suárez, E., Roustán, G., & Vilches, C. (2007). Influence of KIR gene diversity on the course of HSV-1 infection: resistance to the disease is associated with the absence of KIR2DL2 and KIR2DS2. *Tissue Antigens.*, Vol.70, No.1, (July 2007), pp.34-41

Faure, M., & Long, E.O. (2002). KIR2DL4 (CD158d), an NK cell-activating receptor with inhibitory potential. *J Immunol*, Vol.168, No.15, (June 2002), pp. 6208–6214

Felix, NJ, & Allen, PM.(2007). Specificity of T-cell alloreactivity. *Nat Rev Immunol*, Vol.7, No.12, (December 2007), pp. 942-53

Fellay, J., Shianna, K.V., Ge, D., Colombo, S., Ledergerber, B., Weale, M., Zhang, K., Gumbs, C., Castagna, A., Cossarizza, A., Cozzi-Lepri, A., De Luca, A., Easterbrook, P., Francioli, P., Mallal, S., Martinez-Picado, J., Miro, J.M., Obel, N., Smith, JP., Wyniger, J., Descombes, P., Antonarakis, S.E., Letvin, N.L., McMichael, A.J., Haynes, B.F., Telenti, A., & Goldstein, D.B.(2007). A whole-genome association study of major determinants for host control of HIV-1. *Science*, Vol.317, No.5840, (August 2007), pp. 944-7

Feng, B.J., Sun, L-D, Soltani-Arabshahi, R., Bowcock, A.M., Nair, R.P., Sutuart, P., Elder, J.T., Schrodi, S., Begovich, A.B., Abecasis, G.R., Zhang, X-J, Callis-Duffin, K.P., Krueger, G.G, & Goldgar, D.E. (2009). Multiple Loci within the major histocompatibility complex confer risk of psoriasis. *PLoS Genet*, Vol.5, No.8, (August 2009), e1000606

Foley, B.A., De Santis, D., Van Beelen, E., Lathbury, L.J., Christiansen, F.T., & Witt, C.S. (2008). The reactivity of Bw4+ HLA-B and HLA-A alleles with KIR3DL1: implications for patient and donor suitability for haploidentical stem cell transplantations. *Blood*, Vol. 112, No. 2, (July 2008), pp.435-43

Gagne, K., Brizard, G., Gueglio, B., Milpied, N., Herry, P., Bonneville, F., Cheneau, M.L., Schleinitz, N., Cesbron, A., Follea, G., Harrousseau, J.L., & Bignon, J.D. (2002). Relevance of KIR gene polymorphisms in bone marrow transplantation outcome. *Human Immunology*, Vol. 63, No. 4 , (April 2002), pp. 271–280.

Gao, X., Jiao, Y., Wang, L., Liu, X., Sun, W., Cui, B., Chen, Z., & Zhao, Y. (2010). Inhibitory KIR and specific HLA-C gene combinations confer susceptibility to or protection against chronic hepatitis B. *Clin Immunol*, Vol.137, No.1, (October 2010), pp. 139-46

Gillespie, G.M., Bashirova, A., Dong, T., McVicar, D.W., Rowland-Jones, S.L., & Carrington, M.(2007). Lack of KIR3DS1 binding to MHC class I Bw4 tetramers in complex with CD8+ T cell epitopes. *AIDS Res Hu. Retroviruses*, Vol.23, No.3, (March 2007), pp. 451–455

Gonzalez, A., McErlean, C., Meenagh, A., Shovlin, T., & Middleton, D. (2009).Killer cell immunoglobulin-like receptor allele discrimination by high-resolution melting. *Hum Immunol*, Vol.70, No.10, (October 2009), pp. 858-63

Gourraud, P.A., Meenagh, A., Cambon-Thomsen, A., & Middleton, D.(2010). Linkage disequilibrium organization of the human KIR superlocus: implications for KIR data analyses. *Immunogenetics*, Vol.62, No.11-12, (December 2010), pp. 729-40

Graef, T., Moesta, A.K., Norman, P.J., Abi-Rached, L., Vago, L., Older Aguilar, A.M., Gleimer, M., Hammond, J.A., Guethlein, L.A., Bushnell, D.A., Robinson, P.J., & Parham, P. (2009). KIR2DS4 is a product of gene conversion with KIR3DL2 that introduced specificity for HLA-A*11 while diminishing avidity for HLA-C. *J Exp Med*, Vol.206, No.11, (October 2009), pp. 2557–2572

Hansasuta, P., Dong, T., Thananchai, H., Weekes, M., Willberg, C., Aldemir, H., Rowland-Jones, S., & Braud, V.M. (2004). Recognition of HLA-A3 and HLAA11 by KIR3DL2 is peptide-specific. *Eur J Immunol*, Vol.34, No.6, (June 2004), pp. 1673–1679

Harville TO: HLA Typing for Cellular Product Characterization and Identity Testing. In: Cellular Therapy: Principles, Methods, and Regulations. Ed. Areman and Loper. AABB, Bethesda, MD, 2009, pp 627-643

Herberman, R.B., Nunn, M.E., & Lavrin, D.H. (1975). Natural cytotoxic reactivity of mouse lymphoid cells against syngeneic acid allogeneic tumors. I. distribution of reactivity and specificity. *Int J Cancer*, Vol.16, No.2, (August 1975), pp. 216–229

Hiby, S.E., Walker, J.J., O'shaughnessy, K.M., Redman, C.W., Carrington, M., Trowsdale, J., & Moffett, A. (2004). Combinations of maternal KIR and fetal HLA-C genes influence the risk of preeclampsia and reproductive success.*J Exp Med*, Vol.8, (October 2004), pp.957-65

Hiby, S.E., Regan, L., Lo, W., Farrel,l L., Carrington, M., & Moffett, A. (2008). Association of maternal killer-cell immunoglobulin-like receptors and parental HLA-C genotypes with recurrent miscarriage. *Hum Reprod*, Vol.23, No.4, (April 2008), pp. 972-6

Holm, S.J., Sakuraba, K., Mallbris, L., Wolk, K., Ståhle, M., & Sánchez, F.O. (2005). Distinct HLA-C/KIR genotype profile associates with guttate psoriasis. *J Invest Dermatol*, Vol.125, No.4, (October 2005), pp. 721-30

Hsu, KC, Chida, S., Geraghty, DE, Dupont, B & Geraghty, D.E. (2002.). The killer cell immunoglobulin-like receptor (KIR) genomic region: gene-order, haplotypes and allelic polymorphism. *Immunological Review, Vol.*190, No.1, (December 2002), pp. 40-52

Hsu, K.C., Keever-Taylor, C.A., Wilton, A., Pinto, C., Heller, G., Arkun, K., O'Reilly, R.J., Horowitz, M.M., & Dupont, B. (2005). Improved outcome in HLA-identical sibling hematopoietic stem-cell transplantation for acute myelogenous leukemia predicted by KIR and HLA genotypes. *Blood*, Vol. 105, No. 12, (June 2005), pp. 4878–4884

Jenisch, S., Westphal, E., Nair, R.P., Stuart, P., Voorhees, J.J., Christophers, E., Krönke, M., Elder, J.T., & Henseler, T. (1999). Linkage disequilibrium analysis of familial psoriasis: identification of multiple disease-associated MHC haplotypes. *Tissue Antigens*, Vol.53, No.2, (February 1999), pp. 135-46

Jennes, W., Verheyden, S., Demanet, C., Adjé-Touré, C.A., Vuylsteke, B., Nkengasong, J.N., & Kestens, L. (2006). Cutting edge: resistance to HIV-1 infection among African female sex workers is associated with inhibitory KIR in the absence of their HLA ligands. *J Immunol*, Vol.177, No.10, (November 2006), pp.6588-92

Leung, W., Iyengar, R., Turner, V., Lang, P., Bader, P., Conn, P., Niethammer, D., & Handgretinger, R. (2004). Determinants of antileukemia effects of allogeneic NK cells. *Journal of Immunology*, Vol. 172, No. 1, (January 2004), pp. 644–650

Leung, W. (2011). Use of NK cell activity in cure by transplant. *Br J Haematol*, Vol. 155, No.1, (October 2011), pp. 14-29

Ljunggren, HG, & Kärre, K.(1990). In search of the 'missing self': MHC molecules and NK cell recognition. *Immunol Today*, Vol.11, No.7, (July 1990), pp. 237–244

Luszczek, W., Mańczak, M., Cisło, M., Nockowski, P., Wiśniewski, A., Jasek, M., & Kuśnierczyk, P.(2004). Gene for the activating natural killer cell receptor, KIR2DS1, is associated with susceptibility to psoriasis vulgaris. *Hum Immunol*, Vol.65, No.7, (July 2004), pp. 758-66

Karre, K., Ljunggren, H.G., Piontek, G., & Kiessling, R.(1986). Selective rejection of H-2-deficient lymphoma variants suggests alternative immune defence strategy. *Nature,* Vol.319, No.6055, (February 1986), pp. 675–678

Khakoo, S.I., Rajalingam, R., Shum, B.P., Weidenbach, K., Flodin, L., Muir, D.G., Canavez, F., Cooper, S.L., Valiante, N.M., Lanier, L.L., & Parham, P. (2000). Rapid evolution of NK cell receptor systems demonstrated by comparison of chimpanzees and humans. *Immunity,* Vol.12, No.6, (June 2000), pp. 687-698

Khakoo, S.I., Thio, C.L., Martin, M.P., Brooks, CR., Gao, X., Astemborski, J., Cheng, J., Goedert, J.J., Vlahov, D., Hilgartner, M., Cox, S., Little, A.M., Alexander, G.J., Cramp, M.E., O'Brien, S.J., Rosenberg, W.M., Thomas, D.L., & Carrington, M. (2004). HLA and NK cell inhibitory receptor genes in resolving hepatitis C virus infection. Science, Vol.305, No.5685, (August 2004), pp.872-4

Kiessling, R., Klein, E., & Wigzell, H. (1975). "Natural" killer cells in the mouse. I. cytotoxic cells with specificity for mouse Moloney leukemia cells. Specificity and distribution according to genotype. *Eur J Immunol,* Vol.5, No.2, (February 1975), pp. 112–117

Kikuchi-Maki, A., Yusa, S., Catina, T.L., & Campbell, K.S. (2003). KIR2DL4 is an IL-2-regulated NK cell receptor that exhibits limited expression in humans but triggers strong IFN-gamma production. *J Immunol,* Vol.171, No.7, (October 2003), pp. 3415–3425

Kikuchi-Maki, A., Catina, T.L., & Campbell, K.S. (2005). Cutting edge: KIR2DL4 transduces signals into human NK cells through association with the Fc receptor gamma protein. *J Immunol,*Vol.174, No.7, (April 2007), pp. 3859-3863

Kulkarni, S., Martin, M.P., & Carrington, M. (2010). KIR genotyping by multiplex PCR-SSP. *Methods Mol Biol.,* Vol.612, pp. 365-75

Malnati, M.S., Peruzzi, M., Parker, K.C., Biddison, W.E., Ciccone, E., Moretta, A., & Long, E.O. (1995). Peptide specificity in the recognition of MHC class I by natural killer cell clones. *Science,* Vol.267, No.5200, (February 1995),pp. 1016-1018

Martin, M.P., & Carrington, M .(2008). KIR locus polymorphisms: genotyping and disease association analysis. *Methods Mol Biol,* Vol.415, pp. 49-64

Martin, M.P., Gao, X., Lee, J.H., Nelson, G.W., Detels, R., Goedert, J. J., Buchbinder, S., Hoots, K., Vlahov, D., Trowsdale, J., Wilson, M., O'Brien, S.J., & Carrington, M.(2002). Epistatic interaction between KIR3DS1 and HLA-B delays the progression to AIDS. *Nat. Genet,* Vol.31, No.4, (August 2002), pp. 429–434

Martin, M.P., Nelson, G., Lee, J.H., Pellett, F., Gao, X., Wade, J., Wilson, M.J., Trowsdale, J, Gladman, D., & Carrington, M. (2002). Cutting edge: susceptibility to psoriatic arthritis: influence of activating killer Ig-like receptor genes in the absence of specific HLA-C alleles. *J Immunol,* Vol.169, No.6, (September 2002), pp. 2818-22.

McQueen, K.L., Dorighi, K.M., Guethlein, L.A., Wong, R., Sanjanwala, B., & Parham, P. (2007). Donor-recipient combinations of group A and B KIR haplotypes and HLA class I ligand affect the outcome of HLA-matched, sibling donor hematopoietic cell transplantation. *Human Immunology,* Vol. 68, No. 5, (May 2007), pp. 309–323

Middleton, D., & Gonzelez, F. (2010). The extensive polymorphism of KIR genes. *Immunology,* Vol.129, No.1, (January 2010), pp. 8-19

Moesta, A.K., Norman, P.J., Yawata, M., Yawata, N., Gleimer, M., & Parham, P. (2008). Synergistic polymorphism at two positions distal to the ligand-binding site makes KIR2DL2 a stronger receptor for HLA-C than KIR2DL3. *J Immunol.,*Vol.180, No.6, (March 2008), pp. 3969-3979

Moretta, A., Bottino, C., Vitale, M., Pende, D., Biassoni, R., Mingari, MC, & Moretta, L. (1996). Receptors for HLA class-I molecules in human natural killer cells. *Annu Rev Immunol*,Vol.14, pp. 619-48

Nair, R.P., Stuart, P., Henseler, T., Jenisch, S., Chia, N.V., Westphal, E., Schork, N.J., Kim, J., Lim, H.W., Christophers, E., Voorhees, J.J., & Elder, J.T. (2000). Localization of psoriasis-susceptibility locus PSORS1 to a 60-kb interval telomeric to HLA-C. *Am J Hum Genet*, Vol.66, No.6, (June 2000), pp. 1833-44

Nair, R.P., Stuart, P.E., Nistor, I., Hiremagalore, R., Chia, N.V., Jenisch, S., Weichenthal, M., Abecasis, G.R., Lim, H.W., Christophers, E., Voorhees, J.J. & Elder, J.T. (2006). Sequence and haplotype analysis supports HLA-C as the psoriasis susceptibility 1 gene. *Am J Hum Genet*, Vol.78, No.5, (May 2006), pp. 827-51

Nelson, G.W., Martin, M.P., Gladman, D., Wade, J., Trowsdale, J., & Carrington, M. (2004). Cutting edge: heterozygote advantage in autoimmune disease: hierarchy of protection/susceptibility conferred by HLA and killer Ig-like receptor combinations in psoriatic arthritis. *J Immunol*, Vol.173, No.7, (October 2004), pp. 4273-6

Norman, P.J., Abi-Rached, L., Gendzekhadze, K., Korbel, D., Gleimer, M., Rowley, D., Bruno, D.,.Carrington, C.V., Chandanayingyong, D., Chang, Y.H., Crespi, C., Saruhan-Direskeneli, G., Fraser, PA, Hameed, K., Kamkamidze, G., Koram, K.A., Layrisse, Z., Matamoros, N., Mila, J., Park, M.H., Pitchappan, R.M., Ramdath, D.D., Shiau, M.Y., Stephens, H.A., Struik, S., Verity, D.H., Vaughan, R.W., Tyan, D., Davis, R.W., Riley, E.M., Ronaghi, M., & Parham, P. (2007). Unusual selection on the KIR3DL1/S1 natural killer cell receptor in Africans. *Nat. Genet*, Vol.39, No.9, (September 2007), pp. 1092–1099

Nowak, I., Majorczyk, E., Płoski, R., Senitzer, D., Sun, J.Y., & Kuśnierczyk, P. (2011). Lack of KIR2DL4 gene in a fertile Caucasian woman. *Tissue Antigens*, Vol.78, No.2, (August 2011), pp.115-9.

O'Connor, GM, Yamada, E., Rampersaud, A., Thomas, R., Carrington, M., & McVicar, DW. (2011). Analysis of Binding of KIR3DS1*014 to HLA Suggests Distinct Evolutionary History of KIR3DS1. *J Immunol*, Vol.187, No.5, (September 2001), pp. 2162-71

Older Aguilar, A.M., Guethlein, L.A., Adams, E.J., Abi-Rached, L., Moesta, A.K., & Parham, P. (2010). Coevolution of killer cell Ig-like receptors with HLA-C to become the major variable regulators of human NK cells. *J Immunol*, Vol.185, No.7, (October 2010), pp. 4238-51

Parham, P., Norman, P.J., Abi-Rached, L., & Guethlein, L.A. (2011). Variable NK cell receptors exemplified by human KIR3DL1/S1. *J Immunol*, Vol.187, No.1, (July 2011), pp. 11-9

Pende, D., Biassoni, R., Cantoni, C., Verdiani, S., Falco, M., di Donato, C., Accade, L., Bottino, C., Moretta, A., & Moretta, L. (1996). The natural killer cell receptor specific for HLA-A allotypes: a novel member of the p58/p70 family of inhibitory receptors that is characterized by three immunoglobulin-like domains and is expressed as a 140-kD disulphidelinked dimer. *J Exp Med, Vol.*184, No.2, (August 1996), pp. 505-18

Pende, D., Marcenaro, S., Falco, M., Martini, S., Bernardo, M.E., Montagna, D., Romeo, E., Cognet, C., Martinetti, M., Maccario, R., Maria, M.C., Vivier, E., Moretta, L., Locatelli, F., & Moretta, A. (2009). Anti-leukemia activity of alloreactive NK cells in KIR ligand-mismatched haploidentical HSCT for pediatric patients: evaluation of the functional role of activating KIR and redefinition of inhibitory KIR specificity. *Blood,* Vol.113, No.13, (March 2009), pp. 3119-3129

Peruzzi, M., Parker, K.C., Long, E.O., & Malnati, M.S. (1996). Peptide sequence requirements for the recognition of HLA-B* 2705 by specific natural killer cells. *J Immunol,* Vol.157, No.8, (October 1996), pp. 3350-3356

Pyo, C.W., Guethlein, L.A., Vu, Q., Wang, R., Abi-Rached, L., Norman, P.J., Marsh, S.G.E., Miller, J.S., Parham, P., & Geraghty, D.E. (2010). Different patterns of evolution in the centromeric and telomeric regions of group a and B haplotypes of the human killer cell Ig-like receptor locus. *PLoS One,* Vol.5, No.12, (December 2010), e15115

Ponte, M., Cantoni, C., Biassoni, R., Tradori-Cappai, A., Bentivoglio, G., Vitale, C., Bertone, S., Moretta, A, Moretta, L., & Mingari, M.C. (1999). Inhibitory receptors sensing HLA-G1 molecules in pregnancy: decidua-associated natural killer cells express LIR-1 and CD94/NKG2A and acquire p49, an HLA-G1-specific receptor.*Proc Natl Acad Sci USA, Vol.*96, *No.*10, *(May* 1999),*pp.*5674-5679.

Stern, M., Ruggeri, L., Capanni, M., Mancusi, A., & Velardi, A. (2008). Human leukocyte antigens A23, A24, and A32 but not A25 are ligands for KIR3DL1. *Blood,* Vol. 112, No. 3, (August 2008), pp. 708-10

Qi, Y., Martin, M.P., Gao, X., Jacobson, L., Goedert, J.J., Buchbinder, S., Kirk, G.D., O'Brien, S.J., Trowsdale, J., & Carrington, M. (2006). KIR/HLA pleiotropism: protection against both HIV and opportunistic infections. *PLoS Pathos,* Vol.2, No. 8, (August 2006), e79

Rajagopalan, S., & Long, E.O. (1997). The direct binding of a p58 killer cell inhibitory receptor to human histocompatibility leukocyte antigen (HLA)-Cw4 exhibits peptide selectivity. *J Exp Med,* Vol.185,pp. 1523-8

Rajagopalan, S., & Long, E.O. (1999). A human histocompatibility leukocyte antigen (HLA)-G-specific receptor expressed on all natural killer cells. *J Exp Med, Vol.* 189, No.7 , (April 1999), *pp.* 1093-1100

Rajagopalan, S., Fu, J., & Long, E.O. (2001). Cutting edge: induction of IFN-gamma production but not cytotoxicity by the killer cell Ig-like receptor KIR2DL4 (CD158d) in resting NK cells. *J Immunol,* Vol.167, No.4, (August 2001), pp. 1877–1881

Rajagopalan, S., Bryceson, Y.T., Kuppusamy, S.P., Geraghty, D.E., van der Meer, A., Joosten, I., & Long, E.O. (2006). Activation of NK cells by an endocytosed receptor for soluble HLA-G. *PLoS Biol,Vol.* 4, No.1, (January 2006), pp. e9

Rajalingam, R., Parham, P., & Abi-Rached, L. (2004). Domain shuffling has been the main mechanism forming new hominoid killer cell Ig-like receptors. *J Immunol, Vol.*172, No.1, (January 2004), pp.356-69

Ruggeri, L., Capanni, M., Urbani, E., Perruccio, K., Shlomchik, W.D., Tosti, A., Posati, S., Rogaia, D., Frassoni, F., Aversa, F., Martelli, M.F., & Velardi, A. (2002). Effectiveness of donor natural killer cell alloreactivity in mismatched hematopoietic transplants. *Science,* Vol. 295, No. 5562, (March 2002), pp. 2097–2100.

Ruggeri, L., Mancusi, A., Capanni, M., Martelli, M.F., & Velardi, A.(2005). Exploitation of alloreactive NK cells in adoptive immunotherapy of cancer. *Current Opinion in Immunology,* Vol.17, No.2, (April 2005), pp. 211–217

Selvakumar, A., Steffens, U., & Dupont, B. (1996). NK cell receptor gene of the KIR family with two Ig domains but highest homology to KIR receptors with three Ig domains. *Tissue Antigens* ,Vol.48, No.4 Pt 1, (October 1996), pp. 285-295

Shilling, H.G., Guethlein, L.A., Cheng, N.W., Gardiner, C.M., Rodriguez, R., Tyan, D., & Parham, P. (2002). Allelic polymorphism synergizes with variable gene content to individualize human KIR genotype. *J Immunol*, Vol.168, No.4, (March 2002), pp. 2307-15

Sigalov AB(2010). Thc SCHOOL of nature: I. Transmembrane signaling. *Self Nonself*, Vol.1, No.1,(January 2010), pp. 4-39

Stewart, C.A., Laugier-Anfossi, F., Vely, F., Saulquin, X., Riedmuller, J., Tisserant, A., Gauthier, L., Romagne, F., Ferracci, G., Arosa, F.A, Moretta, A., Sun, P.D., Ugolini, S., & Vivier, E. (2005). Recognition of peptide-MHC class I complexes by activating killer immunoglobulin- like receptors. *Proc. Natl. Acad. Sci. USA*, Vol.102, No.37, (September 2005), pp. 13224–13229

Suzuki, Y., Hamamoto, Y., Ogasawara, Y., Ishikawa, K., Yoshikawa, Y., Sasazuki, T., & Muto, M. (2004). Genetic polymorphisms of killer cell immunoglobulin-like receptors are associated with susceptibility to psoriasis vulgaris. *J Invest Dermatol*, Vol.122, No.5, (May 2004), pp. 1133-6

Thananchai, H., Gillespie, G., Martin, M.P., Bashirova, A., Yawata, N., Yawata, M., Easterbrook, P., McVicar, D.W., Maenaka, K., Parham, P., Carrington, M., Dong, T., & Rowland-Jones, S. (2007). Cutting Edge: Allele-specific and peptide-dependent interactions between KIR3DL1 and HLA-A and HLA-B. *J Immunol*, Vol. 178, No. 1 , (January 2007), pp. 33-7

Tiemessen, C.T., Paximadis, M., Minevich, G., Winchester, R., Shalekoff, S., Gray, G.E., Sherman, G.G., Coovadia, A.H., & Kuhn, L. (2011). Natural Killer Cell Responses to HIV-1 Peptides are Associated With More Activating KIR Genes and HLA-C Genes of the C1 Allotype. *J Acquir Immune Defic Syndr*, Vol.57, No.3, (July 2011), pp. 181-189

Tiilikainen, A., Lassun, A., Karvonen, J., Vartainen, P., & Julin, M. (1980). Psoriasis and HLA-Cw6. *Br J Dermatol*, Vol.102, No.2, (February 1980), pp. 179-84

Thomas, R., App,s R., Qi, Y., Gao, X., Male, V., O'hUigin, C., O'Connor, G., Ge, D., Fellay, J., Martin, J.N., Margolick, J., Goedert, J.J., Buchbinder, S., Kirk, G.D., Martin, M.P., Telenti, A., Deeks, S.G., Walker, B.D., Goldstein, D., McVicar, D.W., Moffet,t A., & Carrington M. (2009). HLA-C cell surface expression and control of HIV/AIDS correlate with a variant upstream of HLA-C. *Nat Genet*, Vol.41, No.12, (December 2009), pp.1290-4

Ugolotti, E., Vanni, I., Raso, A., Benzi, F., Malnati, M., & Biassoni, R. (2011). Human leukocyte antigen-B (-Bw6/-Bw4 I(80), T(80)) and human leukocyte antigen-C (-C1/-C2) subgrouping using pyrosequence analysis. *Hum Immunol*, Vol.72, No.10, (October 2011), pp. 859-868

Uhrberg, M., Valiante, N.M., Shum, B.P., Shilling, H.G., Lienert-Weidenbach, K., Corliss, B., Tyan, D., Lanier, L.L., & Parham, P.(1997). Human diversity in killer cell inhibitory receptor genes. *Immunity*, Vol.7, No.6, (December 1997), pp. 753-63

van der Meer, A., Schaap, N.P., Schattenberg, A.V., van Cranenbroek, B., Tijssen, H.J., & Joosten, I. (2008). KIR2DS5 is associated with leukemia free survival after HLA identical stem cell transplantation in chronic myeloid leukemia patients. *Mol Immunol*, Vol.45, No. 13, (August 2008), pp. 3631-8

Velardi, A. (2008). Role of KIRs and KIR ligands in hematopoietic transplantation. *Curr Opin Immunol*. Vol.20, No: 5, (October 2008), pp.581-7

Vilches, C., & Parham, P.(2002). KIR: Diverse, rapidly evolving receptors of innate and adaptive immunity. *Annu. Rev. Immunol*, Vol.20, No.1, (April 2002), pp. 217-251

Wagtmann, N., Biassoni R., Cantoni, C., Verdiani, S., Malnati, M.S., Vitale, M., Bottino, C., Moretta, L., Moretta, A., & Long, E.O. (1995). Molecular clones of the p58 NK cell receptor reveal immunoglobulin-related molecules with diversity in both the extra- and intracellular domains. *Immunity, Vol.* 2, No.5, (May 1995), pp. 439-449

Wang, S., Zhao, Y.R., Jiao, YL., Wang, L.C., Li, J.F., Cui, B., Xu, C.Y., Shi, Y.H., & Chen, Z.J. (2007). Increased activating killer immunoglobulin-like receptor genes and decreased specific HLA-C alleles in couples with recurrent spontaneous abortion. *Biochem Biophys Res Commun*, Vol.360, No.3, (Aug ust 2007), pp. 696-701

Williams, F., Meenagh, A., Sleator, C., Cook, D., Fernandez-Vina, M., Bowcock, A.M., & Middleton, D. (2005). Activating killer cell immunoglobulin-like receptor gene KIR2DS1 is associated with psoriatic arthritis. *Hum Immunol*, Vol.66, No.7, (July 2005), pp. 836-41

Winter, C.C., & Long, E.O. (1997). A single amino acid in the p58 killer cell inhibitory receptor controls the ability of natural killer cells to discriminate between the two groups of HLA-C allotypes. *J Immunol,* Vol. 158, No. 9, (May 1997), pp. 4026–4028

Winter, C.C., Gumperz, J.E., Parham, P., Long, E.O., & Wagtmann, N.(1998). Direct binding and functional transfer of NK cell inhibitory receptors reveal novel patterns of HLA-C allotype recognition. *J Immunol*, Vol.161, No.2, (July 1998), pp. 571–577

Yan, W.H., Lin, A., Chen, B.G., Zhou, MY., Dai, M.Z., Chen, X.J., Gan, L.H., Zhu, M., Shi, W.W., Li, B.(2007)Possible roles of KIR2DL4 expression on uNK cells in human pregnancy.*Am J Reprod Immunol*, Vol.57, No.4, (April 2007), pp.233-42

Zaia, J.A., Sun, J.Y., Gallez-Hawkins, G.M., Thao, L., Oki, A., Lacey, S.F., Dagis, A., Palmer, J., Diamone, D.J., Forman, S.J., & Senitzer, D. (2010). The effect of single and combined activating KIR genotypes on CMV infection and immunity after hematopoietic cell transplantation. *Biol Blood Marrow Transplant*, Vol.15, No.3, (March 2010), pp. 315-25

Zhang, H., Liu, S., Liu, Z., & Li J. (2008). "Expression of iKIR-HLACw in patients with inflammatory bowel disease". *Life Science Journal*, Vol.5, No4, (September 2008), pp. 17–22

Zhi-ming, L., Yu-lian, J., Zhao-lei, F., Chun-xiao, W., Zhen-fang, D., Bing-chang, Z., & Yue-ran, Z. (2007). Polymorphisms of killer cell immunoglobulin-like receptor gene: possible association with susceptibility to or clearance of hepatitis B virus infection in Chinese Han population. *Croat Med J, Vol.*48, No.6, (December 2007), pp.800-6

7

Sequence Analysis of MHC Class II Genes in Cetaceans

Wei-Cheng Yang[1], Lien-Siang Chou[2] and Jer-Ming Hu[2]
[1]*Department of Veterinary Medicine, National Chiayi University*
[2]*Institute of Ecology and Evolutionary Biology, National Taiwan University*
Taiwan

1. Introduction

Genes of the major histocompatibility complex (MHC) offer several assets that make them unique candidates for studies of adaptation in natural populations (Potts & Wakeland, 1990; Hedrick, 1994). The primary role of the MHC is to recognize foreign proteins, present them to specialist immune cells and initiate an immune response (Klein & Figueroa, 1986). The MHC gene family includes highly polymorphic genes encoding a set of transmembrane glycoproteins that are critical to the generation of immune responses (Kennedy et al., 2002). In general, foreign proteins enter cells either by infection or by phagocytosis into antigen-presenting cells such as macrophages. These foreign proteins are broken down into small peptides and loaded onto specific MHC molecules. The MHC molecule comprises an immunoglobulin stalk, which anchors the molecule to the cell surface, and a basket receptor called antigen-recognizing sites (ARS) located in peptide binding region (PBR). A subset of these protein/MHC complexes are then transported to the cell surface and presented for interrogation by the circulating T-cell population. A complex cascade of immune responses is triggered when the T cell binds to the presented peptide. Two major groups of MHC genes can be distinguished. MHC class I genes play an essential role in the immune defense against intracellular pathogens by binding peptides mainly derived from viral proteins and cancer-infected cells. They are expressed on the surface of all nucleated somatic cells. In contrast, MHC class II genes are predominantly involved in monitoring the extracellular environment by presenting peptides mainly derived from parasites (e.g. bacteria, nematodes, cestodes) to the T-cells. They are primarily expressed on antigen-presenting cells of the immune system, such as B cells and macrophages. Although ARS do show a degree of specificity, a single MHC molecule can bind multiple peptides that have common amino acids at particular anchor positions (Altuvia & Margalit, 2004). Genes within the MHC involved in antigen presentation constitute the most polymorphic loci known in vertebrates (Hedrick, 1994). The polymorphism of the MHC-molecules is associated with the diversity of the T-lymphocyte receptors that in turn determine the disease and parasite resistance of an organism and thus may affect the long-term survival rate of populations (Hedrick et al., 1999; Paterson et al., 1998). The ARS show high levels of polymorphism not only in the number of alleles but also in the sequence variation among alleles (Hughes & Yeager, 1998). The general view is that balancing selection is the determinant role in shaping patterns of nucleotide diversity in MHC genes (Bernatchez & Landry, 2003; Hughes & Nei, 1989).

Balancing selection refers to forms of natural selection in which no single allele is absolutely most fit (Hughes & Yeager, 1998, Meyer & Thomson, 2001). It is in contrast to directional selection that favors a few alleles. Balancing selection results not only in the maintenance of large numbers of alleles in populations, but also in greatly enhanced persistence of allelic diversity over extremely long time periods relative to neutral genetic variation (Paterson, 1998). It results in an observation termed 'trans-species evolution of polymorphism (Klein & Figueroa, 1986), which some alleles from a species are more similar to the alleles of different species than each other, rather than the species-specific pattern.

Genetic and antigenic diversity of the MHC could be important in a host's ability to accommodate rapidly evolving infectious agents that periodically afflict natural populations (Klein & Sato, 1998). Exactly how much MHC diversity is required to ensure long-term population viability remains a fundamental question in conservation genetics. A lack of variation at the MHC may increase the susceptibility of an isolated population to infectious disease epidemics, with potentially catastrophic consequences (Bowen et al., 2002). For example, a link between MHC diversity and an effective response to both pathogenic and toxicogenic challenges was proposed (Acevedo-Whitehouse et al., 2003). Therefore, understanding the polymorphism of these genes, and their products, is vital for studying infectious disease ecology at the population level. This is particularly important in marine species whose chemical and microbial environment is increasingly influenced by anthropogenic encroachment, which increases marine species' risk of exposure to novel pathogens (Harvell et al., 1999). However, not all MHC genes show high diversity. The most diverse and extensively studied MHC genes are the *DQB* and *DRB* genes. Diversity of *DQB* or *DRB* genes has been characterized in many mammalian species such as primates (Bontrop et al., 1999), bank vole (Axtner & Sommer, 2004), domestic mammals (Schook & Lamont, 1996, Yuhki & O'Brien, 1997, Mikko et al., 1999, Wagner et al., 1999), and marine mammals (Murray et al., 1999, Bowen et al., 2002, 2004, Baker et al., 2006, Hayashi et al., 2006, Yang et al., 2007, Xu et al., 2007). After these studies on non-model free-ranging species were carried out, intriguing questions were raised about whether and how selection operates on the MHC of natural populations characterized by distinct pathogens and demographic and environmental conditions (Bernatchez & Landry, 2003; Sommer, 2005).

It was suggested that the pathogen environment of marine mammals may provide a diminished selective pressure for maintaining MHC polymorphism (Murray et al., 1995; Murray & White, 1998; Slade, 1992), due to the relatively low prevalence of infectious disease in the marine environment. For example, Murray et al. (1995) found that the genetic variability at the MHC *DQB* loci of the beluga (*Delphinapterus leucas*) was much lower than those of primates. There are several other hypotheses that have been put forward to explain the reduction of MHC diversity in marine mammals, such as population bottlenecks and random drift acting in small populations (Murray & White, 1998; Slade, 1992). In order to discriminate among the hypotheses, it would be most informative to assess MHC variation in delphinids with large populations and no evidence of historic population bottlenecks.

Seventy to fifty five million year ago (Mya), in the warm shallow waters of the Tethy Sea, mammals related to ungulates are thought have begun one of the most successful recolonizations of the marine environment (Arnason & Gullberg, 1996; Bajpai & Gingerich, 1998; Thewissen & Williams, 2002). It is possible that earliest cetaceans were faced with a new range of pathogens associated with the marine environment. The study of the evolution of the MHC in cetaceans presents an exciting opportunity to observe the response of the MHC to the new pressures of the marine environment. We reviewed the relationship between alleles in different cetacean species to evaluate whether certain allele sequences were shared by different cetaceans inhabiting similar or different environments. In addition, phylogenetic analyses revealed that the sequence divergence in several species might reflect different selective pressures between pathogens in oceanic and coastal waters. The information gained from sequence analysis is the essential foundation to analyze variation of MHC genes and study infectious disease ecology.

2. Sequence variation of MHC class II genes in cetaceans

The studies of MHC variation in cetaceans were directed at investigating variation of *DQB* gene exon 2 locus, which has been shown to be highly polymorphic in many terrestrial carnivores and domestic animals (Schook & Lamont, 1996; Wagner et al., 1999; Yuhki & O'Brien, 1997). MHC class II gene investigation in cetacean species presumed that immunogenetic diversity is generated by polymorphism at one or two specific loci (Murray et al., 1999), a reasonable assumption based on established knowledge in terrestrial species (Mikko et al., 1999; Wagner et al., 1999). In most studies, the sequence analysis of amplified 172 bp fragments showed that there are no more than two alleles revealed in each individuals. One single *DQB* locus has been reported in other toothed whales (Hayashi et al., 2003; Hayashi et al., 2006; Murray et al., 1995). However, duplicate *DQB* genes were described in the baleen whales (Baker et al., 2006), baiji (*Lipotes vexillifer*) (Yang et al., 2005), and finless porpoise (*Neophocaena phocaenoides*) (Xu et al., 2007, 2009). It was proposed that bearing multiple *DQB* genes is consistent with the retention of an ancestral condition shared with the ruminants, and it has been lost in the more derived cetaceans such as the true dolphins (Baker et al., 2006). However, this suggestion is not supported by the finless porpoise, which is also supposed to be a derived species.

MHC variation has been examined in some species of cetaceans and revealed different results. Earlier studies demonstrated low level of MHC genetic diversity in fin whales (*Balaenoptera physalus*) and sei whales (*Balaenoptera borealis*) (Trowsdale et al., 1989). However, Nigenda-Morales et al. (2007) reported the PBR of the *DQB* locus in fin whales from Gulf of California has experienced strong positive selection. Sequence analysis of beluga whales MHC-II loci (including *DQB* and *DRB*) revealed low but measurable polymorphism (Murray et al., 1995; Murray & White, 1998). Recent sequencing analysis of cetacean populations revealed considerable sequence variation in some species of the baleen whales and toothed whales (Baker et al., 2006; Hayashi et al., 2003; Xu et al., 2007, 2008, 2009; Vassilakos et al., 2009; Yang et al., 2005; Yang et al., 2007, 2008, 2010; Heimeier et al., 2009). These studies also found evidence of positive selection, as showed by high levels of nonsynonymous substitutions at ARS. For example, the amount of variation of *DQB* in common bottlenose dolphins (*Tursiops truncatus*) (Yang et al., 2008) is significantly higher (6 alleles and 21 nucleotide substitutions in 172 bp found in 42 dolphins) than that in beluga (only 5 alleles and 11 nucleotide substitutions in 172 bp found in 233 beluga) (Murray et al., 1995). Xu et al. (2007) reported that finless porpoises seem to retain considerable MHC genetic variation (14 *DQB* alleles in 195 porpoises) despite population decline in recent years. Moreover, the finding in humpback whales (23 *DQB* alleles from 30 individuals) (Baker et al., 2006) provided a counter example to the expectations of a slow mutation rate for animals with large body size and long generation time. These findings not only suggest a positive selection pressure on the cetacean *DQB* locus but also argue against a reduction in the marine environment selection pressure. Similar arguments were made in the studies on beluga *DRB*1 locus (Murray & White, 1998), North Atlantic right whale (*Eubalaena glacialis*) *DQB* locus (Murray, 1997), Baiji *DQB* locus (Yang et al., 2005), and finless porpoise *DQB* locus (Hayashi et al., 2006). Besides, no deviation from Hardy-Weinberg expectations (i.e. no excess of heterozygotes) was observed in beluga and common bottlenose dolphins, suggesting that the effect of balancing selection for short time periods might be weak and masked by other microevolutionary forces (e.g. gene flow, mutation, drift, and non-random mating). Similar conclusions were reached by Boyce et al. (1997) from bighorn sheep (*Ovis canadensis*), Huang and Yu (2003) from the Southeast Asian house mouse (*Mus musculus castaneus*) in Taiwan, and Miller et al. (2004) from New Zealand robins (*Petroica australis*). Nonetheless, there are other possible explanations, such as spatiotemporal variation of selection and demographic processes acting on small populations (reviewed by Piertney & Oliver, 2006). Hayashi et al. (2006) also found evidence for both balancing selection overall, and genetic drift in small, local populations for the *DQB* locus in the finless porpoise.

The sequence information raises important questions regarding immunologic diversity in cetaceans. While those studies present valuable information, variation at 1 part of a gene, or 1 gene, is not an appropriate measure of variation for the entire MHC (Murray & White, 1998). It is possible that low diversity at the MHC has been observed only because short fragments (usually less than 200 bp) were amplified and the functionality of the alleles was not taken into account (e.g., Sommer, 2003, Amills et al., 2004), which might lead to a misinterpretation of the results (Axtner & Sommer, 2007), with the possible consequence that a severe population bottleneck is inferred (Baker et al., 2006). Besides, the MHC variation in one locus cannot definitely represent the ability of pathogen defense of a species because MHC polymorphism in marine mammals arises from several loci. For example, a moderate to high degree of polymorphism is only found in *DRB* genes, not in *DQB* gene, in beluga and California sea lion (*Zalophus californianus*) (Bowen et al., 2004; Murray and White, 1998), and the situation reverses in humpback whale (*Megaptera novaeangliae*) (Baker et al., 2006). Therefore, characterization of full-length expressed sequences of MHC genes is very important for making valid evolutionary inferences on non-model species like cetaceans. To date, there is only one published article characterizing the full-length *DQB* and *DRB* gene sequences in cetaceans (Yang et al., 2007), which were from the RACE cDNA products of *T. truncatus* and *T. aduncus*. The nucleotide and deduced amino acid sequences of the 780- (*DQB*-primer derived) and 801-bp (*DRB*-primer derived) products were typical of transcripts from mammalian class II genes. The result revealed the presence of 1 *DQB* locus and 2 *DRB* loci in *Tursiops*. The high proportions of non-synonymous nucleotide substitutions in the putative peptide-binding regions of *Tutr-DQB*, *Tuad-DRB*, and *Tutr-DRB* suggest positive selection pressure on these gene loci (Hughes & Yeager, 1998) and imply functional roles for these molecules in pathogen-specific immune responses. In *DRB* of *T. aduncus*, for example, the majority of 44 variable sites were in exon 2 (38/44), with the remainder being distributed in exons 1 (1/44), 3 (4/44), and 4 (1/44). The deduced amino acid sequences indicated that the substitutions clearly tended to be clustered around the ARS. The divergence of non-synonymous substitutions was significant at the codons of the ARS ($p < 0.005$). The polymorphic *Tuad*-DRβ amino acid residues ($n = 25$) were located in the leader peptide (1/25), the $\beta 1$ domain (21/25), the $\beta 2$ domain (2/25), and the transmembrane domain (1/25).

The correlations between MHC alleles and disease resistance (e.g. malaria, hepatitis B, leprosy, tuberculosis) and disease-susceptibility (cancer, parasite infestation) have been reported (reviewed by Sommer, 2005). Human pathologies have also been correlated to specific amino acid replacement and motif changes in ARS among different populations (reviewed by Vassilakos et al., 2009). There are striking differences in the prevalences of some disease-resistance alleles in different human population. MHC associations also show some geographic variation. It seems likely that the same evolutionary selection pressures that have given rise to polymorphisms in genes involved in resisting infectious pathogens have contributed to marked allele frequency differences at the same loci. Gene-environment interactions are likely to introduce another layer of complexity. In marine mammals, for example, MHC genotypes of California sea lions were associated with urogenital cancer (Bowen et al., 2005). One of the *DQB* allele in *T. truncatus* was found being assocaited with strandings although only marginally significant (Yang et al., 2008). In addition, only five individuals carried this allele were fresh enough for pathological examination in that study so that the subsequent statistical analysis of lesions could not be done. Therefore, further studies are needed to identify genes of major to moderate effect in a single population with large sample size and then determine whether a similar effect is found elsewhere, and we may elucidate the potential mechanisms underlying the association between MHC alleles and cetacean strandings.

3. Phylogenetic analyses of MHC class II genes in cetaceans

Recent molecular and morphological studies have suggested that the order Cetacea may be more closely related to even-toed ungulates than to other orders of ungulates (Arnason et al., 2000; Boisserie et al., 2005; Kumar & Hedges, 1998; Murphy et al., 2001). In addition, cetaceans and hippopotamuses (*Hippopotamus amphibius*) form a monophyletic group deeply nested within Cetartiodactyla while camels and pigs are basal to this order (Boisserie et al., 2005; Gatesy 1997; Gatesy et al., 1996; Nikaido et al., 1999). The molecular clock estimate for the divergence of the artiodactyls and cetaceans is about 60 Mya (Arnason and Gullberg 1996). It is believed that early cetaceans initially lived in freshwater habitats as terrestrial quadrupeds and were partly dependent on freshwater at some stages of their life before they gradually adapted to the marine environment and became fully aquatic marine mammals in the end (Thewissen & Williams, 2002). The adaptation of immune response in cetaceans is supposed to be critical to cetaceans in their move from land to water, which is an enormous shift in habitat environment. Since major qualitative differences in microorganisms and infectious diseases are believed to exist between marine and terrestrial environments (McCallum et al., 2004), the immune genes of primitive cetaceans are supposed to be adapted for defending against distinct pathogens in aquatic environment. Several empirical studies showed that heterogeneity in selection pressure directly correlates with MHC gene diversity (Bernatchez & Landry, 2003; Charbonnel & Pemberton, 2005; Wegner et al., 2003).

Both class I and class II MHC gene families have been shown to evolve according to the birth-and-death process (Nei et al., 1997). The MHC class II loci of mammals have homologous relationships and slower rate of birth-and-death evolution than that of class I loci (Takahashi et al., 2000). Takahashi et al. (2000) used long nucleotide sequences (573 bp) including PBR and other regions from vertebrate MHC class II α and β-chain loci to study the time of origin and evolutionary relationships of these loci. Their result showed the definite grouping of sequences from different genes. However, only three species from Cetartiodactyla (pig, cattle, and sheep) were studied while the evolutionary relationships of MHC genes among Cetartiodactyla remain unresolved. We may know how and when the habitat shift, accompanied by the change of foreign antigens, affected the history of co-evolution between MHC genes and pathogens when cetaceans moved from land to water by interpreting the phylogenetic relationship and divergence time estimates of MHC class II genes in cetaceans and their close-related terrestrial species. Yang et al. (2010) constructed phylogenetic trees and estimate the divergence times of clades using cDNA sequences (616 bp) of *DQB* and *DRB* genes that encode the extracellular domain (including PBR), connecting peptide, transmembrane, and part of the cytoplasmic tail from cetaceans (bottlenose dolphins; *T. truncatus* and *T. aduncus*), hippo and other ungulates, together with other MHC class II β-chain genes from fish, frog, chicken, and other mammals. It showed that the phylogenetic relationships in the respective cetartiodactyl group in *DQB* and *DRB* clades in this study do not correspond to that in the previously accepted species tree. It is striking to observe that cetaceans (bottlenose dolphins) and artiodactyls (pig, hippo, and ruminants) form two distinct clades in both *DQB* and *DRB* phylogenies, rather than being of the same clade with hippo and dolphin as the closest relatives. The authors presumed that the sequences of cetaceans and artiodactyls are paralogous in *DQB* and *DRB* genes, respectively. Paralogous genes separated by gene duplication events, which has been proposed to be a major force in MHC evolution, while the orthologous genes separated by speciation events. (Klein et al., 1998). The gene duplication has been observed in the genetic organization of MHC genes in many mammals. In bovine MHC class II genes, for example, two *DQB* genes and nine *DRB* genes were detected, with eight of the *DRB* genes being likely pseudogenes (Ellis & Ballingall, 1999). Since natural selective pressures of infectious diseases between terrestrial and aquatic (especially marine) environments are different (McCallum et al., 2004), the pathogen-driven evolution (Meyer & Thomson, 2001) was supposed to be very likely the driving force of birth-and-death process in the MHC genes for the cetaceans and their terrestrial relatives leading to the paralogy (Yang et al., 2010). Besides, if the MHC genes of cetaceans did evolve in a different direction from their terrestrial relatives, it is important to know when cetaceans entered into the water and how their MHC genes evolved. For estimating the divergence time of MHC genes of cetartiodactyls, Bayesian inference (BI) tree with birth-death clock model provided better estimates of divergence time of MHC genes than neighbor-joining (NJ) tree using Kimura 2-parameter model with linearized tree method (Yang et al., 2010). The result suggested that cetaceans (*T. truncatus* and *T. aduncus*) diverged from artiodactyls (pig, hippo, and ruminants) about 60 Mya or slightly earlier, which is comparable with the first appearances of fossil cetaceans around 53.5 Mya, artiodactyls at 55 Mya, and other molecular estimate of divergence time of cetacean/artiodactyl at 60 Mya (Arnason & Gullberg, 1996; Arnason et al., 2000, 2004; Theodor, 2004). However, only two close-related species of true dolphins were included in this study, and therefore the full-length sequences from other early divergence of cetaceans (such as baleen whales and river dolphins) are needed for confirming the hypothesis. Furthermore, several other mammal groups have also made the evolutionary transition from land to sea, such as pinnipeds, sea otters, polar bears and sirenians. Studying MHC genes of these marine mammals and their terrestrial relatives will provide us further insight into the evolution of MHC genes.

Some MHC alleles from a species are more similar to the alleles of different species than each other, rather than the species-specific pattern. This scenario has been referred to as trans-species evolution (Klein, 1987), which is one of the characteristics of the MHC genes and has been identified in a wide range of taxa including primates, salmonids, ungulates, pinnipeds, rodents, geckos, and warblers (reviewed by Piertney & Oliver, 2006). In cetaceans, most of the phylogenetic analyses of PBR sequences of *DQB* and *DRB* loci also show trans-specific pattern (Baker et al., 2006; Hayashi et al., 2003; Xu et al., 2009; Yang et al., 2008; Heimeier et al., 2009). Involving in 28 species of cetaceans, Xu et al. (2009) shows no or weak support for clades of same family or species in the phylogenetic relationship among *DQB* alleles. For example, no monophyletic groups for two cetacean suborders (Mysticeti and Odontoceti) were found. In addition, some alleles were more closely related with those from other species even from other families rather than with intraspecific alleles. It raised question about whether such pattern of apparent transspecific sharing of alleles is due to common lineages or convergence of independent lineages (Yeager & Hughes, 1999). Coalescent and neutral theories predict that two species will share a proportion of alleles at any given locus immediately following divergence from their ancestral form. Over time, from a phylogenetic perspective one should see a gradual progression from polyphyly, through paraphyly, to monophyly. However, balancing selection, which acts on MHC genes, retains alleles among species for considerably longer periods of time and increases the time over which there is incomplete lineage sorting and delaying the time to monophyly (Piertney and Oliver, 2006). If the trans-species evolutionary pattern in cetaceans described in previous studies is due to common lineage, the sharing of similar alleles by a common ancestry between cetacean families would require their preservation for a considerably long time, such as Delphinidae (dolphins) / Monodontidae (beluga) separating at least 15 Mya (Arnason et al., 2004), or Delphinidae/Lipotidae (baiji) 25 Mya (Nikaido et al., 2001). The result in Yang et al. (2010) supported this assumption. The authors estimated the divergence time of two close-related dolphin species (*Tursiops truncatus* and *T. aduncus*) in *DQB* and *DRB* genes (>20 Mya) is much earlier than the separation date of these two species. The earliest fossils identifiable as *Tursiops* dated to only 4-7 Mya (Barnes 1990), as well as the emergence of oldest delphinid which is possible 11 Mya of latest Miocene (Barnes 1977). The authors postulated these allelic lineages of *Tursiops* MHC genes may emerge by gene duplication during the period of early radiation of small toothed whales (from late Oligocene to early Miocene, 22 Mya (Arnason et al., 2004). Since MHC alleles could be persisted over extremely long time period by balancing selection (Bernatchez and Landry 2003), these lineages were maintained for a long evolutionary period through speciation events of cetaceans and cause the observed scenario of trans-species evolutionary pattern.

Apart from trans-species evolution, several studies on phylogenetic analyses of PBR sequences of *DQB* and *DRB* loci showed other interesting evolutaionay patterns. The first is the homoplasy of PBR in *DQB* and *DRB* genes (Baker et al., 2006; Yang et al., 2010). The *DQB* and *DRB* genes are thought to have arisen early in the placental mammals and evolved independently such that sequences of each gene can be recognized as orthologous across lineages (e.g., Ellis 1999; Groenen et al., 1990). Thus, sequences from either gene of different mammals should group together with their orthologs in phylogenetic reconstruction, exclusive of sequences from paralogous loci. Although this pattern was observed when the longer or full length of the fragment was used (Baker et al., 2006; Yang et al., 2010), it was not the case when only PBR sequences (~170 bp) were for comparison: the *DQB* and *DRB* sequences of *Tursiops* are sistergroups within the clade containing all other *DRB* sequences of mammals (Yang et al., 2010), and cetacean *DQB* sequences grouped with some cetacean *DRB* sequences and appeared most closely related to the primate and ungulate *DQB* (Baker et al., 2006). A similar pattern of *DQB/DRB* convergence is reported in the canids (Seddon & Ellegren, 2002). The best explanation is convergent evolution (Yeager & Hughes, 1999), and small-scale conversion of the *DRB* by *DQB* alleles seems most consistent with the available evidence and is the most potentially responsible for convergence (Baker et al., 2006).

Second, Xu et al. (2008) reported that the *DQB* exon 2 of the baiji revealed striking similarity with those of the finless porpoise. Especially, some identical alleles were shared by both species at the DQB locus. The scenario of total identity amongst MHC alleles from different species have been reported, but most of which are restricted to congeneric species and rarely from above genus level (reviewed by Xu et al., 2008). The two species are highly divergent with each other, with the baiji included in Lipotidae of the superfamily Lipotoidea and the finless porpoise in Phocoenidae of the superfamily Delphinoidea, respectively. It is difficult to explain the identity and high similarity between distantly related species using trans-species evolution. Unlike trans-species evolution, the identity and similarity that are shared in the case of convergent evolution are not the result of evolution from a common ancestor, but typically explained as the result of common adaptive solutions to similarly environmental pressures. It is known that baiji and finless porpoise are sympatric in the Yangtze River and facing similar selection pressure from the similar freshwater environment, shaping the same motifs or alleles in both species in order to adapt to the similar pressures (Xu et al., 2008). Further studies are needed to clarify the convergent evolution with more MHC loci or other molecular data.

The third is adaptive differentiation. Yang et al. (2007) reported that the phylogenetic analyses of the full-length region and exon 2 of *DQB* and *DRB* showed no mixture but a clear division between *T. truncatus* (from Taiwan and Japan) and *T. aduncus* (from Taiwan and Indonesia). This is an intriguing result compared to the general trans-specific pattern of evolution observed for cetacean MHC loci. The species-specific clustering of *DQB* or *DRB* loci has been described in a few species (South African antelope by van der Walt et al. 2001, cotton rats by Pfau et al. 1999). Compared with *T. truncatus* which generally appears in deep, offshore waters, *T. aduncus* inhabits shallow, tropical, coastal waters and its body size is smaller than *T. truncatus* (Zhou & Qian, 1985). Because shallow waters along the coast are influenced by terrestrial runoff, the diversity and abundance of pathogens in the coastal waters likely differ from those in oceanic areas (Hayashi et al., 2006). Moreover, Wang et al. (1994) showed the parasites, Phyllobothrium, Monorhygma, and Crassicauda, are found only in the offshore form of *T. truncatus*, whereas Braunina is found in the coastal population in the western North Atlantic. Since *T. truncatus* and *T. aduncus* have different diets, microflora, and distributions (Wang et al., 1999, Wang 2003), thus it is reasonable to assume that different selective pressures from pathogens exist in oceanic (*T. truncatus*) and coastal (*T. aduncus*) waters. The most likely explanation is that species-specific alleles may have adaptive value for certain species and can be discriminately selected. When the selective advantage of MHC alleles differs among environments that vary in the diversity and abundance of pathogens, pathogen-driven directional selection could act differentially among individuals from distinct populations (Bernatchez and Landry 2003). This would have resulted in sequence divergence of exon 2 in bottlenose dolphins as observed in the study (Yang et al., 2007). The findings in Vassilakos et al. (2009) provided further support of this hypothesis. They showed coastal and offshore samples of *Tursiops* from various sources exhibited significantly different profiles of PBR (Coastal: Western North Atlantic coastal *T. truncatus* and *T. aduncus* off South Africa; offshore: *T. truncatus* from the Mediterranean Sea, Eastern North Atlantic, Western North Atlantic pelagic, and the eastern North Pacific off southern California). Similar functional analysis has been used in human studies (reviewed by Vassilakos et al., 2009). We do not know how similar the pathogen environments are for coastal *T. truncatus* and *T. aduncus*. Although the possible pathogen-specific interactions are not known, it suggested the directional selection in local, differentiated populations because the pattern of differences and similarities is consistent with this interpretation (Vassilakos et al., 2009). Since extant cetacean fauna consists of more than 80 species and live in varied habitats, such as ocean, estuary, polar regions, and river, it is interesting to elucidate the evolution of cetacean MHC genes by obtaining more sequences and loci from a variety of cetacean species.

4. Conclusion

Over the past two decades cetacean MHC immunogenetics has developed from a genetic diversity study to a diverse field exploiting new methodologies to identify the evidence of pathogen-host coevolution. The previous studeis set out to achieve two major goals: (1) to assess levels of MHC variation in cetaceans to elucidate the role of selection in the evolution of cetacean MHC loci; (2) to characterize PBR and full-length MHC class II *DQB* and *DRB* genes in cetaceans and shed light on the evolution of cetacean MHC genes by performing the phylogenetic analyses. Although the information provides aspects for discussing the relationship between emergence of cetaceans and evolutionary pattern of MHC genes, the key questions remain the same. What MHC polymorphisms affect differential susceptibility to infectious diseases in cetaceans? What extent has selection by particular pathogens or enviroment given rise to observed polymorphism in MHC genes? Can the identification of certain allele related to specific environment or population identify loci that are targets for conservation interventions? For these highly mobile marine species, the expectation would be for random-mating across broad geographic ranges, but various studies have shown restricted gene flow over a range of hundreds or even tens of kilometers (Natoli et al. 2005). We could expect, and cannot excluded, the differentiation by drift at MHC loci. However, the stronger indications from previous studies reflect both the long-term unifying effects of balancing selection, and local, differentiated populations that suggest directional selection.

As emerging infectious diseases in the marine environment are becoming more widely recognized (Harvell et al., 1999), investigations into the genetics of host susceptibility are becoming increasingly important. It appears that most new diseases are not caused by new microorganisms, but rather by known agents infecting new or previously unrecognized hosts. Disease outbreaks are favored by the undermining of host resistance (Harvell et al., 1999), by a shift in balance in the microevolution between pathogens and host, or by the introduction of a novel pathogen into an immunogenetically naive host (Paterson 1998). The rise of catastrophic disease epidemics in marine organisms brings into question the balance between pathogen virulence and host resistance in these systems (Harvell et al., 1999). In fact, recent study in marine mammals proposes a link between MHC polymorphism and an effective response to both pathogentic and toxicogenic challenge (Acevedo-Whitehouse et al., 2003). While marine environment is increasingly influenced by anthropogenic encroachment, the risk of exposure to novel pathogens of marine species is increased (Harvell et al., 1999), especially for coastal species such as *T. aduncus.* Yang et al. (2010) clearly show that MHC gene sequences of *T. aduncus* and *T. truncatus* diverged at least 20 Mya that may enable them to bear different assignment for pathogen defense, indicating that *T. aduncus* might be able to survive under the pathogen pressure in coastal waters. The species' near-shore distribution makes it vulnerable to environmental degradation, direct exploitation, and fishery conflicts (Hammond et al., 2008). Still of concern is the potential transmission of novel pathogens into populations of *T. aduncus* not equipped with the specific immunogenetic repertoire necessary for an effective immune response. Dolphin health and population status reflect the effects of natural and anthropogenic stressors on the species (Wells et al., 2004). Monitoring the health of *T. aduncus* could serve as not only sentinels of the health and status of lower trophic levels in the marine system, but also indicators and warning of impacts on human as more humans inhabit coastal regions. Furthermore, previous studies indicate that cetacean MHC genes have been adapted to different marine environments. Their ability to defend against terrestrial pathogens needs investigation and close monitor, especially in these times there are potential risks of epidemics for cetaceans when they have more occasions for encountering terrestrial pathogens through human exploitation of marine environments or, directly, keeping cetaceans in captivity.

5. Acknowledgment

We are grateful to Dr. Terry Harville for inviting us to publish this review, as well as to two anonymous reviewers for their constructive comments. The authors' research is supported by the grant from the Council of Agriculture of Taiwan to L. S. Chou (94AS-9.1.7-FB-e1(8); 95AS-11.1.3-FB-e1(10)).

6. References

Acevedo-Whitehouse, K.; Gulland, F.; Greig, D. & Amos, W. (2003). Inbreeding: Disease susceptibility in California sea lions. *Nature,* Vol.422, (March 2003), pp. 35, ISSN 0028-0836

Altuvia, Y. & Margalit, H. (2004). A structure-based approach for prediction of MHC-binding peptides. *Methods,* Vol.34, No.4, (December 2004), pp. 454-9, ISSN 1046-2023

Amills, M.; Jimenez, N.; Jordana, J.; Riccardi, A.; Fernandez-Arias, A.; Guiral, J.; Bouzat, J. L.; Folch, J. & Sanchez, A. (2004). Low diversity in the major histocompatibility complex class II DRB1 gene of the Spanish ibex, *Capra pyrenaica. Heredity,* Vol.93, No.3, (September 2004), pp. 266-272, ISSN 0018-067X

Arnason, U. & Gullberg, A. (1996). Cytochrome b nucleotide sequences and the identification of five primary lineages of extant cetaceans. *Molecular Biology and Evolution,* Vol.13, No.2, (February 1996), pp. 407-417, ISSN 0737-4038

Arnason, U.; Gullberg, A.; Gretarsdottir, S.; Ursing, B. & Janke, A. (2000). The mitochondrial genome of the sperm whale and a new molecular reference for estimating eutherian divergence dates. *Journal of Molecular Evolution,* Vol.50, No.6, (June 2000). pp. 569-578, ISSN 0022-2844

Arnason, U.; Gullberg, A., & Janke, A. (2004). Mitogenomic analyses provide new insights into cetacean origin and evolution. *Gene,* Vol.333, (May 2004), pp.: 27-34, ISSN 0378-1119

Axtner, J. & Sommer, S. (2007). Gene duplication, allelic diversity, selection processes and adaptive value of MHC class II DRB genes of the bank vole, *Clethrionomys glareolus. Immunogenetics,* Vol.59, No.5, (May 2007), pp. 417-426, ISSN 0093-7711

Bajpai, S. & Gingerich, P. D. (1998). A new Eocene archaeocete (Mammalia, Cetacea) from India and the time of origin of whales. *PNAS,* Vol.*95, No.26, (December 1998), pp.* 15464-15468, ISSN 0027-8424

Baker, C. S.; Vant, M. D.; Dalebout, M. L.; Lento, G. M.; O'Brien S, J. & Yuhki, N. (2006). Diversity and duplication of DQB and DRB-like genes of the MHC in baleen whales (suborder: Mysticeti). *Immunogenetics,* Vol.58, No.4, (May 2006), pp. 283-296, ISSN 0093-7711

Barnes, L. (1977). Outline of eastern north Pacific cetacean assemblages. *Systematic Biology,* Vol.25, No.4, pp. 321-343, ISSN 1063-5157

Barnes, L. (1990). The fossil record and evolutionary relationships of the genus *Tursiops.* In: *The Bottlenose Dolphin,* S. Leatherwood & R. Reeves, (Ed.), 3-26, Academic Press, ISBN 0124402801, San Diego, USA

Bernatchez, L. & Landry, C. (2003). MHC studies in nonmodel vertebrates: what have I learned about natural selection in 15 years? *Journal of Evolutionary Biology,* Vol.16, No.3, (May 2003), pp. 363-377, ISSN 1010-061X

Boisserie, J. R.; Lihoreau, F. & Brunet, M. (2005). The position of Hippopotamidae within Cetartiodactyla. *PNAS,* Vol.102, No.5 (February 2005), pp. 1537-1541, ISSN 0027-8424

Bontrop, R. E.; Otting, N.; de Groot, N. G.; Doxiadis, G. G. (1999). Major histocompatibility complex class II polymorphisms in primates. *Immunological Reviews,* Vol.197, (February 1999), pp. 339-350, ISSN 0105-2869

Bowen, L.; Aldridge, B. M.; Delong, R.; Melin, S.; Buckles, E. L.; Gulland, F.; Lowenstine, L. J.; Stott, J. L. & Johnson, M. L. (2005). An immunogenetic basis for the high prevalence of urogenital cancer in a free-ranging population of California sea lions (*Zalophus californianus*). *Immunogenetics,* Vol.56, No.11, (February 2005), pp. 846-848, ISSN 0093-7711

Bowen, L.; Aldridge, B. M.; Gulland, F.; Van Bonn, W.; DeLong, R.; Melin, S.; Lowenstine, L. J.; Stott, J. L. & Johnson, M. L. (2004). Class II multiformity generated by variable MHC- DRB region configurations in the California sea lion (*Zalophus californianus*). *Immunogenetics,* Vol.56, No.1, (April 2004), pp. 12-27, ISSN 0093-7711

Bowen, L.; Aldridge, B. M.; Gulland, F.; Woo, J.; Van Bonn, W.; DeLong, R.; Stott, J. L. & Johnson, M. L. (2002). Molecular characterization of expressed DQA and DQB genes in the California sea lion (*Zalophus californianus*). *Immunogenetics,* Vol.54, No.5, (August 2002), pp. 332-347, ISSN 0093-7711

Boyce, W. M.; Hedrick, P. W.; Muggli-Cockett, N. E.; Kalinowski, S.; Penedo, M. C. & Ramey, R. R. (1997). Genetic variation of major histocompatibility complex and microsatellite loci: a comparison in bighorn sheep. *Genetics,* Vol.145, No.2, (February 1997), pp. 421-33, ISSN 0016-6731

Charbonnel, N. & Pemberton, J. (2005). A long-term genetic survey of an ungulate population reveals balancing selection acting on MHC through spatial and temporal fluctuations in selection. *Heredity*, Vol.95, No.5, (November 2005), pp. 377-388, ISSN 0022-1503

Ellis, S. A. & Ballingall, K. T. (1999). Cattle MHC: evolution in action? *Immunological Reviews,* Vol.167, (February 1999), pp. 159-168, ISSN 0105-2869

Gatesy, J. (1997). More DNA support for a Cetacea/Hippopotamidae clade: the blood-clotting protein gene gamma-fibrinogen. *Molecular Biology and Evolution,* Vol.14, No.5, (May 1997), pp. 537-543, ISSN 0737-4038

Gatesy, J.; Hayashi, C.; Cronin, M. A. & Arctander, P. (1996). Evidence from milk casein genes that cetaceans are close relatives of hippopotamid artiodactyls. *Molecular Biology and Evolution,* Vol.13, No.7, (September 1996), pp. 954-963, ISSN 0737-4038

Groenen, M. A.; van der Poel, J. J.; Dijkhof, R. J. & Giphart, M. J. (1990). The nucleotide sequence of bovine MHC class II DQB and DRB genes. *Immunogenetics,* Vol. 31, No.1, pp. 37-44, ISSN 0093-7711

Hammond, P. S.; Bearzi, G.; Bjørge, A.; Forney, K.; Karczmarski, L.; Kasuya, T.; Perrin, W. F.; Scott, M. D.; Wang, J. Y.; Wells, R. S. & Wilson, B. (2008). *Tursiops aduncus.* In: *IUCN 2011. IUCN Red List of Threatened Species. Version 2011.1.*

Harvell, C. D.; Kim, K.; Burkholder, J. M.; Colwell, R. R.; Epstein, P. R.; Grimes, D. J.; Hofmann, E. E.; Lipp, E. K.; Osterhaus, A. D.; Overstreet, R. M.; Porter, J. W.; Smith, G. W. & Vasta, G. R. (1999). Emerging marine diseases--climate links and anthropogenic factors. *Science,* Vol.285, No.5433, (September 1999), pp. 1505-1510, ISSN 0036-8075

Hayashi, K.; Nishida, S.; Yoshida, H.; Goto, M.; Pastene, L. & Koike, H. (2003). Sequence variation of the *DQB* allele in the cetacean MHC. *Mammal Study,* Vol.28, No.2, pp. 89-96, ISSN 1343-4152

Hayashi, K.; Yoshida, H.; Nishida, S.; Goto, M.; Pastene, L. A.; Kanda, N.; Baba, Y. & Koike, H. (2006). Genetic variation of the MHC DQB locus in the finless porpoise (*Neophocaena phocaenoides*). *Zoological Science,* Vol.23, No.2, (February 2006), pp.147-153, ISSN 0289-0003

Hedrick, P. W.; Parker, K. M.; Miller, E. L. & Miller, P. S. (1999). Major histocompatibility complex variation in the endangered Przewalski's horse. *Genetics,* Vol.152, (August 1999), pp. 1701-1710, ISSN 0016-6731

Hedrick, P. W. (1994). Evolutionary genetics of the major histo compatibility complex. *American Naturalist,* Vol.143, No.6, (June 1994), pp. 945-964, ISSN 0003-0147

Heimeier, D.; Baker, C. & Russell, K. (2009). Confirmed expression of MHC class I and class II genes in the New Zealand endemic Hector's dolphin (*Cephalorhynchus hectori*). *Marine Mammal Science,* Vol.25, No.1 (January 2009), pp. 68-90. ISSN 0824-0469

Huang, S. W. & Yu, H. T. (2003). Genetic variation of microsatellite loci in the major histocompatibility complex (MHC) region in the southeast Asian house mouse (*Mus musculus castaneus*). *Genetica,* Vol.119, No.2, (October 2003), pp. 201-18, ISSN 0016-6707

Hughes, A. & Yeager, M. (1998). Natural selection at major histocompatibility complex loci of vertebrates. *Annual Review of Genetics,* Vol.32, No. pp. 415-435, ISSN 0066-4197

Hughes, A. L. & Nei, M. (1989). Nucleotide substitution at major histocompatibility complex class II loci: evidence for overdominat selection. *PNAS,* Vol.86, No.3, (February 1989), pp. 948-962, ISSN 0027-8424

Kennedy, L. J., Ryvar, R., Gaskell, R. M., Addie, D. D., Willoughby, K., Carter, S. D., Thomson, W., Ollier, W. E. & Radford, A. D. (2002). Sequence analysis of MHC DRB alleles in domestic cats from the United Kingdom. *Immunogenetics,* Vol.54, No.5, (August 2002), pp. 348-52, ISSN 0093-7711

Klein, J. & Figueroa, F. (1986). Evolution of the major histocompatibility complex. *Critical Reviews in Immunololy,* Vol.6, No.4, pp. 295-386, ISSN 1040-8401

Klein, J. & Sato, A. (1998). Birth of the major histocompatibility complex. *Scandinavian Journal of Immunology,* Vol.47, No.3, (March 1998), pp. 199-209, ISSN 0030-9475

Klein, J. (1987). Origin of major histocompatibility complexes polymorphism: the trans-species hypothesis. *Human Immunology,* Vol.19, No.3, (July 1987), pp. 155-162, ISSN 0198-8859

Kumar, S. & Hedges, S. B. (1998). A molecular timescale for vertebrate evolution. *Nature,* Vol.392, (April 1998), pp. 917-920, ISSN 0022-1767

McCallum, H.; Kuris, A.; Harvell, C.; Lafferty, K.; Smith, G. & Porter, J. (2004). Does terrestrial epidemiology apply to marine systems? *Trends in Ecololgy & Evolution,* Vol.19, No. 11, (November 2004), pp. 585-591, ISSN 0169-5347

Meyer, D. & Thomson, G. (2001). How selection shapes variation of the human major histocompatibility complex: a review. *Annals of Human Genetics,* Vol.65, (April 2001), pp. 1-26, ISSN 0003-4800

Mikko, S.; Roed, K.; Schmutz, S. & Andersson, L. (1999). Monomorphism and polymorphism at Mhc DRB loci in domestic and wild ruminants. *Immunological Reviews,* Vol.167, (February 1999), 169-178, ISSN 0105-2869

Miller, H. C. & Lambert, D. M. (2004). Genetic drift outweighs balancing selection in shaping post-bottleneck major histocompatibility complex variation in New Zealand robins (Petroicidae). *Molecular Ecology,* Vol.13, No.12, (December 2004), pp. 3709-3721, ISSN 0962-1083

Murphy, W. J.; Eizirik, E.; Johnson, W. E.; Zhang, Y. P.; Ryder, O. A. & O'Brien, S. J. (2001). Molecular phylogenetics and the origins of placental mammals. *Nature,* Vol.409, (February 2001), pp. 614-618, ISSN 0022-1767

Murray, B. W. (1997). Major histocompatibility complex class II sequence variation in cetaceans: DQB and DRB variation in beluga (*Delphinapterus leucas*) and DQB variation in North Atlantic right whales (*Eubalaena glacialis*). *PhD thesis of McMaster University,* Hamilton, Ontario, Canada

Murray, B. W.; Malik, S. & White, B. N. (1995). Sequence variation at the major histocompatibility complex locus DQ beta in beluga whales (*Delphinapterus leucas*). *Molecular Biology and Evolution,* Vol.12, No.4, (July 1995), pp. 582-593, ISSN 0737-4038

Murray, B.; Michaud, R. & White, B. (1999). Allelic and haplotype variation of major histocompatibility complex class II DRB1 and DQB loci in the St Lawrence beluga (*Delphinapterus leucas*). *Molecular Ecology,* Vol.8, No.7, (July 1999), pp. 1127-1139, ISSN 0962-1083

Murray, B. W. & White, B. N. (1998). Sequence variation at the major histocompatibility complex DRB loci in beluga (*Delphinapterus leucas*) and narwhal (*Monodon monoceros*). *Immunogenetics,* Vol.48, No.4, (September 1998), pp. 242-252, ISSN 0093-7711

Natoli, A.; Birkun, A.; Aguilar, A.; Lopez, A. & Hoelzel, A. R. (2005). Habitat structure and the dispersal of male and female bottlenose dophins (*Tursiops truncatus*). *Proceedings Biological Sciences / The Royal Society*, Vol.272, No.1569, (June 2005), pp. 1217–1226, ISSN 0962-8452

Nei, M.; Gu, X. & Sitnikova, T. (1997). Evolution by the birth-and-death process in multigene families of the vertebrate immune system. *PNAS*, Vol.94, No.15, (July 1997), pp. 7799-7806, ISSN 0027-8424

Nigenda-Morales, S.; Flores-Ramírez, S.; Urbán-R, J. & Vázquez-Juárez, R. (2007). MHC DQB-1 polymorphism in the Gulf of California fin whale (*Balaenoptera physalus*) population. *Journal of heredity*, Vol.99, No.1, (January 2007), pp. 14-21, ISSN 0022-1503

Nikaido, M.; Matsuno, F.; Hamilton, H.; Brownell, R. L. Jr.; Cao, Y.; Ding, W.; Zuoyan, Z.; Shedlock, A. M.; Fordyce, R. E.; Hasegawa, M. & Okada, N. (2001). Retroposon analysis of major cetacean lineages: the monophyly of toothed whales and the paraphyly of river dolphins. *PNAS*, Vol.98, No.13, (June 2001), pp. 7384-7389, ISSN 0027-8424

Nikaido, M.; Rooney, A. P. & Okada, N. (1997). Phylogenetic relationships among cetartiodactyls based on insertions of short and long interpersed elements: hippopotamuses are the closest extant relatives of whales. *PNAS*, Vol.96, No.18, (August 1999), pp. 10261-10266, ISSN 0027-8424

Paterson, S. (1998). Evidence for balancing selection at the major histocompatibility complex in a free-living ruminant. *Journal of Heredity*, Vol.89, No.4, pp. 289-294, ISSN 0022-1503

Pfau, R. S.; Van Den Bussche, R. A.; McBee, K. & Lochmiller, R. L. (1999). Allelic diversity at the Mhc-DQA locus in cotton rats (*Sigmodon hispidus*) and a comparison of DQA sequences within the family muridae (Mammalia: Rodentia). *Immunogenetics*, Vol.49, No.10, (September 1999), pp. 886-893, ISSN 0093-7711

Piertney, S. B. & Oliver, M. K. (2006). The evolutionary ecology of the major histocompatibility complex. *Heredity*, Vol.96, pp. 7-21, ISSN 0018-067X

Potts, W. K. & Wakeland, E. K. (1990). Evolution of diversity at the major histocompatibility complex. *Trends in Ecololgy & Evolution*, Vol.5, No. 6, (June 1990), pp. 181-186, ISSN 0169-5347

Schook, L. & Lamont, S. (1996). *The Major Histocompatibility Complex Region of Domestic Animal Species*, CRC Press, ISBN 0849380324, Boca Raton, Florida, USA

Seddon, J. M. & Ellegren, H. (2002). MHC class II genes in European wolves: a comparison with dogs. *Immunogenetics*, Vol.54, No.7, (October 2002), pp. 490-500, ISSN 0093-7711

Slade, R. W. (1992). Limited MHC polymorphism in the southern elephant seal: implications for MHC evolution and marine mammal population biology. *Proceedings Biological Sciences / The Royal Society*, Vol.249, No.1325, (August 1992), pp. 163-71, ISSN 0962-8452

Sommer, S. (2003). Effects of habitat fragmentation and changes of dispersal behaviour after a recent population decline on the genetic variability of noncoding and coding DNA of a monogamous Malagasy rodent. *Molecular Ecology*, Vol.12, No.10, (October 2003), pp. 2845-2851, ISSN 0962-1083

Sommer, S. (2005). The importance of immune gene variability (MHC) in evolutionary ecology and conservation. *Frontiers in Zoology,* Vol.2, No.16, (October 2005), ISSN 1742-9994

Takahashi, K.; Rooney, A. P. & Nei, M. (2000). Origins and divergence times of mammalian class II MHC gene clusters. *Journal of Heredity,* Vol.91, No.3, (May 2000), pp. 198-204, ISSN 0022-1503

Theodor, J. M. (2004). Molecular clock divergence estimates and the fossil record of Cetartiodactyla. *Journal of Paleontology,* Vol.78, No.1, (January 2004), pp. 39-44, ISSN 0022-3360

Thewissen, J. G. M. & Williams, E. M. (2002). The early radiations of Cetacea (Mammalia): evolutionary pattern and developmental correlations. *Annual Review of Ecology, Evolution, and Systematics,* Vol.33, (November 2002), pp. 73-90, ISSN 1543-592X

Trowsdale, J.; Groves, V. & Arnason A. (1989). Limited MHC polymorphism in whales. *Immunogenetics,* Vol.29, No.1, (January 1989), pp. 19-24, ISSN 0093-7711

van der Walt, J. M.; Nel, L. H. & Hoelzel, A. R. (2001). Characterization of major histocompatibility complex DRB diversity in the endemic South African antelope *Damaliscus pygargus*: a comparison in two subspecies with different demographic histories. *Molecular Ecology,* Vol.10, No.7, (July 2001), pp. 1679-1688, ISSN 0962-1083

Vassilakos, D.; Natoli, A.; Dahlheim, M. & Hoelzel, A. R. (2009). Balancing and directional selection at exon-2 of the MHC DQB1 locus among populations of odontocete cetaceans. *Molecular biology and evolution,* Vol.26, No.3, (March 2009), pp. 681-689, ISSN 0737-4038

Wagner, J. L.; Burnett, R. C. & Storb, R. (1999). Organization of the canine major histocompatibility complex: current perspectives. *Journal of Heredity,* Vol.90, No.1, (January 1999), pp. 35-38, ISSN 0022-1503

Wang, J. Y.; Chou, L. S. & White, B. N. (1999). Mitochondrial DNA analysis of sympatric morphotypes of bottlenose dolphins (genus: *Tursiops*) in Chinese waters. *Molecular Ecology,* Vol.8, No.10, (October 1999), pp. 1603-1612, ISSN 0962-1083

Wang, K. R.; Payne, P. M. & Thayer, V. G. (1994). Coastal stock(s) of Atlantic bottlenose dolphin: status review and management. *NOAA Technical Memorandums,* NMFSOPR-4, US Department of Commerce.

Wang, M. C. (2003). Feeding habits, food resource partitioning and guild structure of odontocetes in Taiwanese waters. *PhD thesis of Institute of Zoology,* pp. 148, National Taiwan University, Taipei

Wegner, K. M.; Reusch, T. B. & Kalbe, M. (2003). Multiple parasites are driving major histocompatibility complex polymorphism in the wild. *Journal of Evolutionary Biology,* Vol.16, No.2, (March 2003), pp. 224-232, ISSN 1010-061X

Wells, R. S.; Rhinehart, H. L.; Hansen, L. J.; Sweeney, J. C.; Townsend, F. I.; Stone, R.; Casper, D. R.; Scott, M. D.; Hohn, A. A. & Rowles, T. K. (2004). Bottlenose dolphins as marine ecosystem sentinels: developing a health monitoring system. *EcoHealth,* Vol.1, pp. 246-254, ISSN 1612-9202

Xu, S.; Chen, B.; Zhou, K. & Yang, G. (2008). High similarity at three MHC loci between the baiji and finless porpoise: trans-species or convergent evolution? *Molecular phylogenetics and evolution,* Vol.47, No.1, (April 2008), pp. 36-44. ISSN 1055-7903

Xu, S.; Ren, W. H.; Li, S. Z.; Wei, F. W.; Zhou, K. Y. & Yang, G. (2009). Sequence polymorphism and evolution of three cetacean MHC genes. *Journal of molecular evolution*, Vol.69, No.3, (September 2009), pp. 260-275, ISSN 0022-2844

Xu, S.; Sun, P.; Zhou, K. & Yang, G. (2007). Sequence variability at three MHC loci of finless porpoises (*Neophocaena phocaenoides*). *Immunogenetics*, Vol.59, No.7, (July 2007), pp. 581-592, ISSN 0093-7711

Yang, G.; Yan, J.; Zhou, K. & Wei, F. (2005). Sequence variation and gene duplication at MHC *DQB* Loci of Baiji (*Lipotes vexillifer*), a Chinese river dolphin. *Journal of Heredity*, Vol.96, No.4, (July 2005), pp. 310-317, ISSN 0022-1503

Yang, W. C.; Chou, L. S. & Hu, J. M. (2007). Molecular characterization of expressed DRB and DQB genes in the bottlenose dolphins (*T. aduncus & T. truncatus*). *Zoological Studies*,Vol.46, No.6, (November 2007), pp. 664-679, ISSN 1021-5506

Yang, W. C.; Hu, J. M. & Chou, L. S. (2008). Sequence variation of MHC class II DQB gene in bottlenose dolphin (*Tursiops truncatus*) from Taiwanese waters. *Taiwania*, Vol.53, No.1, (January 2008), pp. 42-50, ISSN 0372-333X

Yang, W. C.; Hu, J. M. & Chou, L. S. (2010). Phylogenetic analyses of MHC class II genes in bottlenose dolphins and their terrestrial relatives reveal pathogen-driven directional selection. *Zoological Studies*, Vol.49, No.1, (January 2010), pp. 132-151, ISSN 1021-5506

Yeager, M. & Hughes, A. L. (1999). Evolution of the mammalian MHC: natural selection, recombination, and convergent evolution. *Immunological Reviews*, Vol.167, No.1, (February 1999), pp. 45-58, ISSN 0105-2869

Yuhki, N. & O'Brien, S. J. (1997). Nature and origin of polymorphism in feline MHC class II DRA and DRB genes. *Journal of Immunology*, Vol.158, No.6, (March 1997), pp. 2822-2833, ISSN 0022-1767

Zhou, K. & Qian, W. (1985). Distribution of the dolphins of the genus *Tursiops* in the China Seas. *Aquatic Mammals* Vol.1, 16-19, ISSN 0167-5427

8

Regulation of MHC Class I by Viruses

Shatrah Othman and Rohana Yusof
University of Malaya, Kuala Lumpur
Malaysia

1. Introduction

Originally recognized for their role in triggering T cell responses that caused the rejection of transplanted tissue, it is now known that MHC-encoded molecules are involved in immune-surveillance and antigen presentation to T lymphocytes. These MHC molecules act as "signposts" that displays fragmented pieces of an antigen (viral proteins in virus-infected cells or mutated proteins in tumor cells) on the host cell surface. Because viruses can infect virtually all nucleated cells, class I molecules are constitutively expressed on almost all nucleated cells. The association of antigenic peptides and MHC molecules is a saturable interaction and once formed, persist for a sufficiently long time to be recognized by the few T cells specific for the antigen as they circulate through. The outcome of T_C cells-mediated killing of the virus-infected cells is usually via apoptosis.

2. Antigen processing and presentation

The cellular pathways of antigen processing are designed to generate peptides that have structural characteristics required for associating with MHC molecules and to place these peptides in the same cellular location as the appropriate MHC molecules with the available peptide-binding cleft. Peptide binding to MHC molecules is essential for stable assembly and surface expression of the MHC molecules.

Class I MHC-associated peptides may be the products of viruses or other intracellular microbes that infect cells or protein antigens produced by mutated oncogenes in tumour cells (Rammensee 1995). They are produced by proteolytic degradation of cytosolic proteins in the proteasome, a large multiprotein enzyme complex found in the cytoplasm (Tanaka and Kasahara 1998). Two catalytic subunits of the proteasome, called low molecular weight protein 2 (LMP-2) and LMP-7 are encoded by genes in the MHC locus (York and Rock 1996). Peptides generated in the cytosol are translocated into the endoplasmic reticulum (ER) by specialized transport associated with antigen processing (TAP) proteins encoded by the TAP1 and TAP2 genes, also in the MHC gene complex. They mediate active ATP-dependent ferrying of peptides from the cytosol into the ER lumen (Spiliotis et al. 2000; Momburg et al. 2001).

Class I α chains and β_2-microglobulin are synthesized in the ER and remain attached to the TAP complex by an ER chaperone protein linker called tapasin until they are loaded with high-affinity peptides (Momburg and Tan 2002). These components collectively form the peptide-loading complex. The class I molecules, once loaded, exit the ER at unique exit sites, transit through the Golgi apparatus, and reach the cell surface to display their bound peptides for recognition by specific $CD8^+$ T_C cells. T_C cell-mediated killing is usually via apoptosis, mediated mainly by granule exocytosis, which releases granzymes and perforin. MHC molecules that fail to obtain high affinity peptides are either subjected to immediate degradation or short term expression at the cell surface followed by endocytosis and degradation (Spiliotis et al. 2000).

Antigen presentation via MHC class I is regulated by interferon (IFN)-γ which increases expression of the class I molecules, transporter proteins (TAP1 and TAP2) and immunoproteasome subunits (LMP2 and LMP7) via transcriptional regulation (Momburg et al. 2001). The induction of TAP by IFN-γ is more rapid than that of MHC class I molecules, which is consistent with the view that the constitutive level of TAP expression is insufficient to support inducible increases of MHC class I (Lobigs et al. 2003).

3. Immune evasion strategies of MHC class I antigen presentation by viruses

The ability of the MHC class I molecules to sample intracellular milieu and present antigens to T_C cells poses great threat to viruses. To freely replicate in infected cells, viruses have evolved numerous strategies that target key stages of the MHC class I antigen presentation pathway, with the goal of preventing the presentation of viral peptides to T_C cells. In order to circumvent this problem, many viruses have evolved strategies to interfere with the antigen presentation pathway. If a virus could inhibit the MHC presentation pathway, that virus would become invisible to T_C cells and would be able to replicate.

Since the first descriptions of adenovirus protein binding to MHC Class I molecules over 20 years ago, there have been many reports of virus counter-attack strategies aimed at the cellular immune response. The main aim of immune-evasion strategies by viruses is to *decrease the cell surface expression* of the MHC molecules. Numerous viral proteins have been found to inhibit components of the MHC class I assembly pathway. Several stages of the antigen presentation pathway have been identified as common target sites for these viral proteins.

3.1 Viral interference with gene transcription

Transcription of key players of the class I antigen presentation pathway is commonly targeted by many viruses such as human oncogenic adenovirus 12 (Ad12), human immunodeficiency virus 1 (HIV-1) and bovine papillomavirus (BPV) (Ambagala et al. 2005). Many viral genes which encode proteins that modulate host immune responses have been identified. The E1A viral protein of Ad12 inhibits transcription of nearly all components of the MHC class I pathway, including α-heavy chain, β_2m, TAP1, TAP2, LMP2, LMP7 and tapasin (Friedman and Ricciardi 1988; Rotem-Yehudar et al. 1994). Similarly, the human cytomegalovirus (HCMV) and murine cytomegalovirus (MCMV) also inhibit gene transcription by disrupting the IFN-γ induced up-regulation of the expression of genes encoding many components of the MHC class I heavy complex (Miller et al. 1999).

The E7 protein of oncogenic human papillomavirus (HPV) type-18 has been shown to downregulate the TAP1 gene transcription by repressing its promoter activity. The E1A protein of adenovirus (Ad) type-12 also has similar inhibitory activity on the TAP1 gene transcription (Abele and Tampé 2006). Although both DNA viruses belong to different virus classes, the resemblance in structure and functions of the two proteins may be mediating the effects.

The human immunodeficient virus type 1 (HIV-1) Tat gene encodes a protein that transactivates transcription of the viral long terminal repeat of HIV-1. It is essential for HIV-gene expression, replication and infectivity. The Tat protein is also able to repress several cellular gene promoters including the heavy chain of the class I molecule and the β_2m genes of the MHC class I (Carroll et al. 1998; Cohen et al. 1999). Bovine papillomavirus E5 and E7 proteins also inhibit transcription of class I heavy chain (Ashrafi et al. 2006).

3.2 Viral interference with peptide generation

The central cytoplasmic processing unit for the generation of peptides for the MHC class I antigen presentation pathway is the proteasome. The degradation of viral proteins into short peptides in the proteasome is a highly complex process and proteolysis is regulated in an ATP-dependent manner. The proteasome recognizes and unfolds ubiquitylated proteins through its 19S subunit and target deubiquitylated forms of these substrates to the 20S proteolytic subunit.

Several viruses interfere with the generation of high affinity peptides to be loaded onto and expressed by the MHC class I complex. These include Epstein-Barr virus 1 (EBV), Kaposi's sarcoma herpesvirus (KSHV), murine leukemia virus (MuLV) and again, HIV-1 Tat protein. The EBV genome encodes EBV nuclear antigen 1 (EBNA-1) protein that contains long repeats of glycine and alanine residues that are resistant to proteasomal processing (Dantuma 2002). It was shown that these repeats may interfere with the recognition and unfolding functions of the 19S subunit, rather than inhibiting ubiquitylation or proteolytic activity.

KSHV encodes a protein known as latency-associated nuclear antigen 1 (LANA1) which resembles the inhibitory properties of EBNA1. However, the repetitive acidic sequence is rich in glutamine, glutamic acid and aspartic acid residues; differing from that of EBNA1. As LANA1 and EBNA1 have no sequence homology, one possible explanation may be that the two have similar structural features with related inhibitory properties. Nonetheless, because the mechanism of antigen processing by the proteasome is the least well-characterized event in the MHC class I presentation pathway, it may be that the inhibition is occurring at a step in the proteasomal degradation that is yet to be identified (Hansen and Bouvier 2009).

The Tat regulatory protein produced by HIV-1 very early after infection that is capable of repressing gene transcription, also has a role in inhibiting the generation of peptides. This protein competes with the IFN-γ inducible 11S regulator for binding to the 20S proteasome. Binding of Tat to the 20S proteasome inhibits the peptidase and proteotytic activity of 20S proteasome (Gavioli et al. 2004). The MuLV, an oncogenic retrovirus, takes advantage of the peptide cleavage specificity of the proteasome in order to prevent the generation of specific immunodominant epitopes and this is achieve only via a single amino acid change in a target protein of MuLV (Beekman et al. 2000).

3.3 Viral inhibition of peptide transport mechanisms

The translocation of peptides into the ER by TAP represents a key stage in the assembly of the MHC class I molecule, since only peptide-loaded class I molecules can leave the ER for transport to the cell surface (Paulsson and Wang 2004). The TAP complex is composed of TAP1 and TAP2, each with an amino-terminal transmembrane domain and a carboxy-terminal nucleotide-binding cytoplasmic domain. The two helices form a pore across the ER membrane through which antigenic peptides can be transported. Peptide transport by TAP consists of two basic steps: ATP-free binding of peptide to TAP and ATP-dependent translocation of peptide into the ER lumen (Abele and Tampé 2006). It is thought that binding of prptides to the cytoplasmic domains triggers a conformational change that stimulates ATP hydrolysis, thereby providing energy required for peptide translocation. However, the mechanism underlying this process is not completely understood.

The human herpes simplex virus (HSV)-encoded protein, ICP47 (infected cell protein 47) inhibits the first step of peptide transport (Ambagala et al. 2005). By binding with high affinity to the cytoplasmic domain of human TAP, ICP47 inhibits peptide binding to and thereby ATP hydrolysis of TAP. In addition, evidence also suggests that ICP47 may act as a competitive inhibitor by binding with high affinity and induces a conformational change in TAP. This effect may be sufficient to cause destabilization and inactivation of TAP, thus turning off ATP hydrolysis and peptide translocation (Orr et al. 2005). ICP47 is highly species specific, since it inhibits with high affinity peptide binding to human TAP but not to TAP from mice, rabbit or guinea pigs. The region of TAP that interacts with ICP47 is, however, yet to be determined.

Human cytomegalovirus (HCMV)-encoded protein, US6, also targets the TAP but through a mechanism that differs from that of ICP47. US6 is an ER-resident integral membrane protein that binds to the ER-luminal domain of TAP and inhibits ATP binding. Like ICP47, US6 prevents peptide-stimulated ATP hydrolysis by inducing long range conformational rearrangements in TAP across the ER membrane (Hewitt et al. 2001). This subsequently inhibits peptide translocation and prevents MHC class I assembly. Unlike ICP47, however, interaction of US6 to TAP does not affect the peptide binding.

Another recently identified protein by EBV, BNLF2a, was shown to prevent the binding of peptides and ATP to TAP (Horst et al. 2011). Another HIV-1 protein, Nef, blocks the TAP transport of peptides into the ER (Cohen et al. 1999; Williams et al. 2002b). Despite the different strategies used by ICP47, US6 and BNLF2a to block peptide transport, the common goal of these proteins is to block peptide-dependent, ATP-induced conformational changes in TAP, thereby exploiting the conformational flexibility of TAP, which is normally required for peptide translocation. This will decrease the available peptide for binding to the MHC class I heavy chains that are waiting in the ER; thereby reducing the generation of completely assembled class I molecules.

3.4 Inhibition of tapasin

Tapasin is a transmembrane glycoprotein that is a crucial component of the peptide-loading complex. It has a key role in influencing the generation of peptide repertoire and expression of stable MHC class I molecules on the cell surface. Similar to TAP, tapasin is also targeted by a number of viral immunoevasins. Tapasin has a chaperone-like function that stabilizes peptide transport, facilitates the removal of peptides weakly bound to MHC class I molecules and ensures high affinity peptide access to MHC class I molecules (Williams et al. 2002a). Only those peptides that can form long-lived complexes with MHC class I molecules become part of the presented repertoire at the end of this so-called peptide-editing process.

The mK3 protein of murine gammaherpesvirus-68 interacts with TAP without affecting peptide transport (Boname et al. 2004). The mK3 is located in the ER and Golgi and belongs to a large group of proteins named the K3 family that inhibits the surface expression of glycoproteins such as MHC class I, ICAM-1 and CD4. The mK3 binds via its C-terminal tail to tapasin and TAP, thereby positioning the N-terminal with ubiquitin ligase activity to the cytoplasmic tail of the MHC class I for subsequent ubiquitylation and proteosomal degradation.

In addition, mK3 also induces the degradation of both TAP subunits and tapasin via direct interactions. In fact, the assembly complex proteins TAP and tapasin are absolutely required for mK3's effect on MHC class I. The absence of TAP or tapasin, or MHC class I mutations abrogating interaction with TAP or tapasin, prevents mK3 from binding to MHC class I and down-regulating its surface expression (Lybarger et al. 2003).

The E3/19K protein of the Adenovirus E3 is a transmembrane glycoprotein that inhibits the ability of tapasin to bridge TAP to MHC class I molecules by binding to TAP, without blocking peptide transport (Bennett et al. 1999). The association of E3/19K with TAP inhibits the formation of TAP-tapasin complex and this impairs the inclusion of TAP into the peptide-loading complex. This competitive inhibition of the bridging function of tapasin delays maturation of tapasin-dependent MHC class I molecule. Thus, the disturbance in the MHC-tapasin interaction ultimately prevents the assembly of MHC class I loading complex.

HCMV also encodes another immediate early protein US3 that directly binds to and inhibits the action of tapasin (Park et al. 2004). The association of US3 with tapasin inhibits tapasin-dependent peptide-loading, thereby preventing optimization of the peptide repertoire presented by the class I molecules. This subsequently leads to retention of the MHC class I molecules in the ER, although substantial amounts of the class I molecules can still reach the cell surface (Park et al. 2004).

3.5 Viral interference with cell surface expression

Down-regulation of the cell surface display of class I molecules is an important mechanism of immune evasion. Technically, once loaded with peptides, the class I MHC molecules leave the ER and translocate to the cell surface through the Golgi apparatus. Many viruses have the ability to interfere with these MHC class I trafficking processes (Ambagala et al. 2005).

In addition to inhibition of tapasin activity, the E3/19k adenovirus protein directly associate with the class I heavy chain and this blocks their transport out of the ER (Bennett et al. 1999). This association is mediated by the ER-luminal domains of both proteins and the retention effect is mediated by the cytoplasmic domains of E3/19k. Interaction between E3/19k and residue 56 of the MHC class I that appears to have crucial roles in modulating the association and ER retention of the class I molecule by the E3/19k (Hansen and Bouvier 2009).

MHC class I chaperones are remarkably efficient in only allowing mature MHC molecules to exit the ER. The elimination of incompletely assembled or misfolded nascent glycoproteins, including MHC molecules, occurs by a process collectively called ER-associated degradation (ERAD) (Vembar and Brodsky 2008). During ERAD, misassembled or misfolded proteins are recognized in the ER lumen and retrotranslocated to the cytoplasm, where they are degraded by the ubiquitin-proteasome machinery.

The HCMV invests heavily in products able to interfere with the MHC class I. Apart from US3 and US6 that have abilities to inhibit TAP, there are also other unique short genes encoded by the virus: US2, US11, US8 and US10. The US2 and US11 are small membrane glycoproteins that target human MHC class I molecules for ERAD. US2 and US11 cause ejection of MHC class I heavy chain into the cytoplasm, which results in their proteasomal degradation. The US2 cytoplasmic domain appears to have major involvement in this process. Besides inhibiting TAP functions previously described, the US3 also possesses a novel, non-contagious ER retention sequence that binds to nascent MHC class I heavy chains in the ER and targets it to ERAD. This prevents its egress of the assembled class I molecules to the cell surface (Park et al. 2004).

Another HCMV viral product, US8 binds MHC class I molecules in the ER and influence the MHC class I-restricted antigen presentation via a mechanism that is yet to be identified (Petersen et al. 2003). Lastly, the US10 also shares many features with US3. It associates with MHC class I heavy chain and delays the trafficking of peptide-loaded class I molecules out of the ER.

The p12(I) protein of human T-cell leukemia virus type 1 (HTLV-1) also redirects MHC class I heavy chains into the cytosol. This protein is localized in the ER and/or Golgi compartments, bind to the heavy chain products of the class I molecules, thus preventing association of the heavy chain with β_2m. This reroutes the MHC class I heavy chain into the cytosol for proteasomal degradation (Ambagala et al. 2005).

The mK3 protein encoded by murine herpesvirus-68, that inhibits TAP and tapasin, also induces rapid turnover of MHC class I molecules by a mechanism not involving endocytosis. The mK3 protein has been demonstrated to assist the virus in the escape from T cells during latent phase of infection. It specifically ubiquitylates MHC class I heavy chains and targets them for ERAD. During infection, the expression of mK3 allows the virus to maintain a higher level of latency and reduces the number of antiviral T_C cells. The mK3 associates with nascent MHC class I heavy chains only in the presence of TAP, its main binding partner. Subsequently, the complex awaits entry onto the peptide-loading complex and ubiquitylates the C-terminal tail of the heavy chain, thereby targeting for ERAD (Lybarger et al. 2003).

Apart from downregulating the expression of MHC class I molecules, the HIV-1 Nef protein is also known to disrupt the trafficking of MHC class I molecules via two mechanisms. First, Nef uses the clathrin adaptor AP1 (adaptor protein 1) to divert the trafficking of MHC class I molecules directly from the Golgi network to an endocytic compartment before they reach the cell surface. This ultimately leads to degradation of the assembled class I molecules in the lysosomes (Lorenzo et al. 2001). MCMV m152gene product gp40 protein too may have similar effect on the trafficking of the class I molecules. The second mechanism of Nef-mediated MHC class I down-regulation is enhancement of endocytosis of the class I molecules from the cell surface.

K3 and K5 proteins of KSHV inhibit the transport of class I molecules to the cell surface and induce rapid internalization of class I molecules from the cell surface via endocytosis (Cohen et al. 1999; Coscoy and Ganem 2000). Although the two proteins are predominantly located in the ER, K3 and K5 do not affect the assembly or transport of MHC class I molecules through the secretory pathway. Instead, they mediate ubiquitination of the cell surface MHC class I molecules by an unknown mechanism. Once ubiquitinated, internalized class I chains are then delivered to endolysosomal vesicles where they undergo degradation.

4. Multiple targets versus multiple immunoevasin

While some viruses encode a single immunoevasin to interfere with one or more steps of the MHC class I pathway, others encode multiple immunoevasins, targeting at different stages of the antigen presentation pathway. A good example of this is the US proteins of HCMV that can inhibit gene transcription, TAP and tapasin functions and also the surface expression of the MHC class I molecules. The HIV-1 also has three distinct proteins that target different site of inhibition, namely the Tat protein that inhibits peptide generation, the vpu protein interferes with the synthesis of class I while the Nef protein takes advantage of a cellular sorting pathway to pirate MHC class I molecules away from the cell surface. The likely reason for producing multiple immunoevasins is to overcome the resistance exerted by certain MHC class I alleles. Other reasons could be the cell and/or tissue specific adaptations of immunoevasins or that multiple immunoevasins, when expressed simultaneously, act synergistically to the benefit of the virus.

Considering the fact that the virus genome size is somewhat restricted, it would be advantageous for a virus to encode a single protein that can interfere with more than one mechanism to counter-attack the MHC class I antigen presentation as methods of immune evasion. The E3/19K of adenovirus can cause direct retention of MHC class I in the ER, inhibits TAP and tapasin functions and also inhibits surface expression. The murine herpesvirus mK3 protein also has multiple actions at the peptide generation and TAP functions in addition to its interference of the surface expression step.

5. Consequences of inhibition of MHC class I antigen presentation by viruses

Inhibition of antigen processing and presentation blocks the assembly and expression of stable class I molecules and the display of viral peptides. As a result, cells infected with such viruses cannot be recognized or killed by $CD8^+$ T_C cells. Natural Killer (NK) cells may be a host adaptation to kill these infected cells because NK cells are activated by the absence of class I MHC molecules (Brutkiewicz and Welsh 1995). Viruses try to evade recognition by T_C cells by inhibiting the class I MHC expression, but NK cells have evolved to respond specifically to the absence of class I MHC on virus-infected cells. Not surprisingly, there is emerging evidence that some viruses may produce proteins that act as ligands for NK inhibitory receptors and thus inhibiting NK cell activation.

In many cases, the viral defense strategies against T_C cells and NK cells are intertwined. The ability of NK cells to recognize and kill infected cells arises from its capacity to distinguish dangerous targets from healthy 'self' (Brutkiewicz and Welsh 1995; Biron et al. 1999). This is in turn dependent on the expression of both inhibitory and activating receptors. Inhibitory receptors on NK cells recognize class I molecules, which are constitutively expressed on most healthy cells but are often not expressed by cells infected with virus. The activity of NK cells is down-regulated when inhibitory receptors interact with 'self' MHC class I (Lanier 1998). Activating receptors on NK cells recognize ligands present on both NK-susceptible target cells and normal cells, but the influence of inhibitory pathways dominates when class I MHC is recognized.

6. Regulation of MHC class I by flaviviruses

In contrast to viruses that avoid the host immune response by down-regulating cell surface MHC complex expression, it is now recognized that Flaviviruses such as JEV, DV and WNV increase the cell surface expression of the MHC molecules (Lobigs et al. 2004; Lin et al. 2006; King et al. 2007; Othman et al. 2010). This peculiar phenomenon of the MHC class I immune modulation by Flaviviruses poses potential threats to both the replicating virus and host.

Numerous experiments related to this have been conducted in various cell types and species. One particular experiment on mouse embryonic fibroblasts showed six- to ten-fold increase in the expression of H-2K and H-2D MHC antigens after infection with WNV, MVE and JEV (King 2003). Up-regulation of class I cell surface expression by WNV has also been demonstrated in human skin fibroblast cells, accounted for by both cytokine-dependent and cytokine-independent mechanisms (Arnold 2004; King et al. 2007). The exact mechanism of the up-regulation remains unclear but evidence of increased mRNAs for HLA-A, HLA-B, HLA-C, LMP-2 and TAP-1 have been observed, suggesting viral-induced transcription of genes involved in the MHC class I complex.

An alternate mechanism for the up-regulation of MHC class I cell surface expression in flavivirus-infected cells, is via the TAP-dependent increase in peptide supply for assembly with MHC class I molecules (Momburg et al. 2001; Lobigs et al. 2003). Flavivirus-mediated peptide import into the ER lumen is time- and virus dose-dependent and takes place during the latent or early productive phase of virus replication (Momburg et al. 2001). Recombinant expression of flaviviral proteins in the absence of productive virus replication is unable to mimic this effect, establishing the importance of viral RNA replication in the induction of MHC class I expression, through both TAP-dependent and independent mechanisms (Hershkovitz et al. 2008). The involvement of NFκB, instead of interferons, has been demonstrated (Kesson and King 2001); yet no particular viral protein has been implicated in the mechanism of action of flaviviral-induced MHC class I surface expression.

7. Consequences of MHC class I induction by flaviviruses to the human host

Up-regulation of MHC class I expression by Flaviviruses has obvious potential disadvantage to the human host, that is increased susceptibility to attack by class I restricted cytotoxic T cells (Douglas and Kesson 1994; Lobigs et al. 2003). Increased cell surface expression of MHC class I molecules on infected cells would generally result in more efficient killing by T_C cells, yet this phenomenon is not observed in flaviviral infections. It has been hypothesized that enhancement of MHC class I expression by flaviviruses enhances the avidity of the cytotoxic T cell-target interaction. Nevertheless, the mechanisms are yet unclear.

With the additional up-regulation of co-stimulatory molecules induced by flaviviruses, the increase in avidity would be expected to recruit a wider range of low affinity T cells, which would otherwise be below the recognition threshold with normal expression of such surface molecules. This could therefore result in the generation of larger range of T_C clones than is usual for antiviral responses, with accordingly varying affinities for MHC class I-virus peptide. This may divert the cytotoxic T cells system to infected cells in G_0 of the cell cycle phase (that express high cell surface MHC concentrations) in preference to infected, most-virus-productive cycling cells (with relatively low MHC) (King 2003; King and Kesson 2003). The latter produces more virus and does not up-regulate MHC and adhesion molecules to the same extent, hence resulting in higher viral propagation and poor viral clearance that become part of the viral survival strategy.

Viral evasion from NK cell recognition involves the selective up-modulation of viral MHC class I homologues with structural similarity to endogenous host class I, mimicking 'self' antigens, that bind inhibitory receptors on NK cells (Orange et al. 2002). WNV- and Hepatitis C virus (HCV)-induced up-regulation of MHC class I cell surface expression has a pronounced effect on the susceptibility of target cells to NK cell lysis and may lead to insufficient induction of the adaptive immune response (Momburg et al. 2001; Herzer et al. 2003). DV-infected cells expressing high levels of cell surface class I molecules are capable of evading lysis by NK cells through higher binding of MHC molecules to low-affinity inhibitory receptors of NK cells.

Clearly, such immunopathological response would result in the destruction of uninfected tissues; in virus encephalitis, such damage would exacerbate the encephalitic syndrome (King 2003). In the case of DV infection, T-cell responses seem to have both protective and pathogenic effects in mouse models. Cytotoxic $CD8^+$ T cells that are cross-reactive among DV serotypes are thought to be immunopathological during secondary infections in humans, exacerbating DHF and causing liver damage through cytotoxic effects (An et al. 2004).

8. Conclusions

Viruses and their hosts have coevolved for millions of years. Viruses are obligate intracellular pathogens that enter permissive cells, hijack cellular metabolic pathways to generate progeny viruses that then leave the cells. At the same time, the human hosts have developed an intricate and fine-tuned adaptive immune system designed to combat these invaders. However, viruses have evolved a diverse array of strategies to evade the human's immune responses and these strategies are as diverse as the viruses themselves. The down-regulation of the MHC class I antigen presentation pathway is a strategy used by many viruses and this however, is counter-attacked by the presence of NK cells of the host.

On the other hand, some viruses prefer to up-regulate the cell surface expression of the class I molecules. Although the opposite is expected, this strategy also appears to favour the virus and results in interference of both the T_C cells-mediated cytolysis and the killing by NK cells. As the battle between viruses and human immune system continues, the discovery of novel immunoevasins and revelations of their modes of actions will continue to broaden the horizons of biology.

9. References

Abele, R. and Tampé, R. 2006. Modulation of the antigen transport machinery TAP by friends and enemies. *FEBS Letters* 580(4): 1156-1163.

Ambagala, A.P.N., Solheim, J.C., and Srikumaran, S. 2005. Viral interference with MHC class I antigen presentation pathway: The battle continues. *Veterinary Immunology and Immunopathology* 107(1-2): 1-15.

An, J., Zhou, D.-S., Zhang, J.-L., Morida, H., Wang, J.-L., and Yasui, K. 2004. Dengue-specific CD8+ T cells have both protective and pathogenic roles in dengue virus infection. *Immunology Letters* 95(2): 167-174.

Arnold, S.J., Osvath, S.R., Hall, R.A., King, N.J.C., Sedger, L.M. 2004. Regulation of antigen processing and antigen presentation molecules in West Nile virus-infected human skin fibroblasts. *Virology* 324: 286-296.

Ashrafi, G.H., Brown, D.R., Fife, K.H., and Campo, M.S. 2006. Down-regulation of MHC class I is a property common to papillomavirus E5 proteins. *Virus Research* 120(1-2): 208-211.

Beekman, N.J., van Veelen, P.A., van Hall, T., Neisig, A., Sijts, A., Camps, M., Kloetzel, P.-M., Neefjes, J.J., Melief, C.J., and Ossendorp, F. 2000. Abrogation of CTL Epitope Processing by Single Amino Acid Substitution Flanking the C-Terminal Proteasome Cleavage Site. *J Immunol* 164(4): 1898-1905.

Bennett, E.M., Bennink, J.R., Yewdell, J.W., and Brodsky, F.M. 1999. Cutting Edge: Adenovirus E19 Has Two Mechanisms for Affecting Class I MHC Expression1. *J Immunol* 162(9): 5049-5052.

Biron, C.A., Nguyen, K.B., Pien, G.C., Cousens, L.P., and Salazar-Mather, T.P. 1999. Natural killer cells in antiviral defense: Function and Regulation by Innate Cytokines. *Annual Review of Immunology* 17(1): 189-220.

Boname, J.M., de Lima, B.D., Lehner, P.J., and Stevenson, P.G. 2004. Viral Degradation of the MHC Class I Peptide Loading Complex. *Immunity* 20(3): 305-317.

Brutkiewicz, R.R. and Welsh, R.M. 1995. Major histocompatibility complex class I antigens and the control of viral infections by natural killer cells. *J Virol* 69(7): 3967–3971.

Carroll, I.R., Wang, J., Howcroft, T.K., and Singer, D.S. 1998. Hiv Tat represses transcription of the [beta]2-microglobulin promoter. *Molecular Immunology* 35(18): 1171-1178.

Cohen, G.B., Gandhi, R.T., Davis, D.M., Mandelboim, O., Chen, B.K., Strominger, J.L., and Baltimore, D. 1999. The Selective Downregulation of Class I Major Histocompatibility Complex Proteins by HIV-1 Protects HIV-Infected Cells from NK Cells. *Immunity* 10(6): 661-671.

Coscoy, L. and Ganem, D. 2000. Kaposi's sarcoma-associated herpesvirus encodes two proteins that block cell surface display of MHC class I chains by enhancing their endocytosis *PNAS* 97: 8051-8056.

Dantuma, N.P.S., A.; Masucci, M. G. 2002. Avoiding proteasomal processing: the case of EBNA1. *Current topics in microbiology and immunology* 269: 23-36.

Douglas, M.W. and Kesson, A.M.a.N.J.K. 1994. CTL recognition of west Nile virus-infected fibroblasts is cell cycle dependent and is associated with virus-induced increases in class I MHC antigen expression. *Immunology* 82(4): 561-570.

Friedman, D.J. and Ricciardi, R.P. 1988. Adenovirus type 12 E1A gene represses accumulation of MHC class I mRNAs at the level of transcription. *Virology* 165(1): 303-305.

Gavioli, R., Gallerani, E., Fortini, C., Fabris, M., Bottoni, A., Canella, A., Bonaccorsi, A., Marastoni, M., Micheletti, F., Cafaro, A., Rimessi, P., Caputo, A., and Ensoli, B. 2004. HIV-1 Tat Protein Modulates the Generation of Cytotoxic T Cell Epitopes by

Modifying Proteasome Composition and Enzymatic Activity. *J Immunol* 173(6): 3838-3843.
Hansen, T.H. and Bouvier, M. 2009. MHC class I antigen presentation: learning from viral evasion strategies. *Nat Rev Immunol* 9(7): 503-513.
Hershkovitz, O., Zilka, A., Bar-Ilan, A., Abutbul, S., Davidson, A., Mazzon, M., Kummerer, B.M., Monsoengo, A., Jacobs, M., and Porgador, A. 2008. Dengue virus replicon expressing the nonstructural proteins suffices to enhance membrane expression of HLA class I and inhibit lysis by human NK cells. *J Virol* 82(15): 7666-7676.
Herzer, K., Falk, C.S., Encke, J., Eichhorst, S.T., Ulsenheimer, A., Seliger, B., and Krammer, P.H. 2003. Upregulation of major histocompatibility complex class I on liver cells by hepatitis C virus core protein via p53 and TAP1 impairs natural killer cell cytotoxicity. *J Virol* 77(15): 8299-8309.
Hewitt, E.W., Gupta, S.S., and Lehner, P.J. 2001. The human cytomegalovirus gene product US6 inhibits ATP binding by TAP. *EMBO J* 20(3): 387-396.
Horst, D., Ressing, M.E., and Wiertz, E.J.H.J. 2011. Exploiting human herpesvirus immune evasion for therapeutic gain: potential and pitfalls. *Immunol Cell Biol* 89(3): 359-366.
Kesson, A.M. and King, N.J. 2001. Transcriptional regulation of major histocompatibility complex class I by flavivirus West Nile is dependent on NF-kappaB activation. *J Infect Dis* 184(8): 947-954.
King, N., Shrestha B, Kesson AM. 2003. Immune modulation by flaviviruses. *Adv Virus Res* 60(121-55).
King, N.J., Getts, D.R., Getts, M.T., Rana, S., Shrestha, B., and Kesson, A.M. 2007. Immunopathology of flavivirus infections. *Immunol Cell Biol* 85(1): 33-42.
King, N.J.C. and Kesson, A.M. 2003. Interaction of flaviviruses with cells of the vertebrate host and decoy of the immune response. *Immunol Cell Biol* 81(3): 207-216.
Lanier, L.L. 1998. NK cell receptor. *Annual Review of Immunology* 16: 359-393.
Lin, R.-J., Chang, B.-L., Yu, H.-P., Liao, C.-L., and Lin, Y.-L. 2006. Blocking of Interferon-Induced Jak-Stat Signaling by Japanese Encephalitis Virus NS5 through a Protein Tyrosine Phosphatase-Mediated Mechanism. *J Virol* 80(12): 5908-5918.
Lobigs, M., Müllbacher, A., and Lee, E. 2004. Evidence that a mechanism for efficient flavivirus budding upregulates MHC class I. *Immunology and Cell Biology* 82(2): 184-188.
Lobigs, M., Mullbacher, A., and Regner, M. 2003. MHC class I up-regulation by flaviviruses: Immune interaction with unknown advantage to host or pathogen. *Immunol Cell Biol* 81(3): 217-223.
Lorenzo, M.E., Ploegh, H.L., and Tirabassi, R.S. 2001. Viral immune evasion strategies and the underlying cell biology. *Seminars in Immunology* 13(1): 1-9.
Lybarger, L., Wang, X., Harris, M.R., Virgin, H.W., and Hansen, T.H. 2003. Virus subversion of the MHC class I peptide-loading complex. *Immunity* 18(1): 121-130.
Miller, D.M., Zhang, Y., Rahill, B.M., Waldman, W.J., and Sedmak, D.D. 1999. Human Cytomegalovirus Inhibits IFN-{alpha}-Stimulated Antiviral and Immunoregulatory Responses by Blocking Multiple Levels of IFN-{alpha} Signal Transduction. *J Immunol* 162(10): 6107-6113.
Momburg, F., Mullbacher, A., and Lobigs, M. 2001. Modulation of Transporter Associated with Antigen Processing (TAP)-Mediated Peptide Import into the Endoplasmic Reticulum by Flavivirus Infection. *J Virol* 75(12): 5663-5671.

Momburg, F. and Tan, P. 2002. Tapasin-the keystone of the loading complex optimizing peptide binding by MHC class I molecules in the endoplasmic reticulum. *Mol Immunology* 39: 217-233.

Orange, J.S., Fassett, M.S., Koopman, L.A., Boyson, J.E., and Strominger, J.L. 2002. Viral evasion of natural killer cells. *Nat Immunol* 3(11): 1006-1012.

Orr, M.T., Edelmann, K.H., Vieira, J., Corey, L., Raulet, D.J., and Wilson, C.B. 2005. Inhibition of MHC Class I Is a Virulence Factor in Herpes Simplex Virus Infection of Mice. *Plos Pathogens* 1(1): 62-71.

Othman, S., Yusof, R., and ABd-Rahman, N. 2010. All serotypes of dengue virus induce HLA-A2 MHC Class I promoter activity in human liver cells. *Transactions of the Royal Society of Tropical Medicine and Hygiene* 104: 806-808.

Park, B., Kim, Y., Shin, J., Lee, S., Cho, K., Früh, K., Lee, S., and Ahn, K. 2004. Human Cytomegalovirus Inhibits Tapasin-Dependent Peptide Loading and Optimization of the MHC Class I Peptide Cargo for Immune Evasion. *Immunity* 20(1): 71-85.

Paulsson, K.M. and Wang, P. 2004. Quality control of MHC class I maturation. *FASEB J* 18(1): 31-38.

Petersen, J.L., Morris, C.R., and Solheim, J.C. 2003. Virus Evasion of MHC Class I Molecule Presentation. *J Immunol* 171(9): 4473-4478.

Rammensee, H.-G. 1995. Chemistry of peptides associated with MHC class I and class II molecules. *Current Opinion in Immunology* 7(1): 85-96.

Rotem-Yehudar, R., Winograd, S., Sela, S., Coligan, J.E., and Ehrlich, R. 1994. Downregulation of peptide transporter genes in cell lines transformed with the highly oncogenic adenovirus 12. *J Exp Med* 180(2): 477-488.

Spiliotis, E.T., Osorio, M., Zúñiga, M.C., and Edidin, M. 2000. Selective Export of MHC Class I Molecules from the ER after Their Dissociation from TAP. *Immunity* 13(6): 841-851.

Tanaka, K. and Kasahara, M. 1998. The MHC class I ligand-generating system: roles of immunoproteasomes and the interferon-gamma-inducible proteasome activator PA28. *Immunol Rev* 163: 161-176.

Vembar, S.S. and Brodsky, J.L. 2008. One step at a time: endoplasmic reticulum-associated degradation. *Nat Rev Mol Cell Biol* 9(12): 944-957.

Williams, A.P., Peh, C.A., Purcell, A.W., McCluskey, J., and Elliott, T. 2002a. Optimization of the MHC Class I Peptide Cargo Is Dependent on Tapasin. 16(4): 509-520.

Williams, M., Roeth, J.F., Kasper, M.R., Fleis, R.I., Przybycin, C.G., and Collins, K.L. 2002b. Direct Binding of Human Immunodeficiency Virus Type 1 Nef to the Major Histocompatibility Complex Class I (MHC-I) Cytoplasmic Tail Disrupts MHC-I Trafficking. *J Virol* 76(23): 12173-12184.

York, I.A. and Rock, K.L. 1996. Antigen processing and presentation by the class i major histocompatibility complex. *Annual Review of Immunology* 14: 369-396.

9

Major and Minor Histocompatibility Antigens to Non-Inherited Maternal Antigens (NIMA)

Masahiro Hirayama, Eiichi Azuma* and Yoshihiro Komada
Mie University Graduate School of Medicine
Japan

1. Introduction

Immunological reactivity results from differences between the transplant host and donor for cell surface determinants known as histocompatibility antigens. Histocompatibility antigens that provoke the most severe transplant reactions are encoded by a series of genes that reside in a discrete chromosomal region termed the major histocompatibility complex (MHC) (Amos 1968). Genes of the human leukocyte antigen (HLA) system encode a complex array of histocompatibility molecules that play a central role in immune responsiveness and in determining the outcome of hematopoietic stem cell transplantation (HSCT) (Beatty, Anasetti et al. 1993; Petersdorf, Longton et al. 1995). The primary goal of histocompatibility testing for patients who are undergoing HSCT is the identification of a suitable HLA-matched donor to reduce the risk of post-transplant complications, which may result from HLA incompatibility. The extensive polymorphism of the HLA system, however, makes the selection of a comprehensively, optimally-matched donor a challenging endeavor, particularly when donors outside of the patient's immediate family are sought. If a suitable donor is not found, clinicians need to explore the possibility of permissive HLA mismatches.

Haploidentical HSCT is curative treatment for patients lacking an HLA-compatible donor or cannot wait until a suitable donor can be found (Reisner, Kapoor et al. 1981; Buckley, Schiff et al. 1999). Haploidentical HSCT is usually employed with T-cell depletion or positive selection of $CD34^+$ cells to avoid severe graft-versus-host disease (GVHD) (Aversa, Tabilio et al. 1994). However there are disadvantages, such as potential for graft failure, fatal opportunistic infections, and relapse of the treated malignancy. To deal with those problems, T-cell "replete" haploidentical HSCT have been performed by researchers in Japan (Ichinohe, Uchiyama et al. 2004). These are based on the hypothesis that long-term maternal microchimerism (MMc) is associated with acquired immunologic hyporesponsiveness to non-inherited maternal antigen (NIMA) (Andrassy, Kusaka et al. 2003; Dutta, Molitor-Dart et al. 2009). T-cell replete HSCT, without GVHD, could be accomplished by using this phenomenon of feto-maternal tolerance. Unfortunately, graft rejection and hyperacute GVHD have been reported in HSCT from NIMA-mismatched siblings, despite detecting of MMc (Okumura, Yamaguchi et al. 2007). Therefore,

* Corresponding Author

development of a predictable method for GVHD in NIMA-mismatched HSCT is needed. We have produced a novel prediction assay, using MLR-ELISPOT (mixed lymphocyte reaction; enzyme-linked immunospot) assay, for detecting reactivity to NIMA (Araki, Hirayama et al. 2010). In this review, we discuss acute GVHD in T-cell depleted and T-cell replete HSCT, the role of major and minor histocompatibility in NIMA tolerance, and prediction of acute GVHD in T-cell replete HSCT via our model assay.

2. Minor histocompatibility antigens in mouse and human

Alloantigens can be divided into major histocompatibility complex (MHC) antigen and minor histocompatibility antigen (MiHA), the former responsible for eliciting the strongest immune responses to allogeneic tissues. The MHC is referred to as the H-2 complex in mice and as the HLA complex in humans.

MHC identity of donor and host is not the sole factor determining immunological reactivity in HSCT. When transplantation is performed in an unrelated setting (MUD, matched-unrelated donor), even if MHC antigens of donor are identical to recipient, considerable transplant reactions may occur because of differences at various minor histocompatibility loci. MiHAs are capable of eliciting cellular alloimmune responses in vitro and in vivo. They are peptides derived from polymorphic proteins. Their immunogenicity arises as a result of their presentation in the context of MHC class I or II, where they are recognized by alloreactive MHC-restricted T cells. The most important immune reactions elicited by in vivo alloreactivity to MiHA are graft rejection and GVHD.

To date, human MiHAs have not been fully characterized. Some murine MiHAs have been compared with human counterparts though (see, HY antigens in Table 1). Immunological targeting of HY proteins results in a relatively high incidence of acute GVHD when male recipients receive HSCT from female donors (Stern, Passweg et al. 2006). While approximately one third of the known MiHAs are encoded in Y chromosome, many MiHAs are located on autosomal chromosomes (Table 1). Genetic linkage analysis has been used to define the genomic regions encoding the MiHAs (Akatsuka, Nishida et al. 2003; de Rijke, van Horssen-Zoetbrood et al. 2005). With these more recent advanced techniques, more human MiHAs epitopes have been identified (van Bergen, Kester et al. 2007; Kawase, Akatsuka et al. 2007; Tykodi, Fujii et al. 2008; Griffioen, van der Meijden et al. 2008; Spaapen, Lokhorst et al. 2008; Spaapen, de Kort et al. 2009; Kamei, Nannya et al. 2009; Stumpf, van der Meijden et al. 2009; Bleakley, Otterud et al. 2010; Van Bergen, Rutten et al. 2010; Sellami, Kaabi et al. 2011).

MiHA	Species	Chromosome	Gene	MHC restriction	Tissue specificity	References
Y chromosome						
HY	Mouse	Y	Smcy	$H\text{-}2K^k$, $H\text{-}2D^b$	Ubiquitous	(Markiewicz et al. 1998)
HY	Mouse	Y	Uty	$H\text{-}2D^b$	Ubiquitous	(Greenfield et al. 1996)
HY	Mouse	Y	Dby	$H\text{-}2A^b$, $H\text{-}2E^k$	Ubiquitous	(Scott et al. 2000)
SMCY	Human	Yq11	JARID1D	HLA-A*02:01, B*07:02	Ubiquitous	(Wang et al. 1995)

MiHA	Species	Chromosome	Gene	MHC restriction	Tissue specificity	References
UTY	Human	Yq11	UTY	HLA-B8, B60	Ubiquitous	(Vogt et al. 2000)
DBY	Human	Yq11	DDX3Y	HLA-B*27:05, DRB1*15:01, DQ5	Hematopoietic	(Zorn et al. 2004)
DFFRY	Human	Yq11.2	USP9Y	HLA-A*01:01	Ubiquitous	(Pierce et al. 1999)
RPS4Y	Human	Yp11.3	RPS4Y1	HLA-B*52:01, DRB3*03:01	Ubiquitous	(Spierings et al. 2003)
TMSB4Y	Human	Yq11.221	TMSB4Y	HLA-A*33:03	Ubiquitous	(Torikai et al. 2004)
Autosomal chromosome						
H3	Mouse	2	Zfp106	$H\text{-}2D^b$	Ubiquitous	(Zuberi et al. 1998)
H4	Mouse	7	Emp3	$H\text{-}2K^b$	Ubiquitous	(Luedtke et al. 2003)
H7	Mouse	9	D9Mit182	$H\text{-}2D^b$	Ubiquitous	(Perreault et al. 1996)
H13	Mouse	2	47c1 cDNA	$H\text{-}2D^b$	Ubiquitous	(Mendoza et al. 1997)
H28	Mouse	3	NS1178	$H\text{-}2K^b$	Ubiquitous	(Malarkannan et al. 2000)
H46	Mouse	7	Il4i1	$H\text{-}2A^b$	Hematopoietic	(Sahara et al. 2003)
H47	Mouse	7	H47	$H\text{-}2D^b$	Ubiquitous	(Mendoza et al. 2001)
H60	Mouse	10	Rae1	$H\text{-}2K^b$	Hematopoietic	(Choi et al. 2001)
HA-1	Human	19p13.3	HMHA1	HLA-A*02:01, A*02:06, B60	Hematopoietic	(Mommaas et al. 2002)
HA-2	Human	7p13-p11.2	MYO1G	HLA-A*02:01	Hematopoietic	(den Haan et al. 1995)
HA-3	Human	15q24-q25	AKAP13	HLA-A*01:01	Ubiquitous	(Spierings et al. 2003)
HA-8	Human	9p24.2	KIAA0020	HLA-A*02:01	Ubiquitous	(Brickner et al. 2001)
HB-1	Human	5q31.3	HMHB1	HLA-B*44:02, B*44:03	B-cell	(Dolstra et al. 1999)
ACC-1, 2	Human	15q24.3	BCL2A1	HLA-A*24:02, B*44:03	Hematopoietic	(Akatsuka et al. 2003)
UGT2B17	Human	4q13	UGT2B17	HLA-A*02:06, A*29:02, B*44:03	Ubiquitous	(Murata et al. 2003)
LRH-1	Human	17p13.3	P2RX5	HLA-B*07:02	Hematopoietic	(de Rijke et al. 2005)
CTSH	Human	15q25.1	CTSH	HLA-A*31:01, A*33:03	Ubiquitous	(Torikai et al. 2006)
LB-ECGF1-1H	Human	2q13.33	ECGF1	HLA-B*07:02	Hematopoietic	(Slager et al. 2006)
PANE1	Human	22q13.2	CENPM	HLA-A*03:01	Hematopoietic	(Brickner et al. 2006)
SP110	Human	2q37.1	SP110	HLA-A*03:01	Hematopoietic	(Warren et al. 2006)

Table 1. Minor histocompatibility antigens in mouse and human

3. Acute GVHD in T-cell depleted or replete haploidentical transplantation

Haploidentical HSCT has made progress over the past 30 years and has become a feasible option for patients without an HLA-identical sibling donor. This is especially true for reconstitution of immunity in infants with severe combined immunodeficiency, where use of rigorously T-cell depleted marrow has been quite successful (Buckley, Schiff et al. 1999). In early trials of haploidentical HSCT, ex vivo T-cell depletion method of haploidentical bone marrow cells was an effective method reported by Reisner et al (Reisner, Kapoor et al. 1981). This procedure without immunosuppressive prophylaxis allowed durable engraftment rate about 75% with acceptable incidence of acute GVHD (36%) in patients with severe combined immunodeficiency (Buckley, Schiff et al. 1999). However, its application to haploidentical HSCT for leukemia was less encouraging due to the high incidence of graft failure (30%) and infectious complications (80%) (O'Reilly, Keever et al. 1987). In a trial from the University of Perugia, the use of T-cell depletion in combination with a high dose of stem cells overcame graft rejection as well as acute GVHD (Aversa, Tabilio et al. 1994). Improved positive selection of $CD34^+$ cells was accomplished by depletion of B cells, in addition to T cells, which resulted in a lower incidence of EBV-associated lymphoproliferative disease (LPD) (Aversa, Terenzi et al. 2005). Another method using ex vivo T-cell depletion of bone marrow cells with anti-T-cell monoclonal antibodies, followed by treatment with cyclosporine and ATG, was encouraging for the use of haploidentical marrow (Henslee-Downey, Abhyankar et al. 1997). Over 95% durable engraftment and low incidence of acute GVHD (13%) were obtained, and accompanied with an acceptable relapse rate (31%) (Mehta, Singhal et al. 2004). Although these various depletion techniques achieved benefit, to truly achieve more acceptable results, further improvement is necessary to address the high rate of malignancy relapses, acute and chronic GVHD, and otherwise, treatment-related morbidity and mortality.

As an alternative to ex vivo T-cell depletion, in vivo T-cell depletion methods have been undertaken for improving relapse rates and treatment-related mortality. Lu et al. from Peking University described the transplantation of combination of G-CSF-primed bone marrow and peripheral blood with intensive immunosuppression using ATG (Lu, Dong et al. 2006). Although the cumulative incidence of grade II to IV acute GVHD was comparatively high, 40%, two-year incidences of relapses and treatment-related mortality were low, 22% and 18%, respectively. More recently, Huang et al., in the same group reported encouraging clinical outcomes in 250 patients with haploidentical HSCT. The 3-year of leukemia free survival in standard and high-risk AML was 70.7% and 55.9%, respectively, and 59.7% and 24.8% for ALL (Huang, Liu et al. 2009). In another approach, Rizzieri et al. reported that alemtuzumab was used for in vivo depletion of both recipient and donor T-cells, in order to allow for more reliable engraftment and decreased GVHD (Rizzieri, Koh et al. 2007).

Sibling-related NIMA-mismatched transplantation, as an approach to T-cell replete haploidentical HSCT, was introduced as an alternative to ex vivo or in vivo T-cell depleted haploidentical HSCT. Van Rood et al. first showed that the incidence of acute GVHD was lower in patients who received T-cell replete grafts from an NIMA-mismatched sibling than those from non-inherited paternal antigen (NIPA) -mismatched sibling (van Rood, Loberiza et al. 2002). This indicated that the presence of immunological hyporesponsiveness against

NIMA in haploidentical transplantation could be important for prevention of GVHD and other immunologic comorbidities. Ichinohe et al. also showed that T-cell replete haploidentical HSCT from NIMA-mismatched family donor was feasible in selected patients with poor-risk hematologic malignancies using standard GVHD prophylaxis (Ichinohe, Maruya et al. 2002). However, 10% of patients still experienced severe acute GVHD, and there was not a useful method to predict acute GVHD in these patients. Thus, both T-cell depleted and T-cell replete haploidentical HSCT have benefits and drawbacks (Table 2). The problems of T-cell depleted HSCT were relatively high rate of graft failure, delayed immune reconstitution resulting in infections, and relapse of malignancies (Henslee-Downey, Abhyankar et al. 1997; Guinan, Boussiotis et al. 1999; Mehta, Singhal et al. 2004; Lu, Dong et al. 2006; Huang, Liu et al. 2009). On the other hand, the problems of T-cell replete haploidentical HSCT were relatively high rates of acute GVHD and treatment-related mortality (Ichinohe, Maruya et al. 2002; van Rood, Loberiza et al. 2002; Kanda, Ichinohe et al. 2009). Therefore, if an effective method to predict GVHD is available, T-cell replete haploidentical HSCT may be feasible with relative safety; lower risk of GVHD, lower risk of infections, and lower risk of malignancy relapse.

Type of HSCT	Age	Source	ATG	Acute GVHD (Grade II-IV)	Graft failure	TRM	Relapse	DFS
T-cell depleted								
(Ex vivo)	0-33	BM	+	5-8 %	3-5 %	17-47 %	11-25 %	35-38 %
(In vivo)	16-25	BM ± PB	+	13-46 %	0-13 %	22-51 %	18-31 %	18-64 %
T-cell replete								
(NIMA/ Mother)	15-28	BM or PB	-*	41-58 %	0-20 %	18-57 %	6-25 %	30-81 %
(NIPA/ Father)	17-20	BM	-*	55-63 %	13-29 %	36-45 %	Unknown	24-44 %

*More than 90% of patients were not used.
Abbreviations: ATG, anti-thymocyte globulin; TRM, treatment-related mortality; DFS, disease-free survival; BM, bone marrow; PB, peripheral blood.

Table 2. Frequency of acute GVHD in T-cell depleted and T-cell replete HSCT

4. Tolerance to non-inherited maternal antigen in murine studies

Maternal cells and fetal cells, most notably lymphocytes, are known to reciprocally traffic across the placenta during fetal development (Hall, Lingenfelter et al. 1995; Lo, Lo et al. 1996), and can result in life-long MMc in the offspring (Maloney, Smith et al. 1999). Prenatal exposure to NIMA affects the neonate's developing immune system, producing some tolerization to the non-inherited MHC components. There have been several previously reported investigations of NIMA (Burlingham, Grailer et al. 1998; Andrassy, Kusaka et al. 2003), as illustrated in Figure 1.

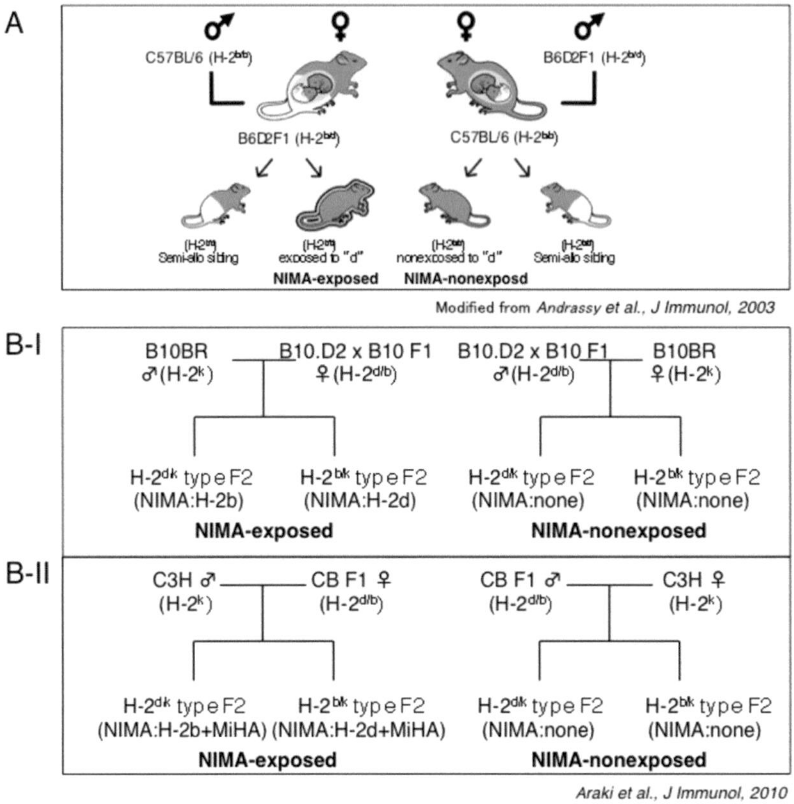

C

Mating combination	Offspring	$NIMA^{H-2}$	$NIMA^{MiHA}$
A B6 ♂ x B6D2F1 ♀ (major + minor)	$H-2^{b/b}$	$H-2^{d}$	Noninherited MiHA of DBA/2
B-I B10.BR ♂ x [B10.D2 x B10] F1 ♀	$H-2^{d/k}$	$H-2^{b}$	none
(major only)	$H-2^{b/k}$	$H-2^{d}$	none
B-II C3H ♂ x [BALB/c x B6] F1 ♀	$H-2^{d/k}$	$H-2^{b}$	Noninherited MiHA of B6 and BALB/c
(major + minor)	$H-2^{b/k}$	$H-2^{d}$	Noninherited MiHA of B6 and BALB/c

Hirayama et al., Chimerism, 2011

A-Left, C57BL/6 (B6) males ($H-2^{b/b}$) were mated with (B6 x DBA/2) F1 female ($H-2^{b/d}$), thus exposing the $H-2^{b/b}$ offspring in utero and via breast feeding to $NIMA^{d}$ antigens. Right, (B6 x DBA/2) F1 males were mated with B6 female, creating $H-2^{b/b}$ backcross offspring that had not been exposed to "d" as reported by Andrassy et al. B-I-Left, B10.BR males ($H-2^{k}$) were mated with (B10.D2 x B10) F1 females ($H-2^{d/b}$), thus exposing the $H-2^{d/k}$ type offspring to $NIMA^{b}$, and $H-2^{b/k}$ type offspring to $NIMA^{d}$ Right, (B10.D2 x B10) F1 males ($H-2^{d/b}$) were mated with B10.BR females ($H-2^{k}$), creating the controls; both $H-2^{d/k}$ and $H-2^{b/k}$ type offsprings that had not been exposed to b and d, respectively. These mice have B10 background, in other words, their MiHA (i.e. H-4, H-13, H-60, etc) are matched, and H-2 antigens are mismatched in both class I and II. B-II-Left, C3H males ($H-2^{k}$) were mated with CB (BALB/c x B6) F1 females ($H-2^{d/b}$), thus exposing the $H-2^{d/k}$ type offspring to NIMA b antigens and MiHA ($NIMA^{H-2b+MiHA}$), and $H-2^{b/k}$ type offspring to $NIMA^{H-2d+MiHA}$. Right, CB F1 males ($H-2^{d/b}$) were mated with C3H females ($H-2^{k}$), creating the controls; both $H-2^{d/k}$ and $H-2^{b/k}$ type offspring that had not been exposed to H-2b+MiHA and H-2d+MiHA, respectively. C, Breeding pattern were summarized in terms of major and minor histocompatibility Ags to NIMA.

Fig. 1. Murine models for non-inherited maternal antigens.

In addition, maternal cells and MHC/HLA proteins are ingested by the baby during nursing, possibly stimulating oral tolerance (Verhasselt, Milcent et al. 2008; Aoyama, Koyama et al. 2009). The clinical benefits of developmentally acquired tolerance to NIMA were first noted by Owen et al. more than 50 years ago (Owen, Wood et al. 1954). Since then, tolerogenic effects of NIMA have been documented at both T- and B-cell levels in a variety of clinical settings (Claas, Gijbels et al. 1988; van Rood and Claas 1990; Burlingham, Grailer et al. 1998). Presence of feto-maternal tolerance was anticipated due to the presence of MMc (Andrassy, Kusaka et al. 2003), and the concept has been used in clinical studies (Ichinohe, Uchiyama et al. 2004). On the basis of this hypothesis, several transplantation centers in Japan have performed clinical trials to test the feasibility of HLA-haploidentical HSCT from a NIMA mismatched relative, without using either T-cell depletion or intensive post-transplant immunosuppression (Ichinohe, Uchiyama et al. 2004; Kanda, Ichinohe et al. 2009).

Persistent MMc is associated with antigen-specific suppression of the associated T-cell responses (van Rood, Loberiza et al. 2002). With the help of highly sensitive polymerase chain reaction (PCR)-based techniques, long-term MMc can be detected from the peripheral blood, or various tissues including liver, skin, and thyroid gland (Ichinohe, Maruya et al. 2002). Several investigators have suggested the association of long-term MMc with the development of tolerance to NIMA (Kodera, Nishida et al. 2005). Thus, successful NIMA-mismatched haploidentical HSCT have been performed confirming long-term MMc as an indication of tolerance induction, in agreement with the correlation between MMc and tolerance in mice, which has been described recently (Dutta, Molitor-Dart et al. 2009). However, in some individuals unsuccessful NIMA-mismatched haploidentical HSCT have occurred, when the concept of MMc would have predicted otherwise.

The relevance of MiHA in tolerance to NIMA has not been reported. In both MHC-identical and MHC-haploidentical transplants, MiHA alloreactivities may be induced (Verdijk, Kloosterman et al. 2004). Therefore, maintaining the focus on the tolerance-induction of NIMA to MHC may have greater clinically relevance. In accord with this, we have shown differences in the NIMA tolerogenic effect in different individuals, divided into high responder (HR) or low responder (LR) categories, depending on the magnitude of the MLR of donor against recipient NIMA (Araki, Hirayama et al. 2010). The magnitude of the responses was associated with the extent of regulatory T cells (Treg) and Foxp3 expression in MHC-mismatched, MiHA-matched HSCT (Figure 2). This, with other reports, describe that Treg mediate tolerance to NIMA (Aluvihare, Kallikourdis et al. 2004; Matsuoka, Ichinohe et al. 2006). Survival rates and GVHD clinical scores of NIMA-exposed LR mice were significantly better than those of NIMA-exposed HR mice (Figure 3). Moreover, the level of MMc was correlated with the tolerogenic effect of the NIMA (Araki, Hirayama et al. 2010).

The mouse MiHA loci confers a wide range of immunogenicity, ranging from weakly to strongly immunogenic (Roopenian, Choi et al. 2002). Several studies have provided evidence that GVHD could be caused by only a limited number of mouse MiHA as described above (Choi, Yoshimura et al. 2001; Yang, Jaramillo et al. 2003; Eden, Christianson et al. 1999). The specific MiHA immunodominance was manifested on genetically varied backgrounds among B10, BALB/c, and DBA/2 strains (Sanderson and Frost 1974; Mendoza, Paz et al. 1997;

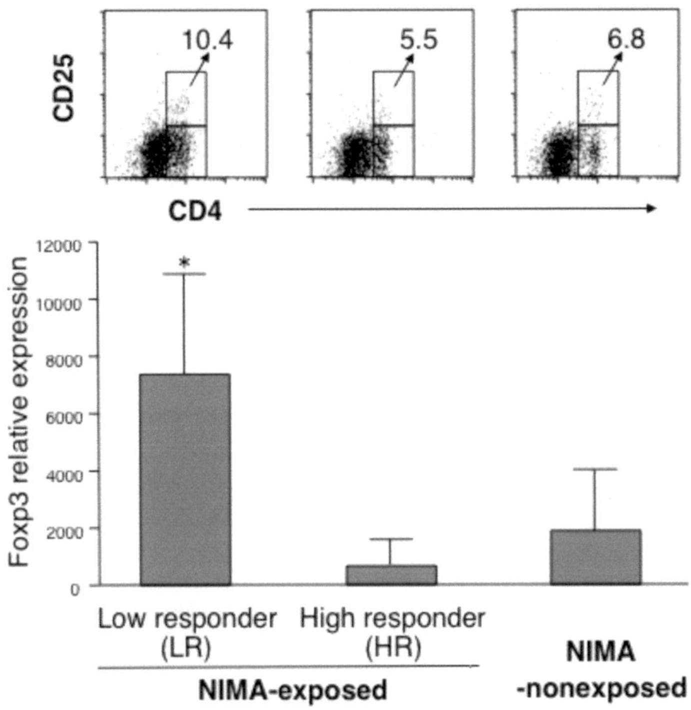

We have shown a difference of proliferative response to NIMA in NIMA-exposed and NIMA-non-exposed mice. The mice were classified into two groups by MLR, based on their reactivity to NIMA; the high responder (HR ≥ mean+1SD in NIMA-nonexposed) or the low responder (LR < mean+1SD) group (Araki, Hirayama et al. 2010). Upper, The percentage of $CD4^+CD25^+$ cells in $CD4^+$ cell population was analyzed by flow cytometry. Lower, The relative expression of Foxp3 compared with GAPDH is presented as the mean + SE. Samples were obtained 21 days after GVHD induction from recipients injected with cells from NIMA-exposed LR, HR, and NIMA-nonexposed mice (n=5 in each group). *p<0.05.

Fig. 2. Regulatory T cells and Foxp3 expression correlated with reactivity to MHC.

Malarkannan, Horng et al. 2000). Previously, there has been no report distinguishing the reactivities of MHC and MiHA from the tolerogenic effect of NIMA. We have proposed to classify the murine models of NIMA based on major and minor histocompatibility antigens to NIMA (Hirayama and Azuma 2011) (Figure 1C). In our study, all B10 congenic mice were used as the former NIMA model, "major only" (Figure 1B-I), and those MiHA had matched entirely in this system (Araki, Hirayama et al. 2010). On the other hand, the previous model (Andrassy, Kusaka et al. 2003; Matsuoka, Ichinohe et al. 2006) (Figure 1A) and the latter our model, "major + minor" (Figure 1B-II) were mismatched at both H-2 and MiHA. Therefore, we need to consider an influence of both major and minor histocompatibility when NIMA tolerance is evaluated (Hirayama and Azuma 2011) (Figure 1C).

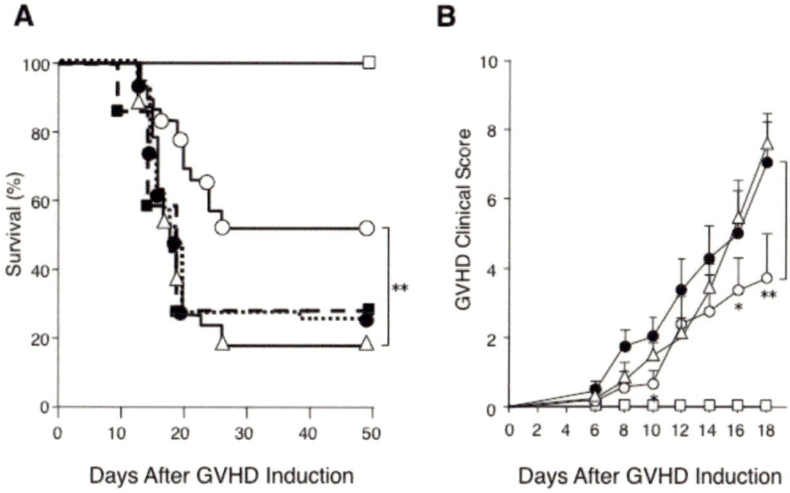

A, The survival of sublethally irradiated recipient B10 female mice injected with vehicle (□, n = 14), cells from NIMA-exposed LR mice (H-2[d/k], NIMA[b]) (○, n = 30), HR mice (NIMA[b]) (Δ, n = 33), NIMA-nonexposed mice (H-2[d/k], NIMA[none]) (•, n = 39), and allogeneic B10.D2 mice (▪, n =14). B, The GVHD clinical score was determined in recipients injected with cells from NIMA-exposed LR mice (○, n = 48), HR mice (Δ, n = 45), allogeneic mice (•, n = 47), and vehicle (□, n = 12). The degree of clinical GVHD was assessed by the scoring system that incorporates five clinical parameters: weight loss, posture, activity, fur texture, and skin integrity, grading from 0 to 2 for each parameter. A clinical index was subsequently generated by summation of the five criteria scores (maximum index=10). Data are expressed as the means + SE of individual animals. **p<0.01, *p<0.05.

Fig. 3. Two distinct reactivities to H-2 in NIMA-exposed mice resulted in differences in GVHD induction.

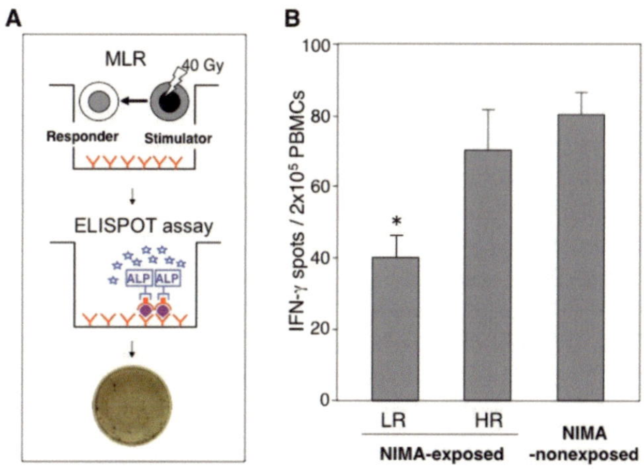

A, ELISPOT assay combining with MLR (MLR-ELISPOT) is a sensitive functional assay to detect alloreactivity for both major and minor histocompatibility antigens in mice. B, The IFN-γ-producing ability before GVHD induction was presented by MLR-ELISPOT. Peripheral blood mononuclear cells from NIMA-exposed LR mice (H-2[d/k], NIMA[b], n=8), HR mice (n=7), and nonexposed mice (n=6) were stimulated with B10 mice peripheral blood mononuclear cells. Data are expressed as the means + SE of individual animals. *p<0.05.

Fig. 4. Prediction of reactivity to NIMA by MLR-ELISPOT assay.

5. Reactivity to mismatched histocompatibility antgens; Tolerogenic or immunogenic?

The mechanisms by which NIMA drive the immune system toward tolerance or rejection of the allograft are still unclear. Although mismatch at MiHA can provoke severe immune responses against host cells upon transplantation (Goulmy, Schipper et al. 1996), the role of MiHA in the NIMA effects has not been described. Recently, naturally acquired tolerance and sensitization to MiHA have been reported (van Halteren, Jankowska-Gan et al. 2009). The presence of MiHA-specific Treg was shown in healthy adult women and men. In addition, it remains to be studied whether or not particular microchimeric cell types are associated with either a sensitized or a tolerized MiHA effect. Our study showed the difference of individual reactivities toward MHC, not MiHA, was critically influenced by the amount of MMc expression (Araki, Hirayama et al. 2010). The relationship between tolerogenic effect and MMc are consistent with a report of Dutta et al. They described the correlation between MMc and NIMA-specific Treg capable of suppressing both delayed type hypersensitivity and lymphoproliferative responses of effector T cells in a conventional NIMA mouse model (van Rood and Claas 1990; Andrassy, Kusaka et al. 2003). Opiela et al. described that transient exposure to low levels of NIMA alloantigens in early life may lead to long-term priming for both cytotoxic and helper T cell functions (Opiela, Levy et al. 2008). On the other hand, Aoyama et al. showed that both oral and in utero exposures to NIMA are required for the maximum induction of tolerance (Aoyama, Koyama et al. 2009). In any case, the mechanism underlying the development of tolerance versus priming to NIMA alloantigens remains to be clarified.

6. Prediction of acute GVHD in mismatched HSCT

Prediction of acute GVHD by in vitro assays prior to transplantation have not be very successful until now. In vitro detection of the frequencies of cytotoxic T-lymphocyte precursors (CTLp) and helper T-lymphocyte precursors (HTLp), in conjunction with MLR have been used as a method to detect individual reactivity to NIMA (Falkenburg, van Luxemburg-Heijs et al. 1996; Moretta, Locatelli et al. 1999; Tsafrir, Brautbar et al. 2000). Moretta et al. described that the frequency of NIMA-specific CTLp in cord blood samples were measured in order to better define the phenomenon of NIMA tolerance (Moretta, Locatelli et al. 1999). NIMA-reactive cord blood cells are detectable, but they were unable to detect differences between CTLp frequencies towards NIMA or NIPA. Falkenburg et al. investigated whether NIMA tolerance could allow transplantation over certain HLA barriers. Both CTLp and HTLp frequencies against NIPA were not statistically different than those directed against NIMA (Falkenburg, van Luxemburg-Heijs et al. 1996). Indeed, Kircher et al. showed that CTLp and HTLp frequencies were not predictive for the risk of acute GVHD in patients received allogeneic HSCT (Kircher, Niederwieser et al. 2004). Established test systems are therefore not available for the prediction of alloreactions and outcome after HSCT. Originally, it was predicted that CTLp reflects alloreactivity of class I mismatch, and HTLp reflect alloreactivity of class II mismatch. Levitsky et al. reported an evaluation of allogeneic reaction that used Treg (Levitsky, Miller et al. 2009). They generated carboxy-fluorescein diacetate succinimidyl ester-labeled $CD4^{+}CD25^{high}$ $FOXP3^{+}$ cells in MLR, which they called "Treg MLR". These cells had varying HLA disparities and varying reactivities to cell components. However, this method reflects only a difference related to MHC class II. Thus, the above-mentioned methods can detect MHC class I or class II separately, but it is difficult to detect them simultaneously. Recently, we reported a novel method, MLR-ELISPOT, to overcome these difficulties, as shown in Table 3.

Assay	Target antigen	References
Frequency of CTLp	MHC class I	(Hadley et al. 1990; Falkenburg et al. 1996; Moretta et al. 1999)
Frequency of HTLp	MHC class II	(Falkenburg et al. 1996; Kircher et al. 2004)
MLR, modified MLR	MHC class II	(Tsafrir, Brautbar et al. 2000)
Treg MLR	MHC class II	(Levitsky, Miller et al. 2009)
MLR-ELISPOT for IFN-γ	MHC class I and II (MiHA)	(Araki, Hirayama et al. 2010)

Table 3. Detection assay to allogeneic antigen

Alloreactivity of NIMA-exposed mice and NIMA-nonexposed mice were evaluated by MLR, and we found quite wider range of reactivity in the former compared with the latter. This helps to indicate that feto-maternal interaction acts on both tolerance (low responder) and sensitization (high responder) (Molitor-Dart, Andrassy et al. 2008; van Halteren, Jankowska-Gan et al. 2009). The reports from Tsafrir et al. and Falkenburg et al. detected a reactivity to NIMA by MLR (Falkenburg, van Luxemburg-Heijs et al. 1996), and CTLp and HTLp (Tsafrir, Brautbar et al. 2000), respectively. Interestingly, when we scrutinized the figures in their articles, individual reactivities of NIMA-exposed group showed a wider range than the control group, and those reactivities seem to be divided into low and high reactions, although they did not discuss these observations. This was further indication that reactivity to NIMA could be detected in vitro, and the condition of feto-maternal interaction promoted either tolerance (low-responder) or sensitization (high-responder).

Several investigators have reported that evaluations of reactivity to NIMA can be assessed, but the clinical relevance remains unknown. Presence of feto-maternal tolerance was anticipated due to MMc (Andrassy, Kusaka et al. 2003), and this concept has been used in clinical studies (Ichinohe, Maruya et al. 2002). Functional importance of MMc in humans has been further studied (Carter, Cerundolo et al. 1999; Cho, Choi et al. 2006). The majority of assays used to detect donor-derived cells in a recipient's blood exploit sex-mismatch between donor and recipient or the polymorphism of the HLA-DR region of the MHC, determined with sequence specific primer PCR (SSP-PCR). SSP-PCR is commonly used for HLA typing the extent of match between donors and recipients prior to transplantation, but may not work well for detection of MMc. The sensitivity of detection of this technique can range from 0.5% to 0.01%, more than adequate for routine HLA-typing, but MMc levels may be from 0.01% to 0.001%, well below the sensitivity of the assay. Therefore, the sensitivity of SSP-PCR for HLA-DR alleles has been increased by the introduction of a nested priming of exon 2 SSP-PCR approached. Most of NIMA-mismatched haploidentical HSCT in Japan require positive MMc of the donor by using the nested SSP-PCR (Ichinohe, Maruya et al. 2002; Carter, Cerundolo et al. 1999).

Although detection of MMc was clinically used for an indication of probable tolerance to NIMA, severe acute cases of GVHD developed (Okumura, Yamaguchi et al. 2007; Kanda, Ichinohe et al. 2009). Studies indicate that NIMA allografts do better than NIPA allografts in vivo (Burlingham, Grailer et al. 1998), and in vitro T-cell responses to NIMA are significantly reduced in IL-2 and IFN-γ production assays, compared with NIPA (Andrassy,

Kusaka et al. 2003). Tsafrir et al. demonstrated this NIMA effect using umbilical cord blood mononuclear cells by a MLR assay (Tsafrir, Brautbar et al. 2000), but Hadley et al. could not detect the NIMA effect using peripheral blood mononuclear cells from healthy individuals (Hadley, Phelan et al. 1990). Thus, there is not a useful method to predict a tolerogenic effect for NIMA, although these studies may suggest that newborns are more tolerogenic to NIMA than older individuals. Recently, we demonstrated that the level of cells producing IFN-γ, but not IL-4 and IL-10, were significantly lower in NIMA-exposed group than NIMA-nonexposed group by using an MLR-ELISPOT assay in a murine model (Araki, Hirayama et al. 2010) (Figure 4). This assay should be easily applicable to humans, and is a versatile method to detect reactivities to MHC class I as well as class II. And, it may also detect reactivity to MiHA (Table 3). In other words, this assay might be useful to predict the total immunological reaction of donor T cells to recipient in mismatched HSCT.

7. Conclusions

The risk of acute GVHD might be influenced by various genetic factors HLA, MiHA, or others (Hsu, Chida et al. 2002; Lin, Storer et al. 2003). NIMA-mismatched haploidentical HSCT has been improving with sustained engraftment, lower early treatment-related mortality, and acceptable rates of GVHD. However, it has been difficult to predict severe GVHD prior to transplantation. Our recent report has addressed the issue (Araki, Hirayama et al. 2010; Hirayama and Azuma 2011). NIMA effects directed toward MHC antigen were divided into high (immunogenic) and low (tolerogenic) reactivities. Our results in mice demonstrated that there was an unevenness in the acquisition and maintenance of MMc in the offspring. Further differential inheritance of MiHA did not influence our results, i.e., the variability amongst offspring was not due to solely to differences in MiHA gene inheritance. The variability seemed intrinsic to chance events in mammalian reproduction; i.e. allogeneic pregnancy and nursing itself (Aoyama, Koyama et al. 2009; Dutta, Molitor-Dart et al. 2009). To date, T-cell replete haploidentical transplantation is performed only in the presence of detected MMc in the recipient, although individual reactivity of donor to the receipient has not been evaluated. Could the pairing result in a low-responder/tolergenic or high-responder/immunogenic situation? Therefore, our recent study is clinically relevant. T-cell replete NIMA-mismatched haploidentical transplantation could be performed more safely by using our assay to evaluate IFN-γ-producing cells of donor against NIMA as a way to further reduce graft failure, prevent transplant mortality, and prevent severe GVHD.

8. Acknowledgments

This study was supported in part by a Research Grant for Tissue Engineering (H17-014) and a Research Grant for Allergic Disease and Immunology (H20-015) from the Japanese Ministry of Health, Labor, and Welfare.

9. References

Akatsuka, Y., T. Nishida, et al. (2003). Identification of a polymorphic gene, BCL2A1, encoding two novel hematopoietic lineage-specific minor histocompatibility antigens.*The Journal of experimental medicine* 197(11): 1489-1500.

Aluvihare, V. R., M. Kallikourdis, et al. (2004). Regulatory T cells mediate maternal tolerance to the fetus.*Nat Immunol* 5(3): 266-271.

Amos, D. B. (1968). Human histocompatibility locus HL-A.*Science* 159(815): 659-660.

Andrassy, J., S. Kusaka, et al. (2003). Tolerance to noninherited maternal MHC antigens in mice.*J Immunol* 171(10): 5554-5561.

Aoyama, K., M. Koyama, et al. (2009). Improved outcome of allogeneic bone marrow transplantation due to breastfeeding-induced tolerance to maternal antigens.*Blood* 113(8): 1829-1833.

Araki, M., M. Hirayama, et al. (2010). Prediction of reactivity to noninherited maternal antigen in MHC-mismatched, minor histocompatibility antigen-matched stem cell transplantation in a mouse model.*J Immunol* 185(12): 7739-7745.

Aversa, F., A. Tabilio, et al. (1994). Successful engraftment of T-cell-depleted haploidentical "three-loci" incompatible transplants in leukemia patients by addition of recombinant human granulocyte colony-stimulating factor-mobilized peripheral blood progenitor cells to bone marrow inoculum.*Blood* 84(11): 3948-3955.

Aversa, F., A. Terenzi, et al. (2005). Full haplotype-mismatched hematopoietic stem-cell transplantation: a phase II study in patients with acute leukemia at high risk of relapse.*J Clin Oncol* 23(15): 3447-3454.

Beatty, P. G., C. Anasetti, et al. (1993). Marrow transplantation from unrelated donors for treatment of hematologic malignancies: effect of mismatching for one HLA locus.*Blood* 81(1): 249-253.

Bleakley, M., B. E. Otterud, et al. (2010). Leukemia-associated minor histocompatibility antigen discovery using T-cell clones isolated by in vitro stimulation of naive CD8+ T cells.*Blood* 115(23): 4923-4933.

Brickner, A. G., A. M. Evans, et al. (2006). The PANE1 gene encodes a novel human minor histocompatibility antigen that is selectively expressed in B-lymphoid cells and B-CLL.*Blood* 107(9): 3779-3786.

Brickner, A. G., E. H. Warren, et al. (2001). The immunogenicity of a new human minor histocompatibility antigen results from differential antigen processing.*The Journal of experimental medicine* 193(2): 195-206.

Buckley, R. H., S. E. Schiff, et al. (1999). Hematopoietic stem-cell transplantation for the treatment of severe combined immunodeficiency.*N Engl J Med* 340(7): 508-516.

Burlingham, W. J., A. P. Grailer, et al. (1998). The effect of tolerance to noninherited maternal HLA antigens on the survival of renal transplants from sibling donors.*N Engl J Med* 339(23): 1657-1664.

Carter, A. S., L. Cerundolo, et al. (1999). Nested polymerase chain reaction with sequence-specific primers typing for HLA-A, -B, and -C alleles: detection of microchimerism in DR-matched individuals.*Blood* 94(4): 1471-1477.

Cho, B. S., H. B. Choi, et al. (2006). Typing by nested PCR-SSP approach raises a question about the feasibility of using this technique for detecting feto-maternal microchimerism.*Leukemia* 20(5): 896-898.

Choi, E. Y., Y. Yoshimura, et al. (2001). Quantitative analysis of the immune response to mouse non-MHC transplantation antigens in vivo: the H60 histocompatibility antigen dominates over all others.*Journal of immunology* 166(7): 4370-4379.

Claas, F. H., Y. Gijbels, et al. (1988). Induction of B cell unresponsiveness to noninherited maternal HLA antigens during fetal life.*Science* 241(4874): 1815-1817.

de Rijke, B., A. van Horssen-Zoetbrood, et al. (2005). A frameshift polymorphism in P2X5 elicits an allogeneic cytotoxic T lymphocyte response associated with remission of chronic myeloid leukemia.*The Journal of clinical investigation* 115(12): 3506-3516.

den Haan, J. M., N. E. Sherman, et al. (1995). Identification of a graft versus host disease-associated human minor histocompatibility antigen.*Science* 268(5216): 1476-1480.

Dolstra, H., H. Fredrix, et al. (1999). A human minor histocompatibility antigen specific for B cell acute lymphoblastic leukemia.*The Journal of experimental medicine* 189(2): 301-308.

Dutta, P., M. Molitor-Dart, et al. (2009). Microchimerism is strongly correlated with tolerance to noninherited maternal antigens in mice.*Blood* 114(17): 3578-3587.

Eden, P. A., G. J. Christianson, et al. (1999). Biochemical and immunogenetic analysis of an immunodominant peptide (B6dom1) encoded by the classical H7 minor histocompatibility locus.*Journal of immunology* 162(8): 4502-4510.

Falkenburg, J. H., S. A. van Luxemburg-Heijs, et al. (1996). Umbilical cord blood contains normal frequencies of cytotoxic T-lymphocyte precursors (ctlp) and helper T-lymphocyte precursors against noninherited maternal antigens and noninherited paternal antigens.*Ann Hematol* 72(4): 260-264.

Goulmy, E., R. Schipper, et al. (1996). Mismatches of minor histocompatibility antigens between HLA-identical donors and recipients and the development of graft-versus-host disease after bone marrow transplantation.*N Engl J Med* 334(5): 281-285.

Greenfield, A., D. Scott, et al. (1996). An H-YDb epitope is encoded by a novel mouse Y chromosome gene.*Nature genetics* 14(4): 474-478.

Griffioen, M., E. D. van der Meijden, et al. (2008). Identification of phosphatidylinositol 4-kinase type II beta as HLA class II-restricted target in graft versus leukemia reactivity.*Proceedings of the National Academy of Sciences of the United States of America* 105(10): 3837-3842.

Guinan, E. C., V. A. Boussiotis, et al. (1999). Transplantation of anergic histoincompatible bone marrow allografts.*N Engl J Med* 340(22): 1704-1714.

Hadley, G. A., D. Phelan, et al. (1990). Lack of T-cell tolerance of noninherited maternal HLA antigens in normal humans.*Hum Immunol* 28(4): 373-381.

Hall, J. M., P. Lingenfelter, et al. (1995). Detection of maternal cells in human umbilical cord blood using fluorescence in situ hybridization.*Blood* 86(7): 2829-2832.

Henslee-Downey, P. J., S. H. Abhyankar, et al. (1997). Use of partially mismatched related donors extends access to allogeneic marrow transplant.*Blood* 89(10): 3864-3872.

Hirayama, M. and E. Azuma (2011). Major and minor histocompatibility antigens to NIMA: Prediction of a tolerogenic NIMA effect.*Chimerism* 2(1): 23-24.

Hsu, K. C., S. Chida, et al. (2002). The killer cell immunoglobulin-like receptor (KIR) genomic region: gene-order, haplotypes and allelic polymorphism.*Immunol Rev* 190: 40-52.

Huang, X. J., D. H. Liu, et al. (2009). Treatment of acute leukemia with unmanipulated HLA-mismatched/haploidentical blood and bone marrow transplantation.*Biol Blood Marrow Transplant* 15(2): 257-265.

Ichinohe, T., E. Maruya, et al. (2002). Long-term feto-maternal microchimerism: nature's hidden clue for alternative donor hematopoietic cell transplantation?*Int J Hematol* 76(3): 229-237.

Ichinohe, T., T. Uchiyama, et al. (2004). Feasibility of HLA-haploidentical hematopoietic stem cell transplantation between noninherited maternal antigen (NIMA)-mismatched family members linked with long-term fetomaternal microchimerism.*Blood* 104(12): 3821-3828.

Kamei, M., Y. Nannya, et al. (2009). HapMap scanning of novel human minor histocompatibility antigens.*Blood* 113(21): 5041-5048.

Kanda, J., T. Ichinohe, et al. (2009). Long-term survival after HLA-haploidentical SCT from noninherited maternal antigen-mismatched family donors: impact of chronic GVHD.*Bone Marrow Transplant* 44(5): 327-329.Kawase, T., Y. Akatsuka, et al. (2007). Alternative splicing due to an intronic SNP in HMSD generates a novel minor histocompatibility antigen.*Blood* 110(3): 1055-1063.

Kircher, B., D. Niederwieser, et al. (2004). No predictive value of cytotoxic or helper T-cell precursor frequencies for outcome when analyzed from the graft after stem cell transplantation.*Ann Hematol* 83(9): 566-572.

Kodera, Y., T. Nishida, et al. (2005). Human leukocyte antigen haploidentical hematopoietic stem cell transplantation: indications and tentative outcomes in Japan.*Semin Hematol* 42(2): 112-118.

Levitsky, J., J. Miller, et al. (2009). The human "Treg MLR": immune monitoring for FOXP3+ T regulatory cell generation.*Transplantation* 88(11): 1303-1311.

Lin, M. T., B. Storer, et al. (2003). Relation of an interleukin-10 promoter polymorphism to graft-versus-host disease and survival after hematopoietic-cell transplantation.*N Engl J Med* 349(23): 2201-2210.

Lo, Y. M., E. S. Lo, et al. (1996). Two-way cell traffic between mother and fetus: biologic and clinical implications.*Blood* 88(11): 4390-4395.

Lu, D. P., L. Dong, et al. (2006). Conditioning including antithymocyte globulin followed by unmanipulated HLA-mismatched/haploidentical blood and marrow transplantation can achieve comparable outcomes with HLA-identical sibling transplantation.*Blood* 107(8): 3065-3073.

Luedtke, B., L. M. Pooler, et al. (2003). A single nucleotide polymorphism in the Emp3 gene defines the H4 minor histocompatibility antigen.*Immunogenetics* 55(5): 284-295.

Malarkannan, S., T. Horng, et al. (2000). Differences that matter: major cytotoxic T cell-stimulating minor histocompatibility antigens.*Immunity* 13(3): 333-344.

Maloney, S., A. Smith, et al. (1999). Microchimerism of maternal origin persists into adult life.*J Clin Invest* 104(1): 41-47.

Markiewicz, M. A., C. Girao, et al. (1998). Long-term T cell memory requires the surface expression of self-peptide/major histocompatibility complex molecules.*Proceedings of the National Academy of Sciences of the United States of America* 95(6): 3065-3070.

Matsuoka, K., T. Ichinohe, et al. (2006). Fetal tolerance to maternal antigens improves the outcome of allogeneic bone marrow transplantation by a CD4+ CD25+ T-cell-dependent mechanism.*Blood* 107(1): 404-409.

Mehta, J., S. Singhal, et al. (2004). Bone marrow transplantation from partially HLA-mismatched family donors for acute leukemia: single-center experience of 201 patients.*Bone Marrow Transplant* 33(4): 389-396.

Mendoza, L. M., P. Paz, et al. (1997). Minors held by majors: the H13 minor histocompatibility locus defined as a peptide/MHC class I complex.*Immunity* 7(4): 461-472.

Mendoza, L. M., G. Villaflor, et al. (2001). Distinguishing self from nonself: immunogenicity of the murine H47 locus is determined by a single amino acid substitution in an unusual peptide.*Journal of immunology* 166(7): 4438-4445.

Molitor-Dart, M. L., J. Andrassy, et al. (2008). Tolerance induction or sensitization in mice exposed to noninherited maternal antigens (NIMA).*Am J Transplant* 8(11): 2307-2315.

Mommaas, B., J. Kamp, et al. (2002). Identification of a novel HLA-B60-restricted T cell epitope of the minor histocompatibility antigen HA-1 locus.*Journal of immunology* 169(6): 3131-3136.

Moretta, A., F. Locatelli, et al. (1999). Characterisation of CTL directed towards non-inherited maternal alloantigens in human cord blood.*Bone Marrow Transplant* 24(11): 1161-1166.

Murata, M., E. H. Warren, et al. (2003). A human minor histocompatibility antigen resulting from differential expression due to a gene deletion.*The Journal of experimental medicine* 197(10): 1279-1289.

O'Reilly, R. J., C. Keever, et al. (1987). HLA nonidentical T cell depleted marrow transplants: a comparison of results in patients treated for leukemia and severe combined immunodeficiency disease.*Transplant Proc* 19(6 Suppl 7): 55-60.

Okumura, H., M. Yamaguchi, et al. (2007). Graft rejection and hyperacute graft-versus-host disease in stem cell transplantation from non-inherited maternal-antigen-complementary HLA-mismatched siblings.*Eur J Haematol* 78(2): 157-160.

Opiela, S. J., R. B. Levy, et al. (2008). Murine neonates develop vigorous in vivo cytotoxic and Th1/Th2 responses upon exposure to low doses of NIMA-like alloantigens.*Blood* 112(4): 1530-1538.

Owen, R. D., H. R. Wood, et al. (1954). EVIDENCE FOR ACTIVELY ACQUIRED TOLERANCE TO Rh ANTIGENS.*Proc Natl Acad Sci U S A* 40(6): 420-424.

Perreault, C., J. Jutras, et al. (1996). Identification of an immunodominant mouse minor histocompatibility antigen (MiHA). T cell response to a single dominant MiHA causes graft-versus-host disease.*The Journal of clinical investigation* 98(3): 622-628.

Petersdorf, E. W., G. M. Longton, et al. (1995). The significance of HLA-DRB1 matching on clinical outcome after HLA-A, B, DR identical unrelated donor marrow transplantation.*Blood* 86(4): 1606-1613.

Pierce, R. A., E. D. Field, et al. (1999). Cutting edge: the HLA-A*0101-restricted HY minor histocompatibility antigen originates from DFFRY and contains a cysteinylated cysteine residue as identified by a novel mass spectrometric technique.*Journal of immunology* 163(12): 6360-6364.

Reisner, Y., N. Kapoor, et al. (1981). Transplantation for acute leukaemia with HLA-A and B nonidentical parental marrow cells fractionated with soybean agglutinin and sheep red blood cells.*Lancet* 2(8242): 327-331.

Rizzieri, D. A., L. P. Koh, et al. (2007). Partially matched, nonmyeloablative allogeneic transplantation: clinical outcomes and immune reconstitution.*J Clin Oncol* 25(6): 690-697.

Roopenian, D., E. Y. Choi, et al. (2002). The immunogenomics of minor histocompatibility antigens.*Immunol Rev* 190: 86-94.

Sahara, H. and N. Shastri (2003). Second class minors: molecular identification of the autosomal H46 histocompatibility locus as a peptide presented by major histocompatibility complex class II molecules.*The Journal of experimental medicine* 197(3): 375-385.

Sanderson, C. J. and P. Frost (1974). The induction of tumour immunity in mice using glutaraldehyde-treated tumor cells.*Nature* 248(450): 690-691.

Scott, D., C. Addey, et al. (2000). Dendritic cells permit identification of genes encoding MHC class II-restricted epitopes of transplantation antigens.*Immunity* 12(6): 711-720.

Sellami, M. H., H. Kaabi, et al. (2011). Minor histocompatibility antigens in Tunisians: could platelet endothelial cell adhesion molecule 1 marker be one of them?*Tissue antigens* 77(1): 68-73.

Slager, E. H., M. W. Honders, et al. (2006). Identification of the angiogenic endothelial-cell growth factor-1/thymidine phosphorylase as a potential target for immunotherapy of cancer.*Blood* 107(12): 4954-4960.

Spaapen, R. M., R. A. de Kort, et al. (2009). Rapid identification of clinical relevant minor histocompatibility antigens via genome-wide zygosity-genotype correlation analysis.*Clinical cancer research : an official journal of the American Association for Cancer Research* 15(23): 7137-7143.

Spaapen, R. M., H. M. Lokhorst, et al. (2008). Toward targeting B cell cancers with CD4+ CTLs: identification of a CD19-encoded minor histocompatibility antigen using a novel genome-wide analysis.*The Journal of experimental medicine* 205(12): 2863-2872.

Spierings, E., A. G. Brickner, et al. (2003). The minor histocompatibility antigen HA-3 arises from differential proteasome-mediated cleavage of the lymphoid blast crisis (Lbc) oncoprotein.*Blood* 102(2): 621-629.

Spierings, E., C. J. Vermeulen, et al. (2003). Identification of HLA class II-restricted H-Y-specific T-helper epitope evoking CD4+ T-helper cells in H-Y-mismatched transplantation.*Lancet* 362(9384): 610-615.

Stern, M., J. R. Passweg, et al. (2006). Influence of donor/recipient sex matching on outcome of allogeneic hematopoietic stem cell transplantation for aplastic anemia.*Transplantation* 82(2): 218-226.

Stumpf, A. N., E. D. van der Meijden, et al. (2009). Identification of 4 new HLA-DR-restricted minor histocompatibility antigens as hematopoietic targets in antitumor immunity.*Blood* 114(17): 3684-3692.

Torikai, H., Y. Akatsuka, et al. (2006). The human cathepsin H gene encodes two novel minor histocompatibility antigen epitopes restricted by HLA-A*3101 and -A*3303.*British journal of haematology* 134(4): 406-416.

Torikai, H., Y. Akatsuka, et al. (2004). A novel HLA-A*3303-restricted minor histocompatibility antigen encoded by an unconventional open reading frame of human TMSB4Y gene.*Journal of immunology* 173(11): 7046-7054.

Tsafrir, A., C. Brautbar, et al. (2000). Alloreactivity of umbilical cord blood mononuclear cells: specific hyporesponse to noninherited maternal antigens.*Hum Immunol* 61(6): 548-554.

Tykodi, S. S., N. Fujii, et al. (2008). C19orf48 encodes a minor histocompatibility antigen recognized by CD8+ cytotoxic T cells from renal cell carcinoma patients.*Clinical cancer research : an official journal of the American Association for Cancer Research* 14(16): 5260-5269.

van Bergen, C. A., M. G. Kester, et al. (2007). Multiple myeloma-reactive T cells recognize an activation-induced minor histocompatibility antigen encoded by the ATP-dependent interferon-responsive (ADIR) gene.*Blood* 109(9): 4089-4096.

Van Bergen, C. A., C. E. Rutten, et al. (2010). High-throughput characterization of 10 new minor histocompatibility antigens by whole genome association scanning.*Cancer research* 70(22): 9073-9083.

van Halteren, A. G., E. Jankowska-Gan, et al. (2009). Naturally acquired tolerance and sensitization to minor histocompatibility antigens in healthy family members.*Blood* 114(11): 2263-2272.

van Rood, J. J. and F. H. Claas (1990). The influence of allogeneic cells on the human T and B cell repertoire.*Science* 248(4961): 1388-1393.

van Rood, J. J., F. R. Loberiza, Jr., et al. (2002). Effect of tolerance to noninherited maternal antigens on the occurrence of graft-versus-host disease after bone marrow transplantation from a parent or an HLA-haploidentical sibling.*Blood* 99(5): 1572-1577.

Verdijk, R. M., A. Kloosterman, et al. (2004). Pregnancy induces minor histocompatibility antigen-specific cytotoxic T cells: implications for stem cell transplantation and immunotherapy.*Blood* 103(5): 1961-1964.

Verhasselt, V., V. Milcent, et al. (2008). Breast milk-mediated transfer of an antigen induces tolerance and protection from allergic asthma.*Nat Med* 14(2): 170-175.

Vogt, M. H., E. Goulmy, et al. (2000). UTY gene codes for an HLA-B60-restricted human male-specific minor histocompatibility antigen involved in stem cell graft rejection: characterization of the critical polymorphic amino acid residues for T-cell recognition.*Blood* 96(9): 3126-3132.

Wang, W., L. R. Meadows, et al. (1995). Human H-Y: a male-specific histocompatibility antigen derived from the SMCY protein.*Science* 269(5230): 1588-1590.

Warren, E. H., N. J. Vigneron, et al. (2006). An antigen produced by splicing of noncontiguous peptides in the reverse order.*Science* 313(5792): 1444-1447.

Yang, J., A. Jaramillo, et al. (2003). Chronic rejection of murine cardiac allografts discordant at the H13 minor histocompatibility antigen correlates with the generation of the H13-specific CD8+ cytotoxic T cells.*Transplantation* 76(1): 84-91.

Zorn, E., D. B. Miklos, et al. (2004). Minor histocompatibility antigen DBY elicits a coordinated B and T cell response after allogeneic stem cell transplantation.*The Journal of experimental medicine* 199(8): 1133-1142.

Zuberi, A. R., G. J. Christianson, et al. (1998). Positional cloning and molecular characterization of an immunodominant cytotoxic determinant of the mouse H3 minor histocompatibility complex.*Immunity* 9(5): 687-698.

10

MHC Class I Quality Control

Gustav Røder, Linda Geironson, Elna Follin,
Camilla Thuring and Kajsa Paulsson
Lund University
Sweden

1. Introduction

The immune system of higher organisms has the unique capability of mounting a specific and adaptive response against invading pathogens. *Specific* in the sense that immune cells recognize molecular features from foreign pathogens, and *adaptive* in the sense that upon re-encounter of the foreign pathogen the immune system respond faster and more efficiently, which is the basic principle used in vaccination. In addition, the immune system has evolved the innate capability of recognizing common, slow mutating features on pathogens by using several different pattern recognition receptors. These defense mechanisms are important, but just like any other organisms pathogens also mutate to adapt to selection pressures thereby escaping immune surveillance. Likewise, the immune system of higher organisms is not a static system, but rather a dynamic ever-changing defense system continuously evolving over millions of years to constantly battle pathogens trying to overcome immune defense barriers and take over the host protein translation machinery. Furthermore, the immune system needs to be in balance with its host, but sometimes the line between functional immunity and auto-reactivity becomes hard to draw. Importantly, it is now a firmly established concept that the immune system eradicates host cells undergoing malignant transformation to prevent tumor formation. With these functions in mind, it is reasonable to claim the adaptive immune system as highly essential in the protection of pathogenic infections and malignant cells. The adaptive immune system contains a variety of T cells; two major groups are the $CD4^+$ T cells that interact with MHC class II (MHC-II) cell surface receptors, and $CD8^+$ T cells, also termed cytotoxic T cells (CTLs) that interact with MHC class I (MHC-I) cell surface receptors. The CTLs kill malignant host cells or host cells infected with foreign pathogens. This chapter focuses on the immunology concerning CTLs and MHC-I. Specifically, we focus on the multi-step, intracellular maturation of MHC-I.

CTLs continuously re-circulate throughout our body and secondary lymphoid organs to scan our cells for peptides presented on MHC-I. These peptides are derived from the interior of the cell, and presented on MHC-I outside the cell on its membrane surface. Each MHC-I receptor binds and presents one small endogenous or foreign peptide, which is derived from within the cell, (Roder, Geironson et al. 2008) and the entire ligand-receptor complex is termed a peptide-MHC-I complex (pMHC-I). Essentially, through their T cell receptor (TcR) the CTLs may recognize a particular pMHC-I on the cell surface of the presenting cell. The strength and outcome of this recognition depends on the identity of both the TcR and the pMHC-I, and occurs normally only when a foreign peptide is bound in the pMHC-I. This is the exact purpose of MHC-I defense system: use peptides to report any intracellular abnormalities such as infections or malignant states, and make the CTLs kill these cells. In the secondary lymphoid organs naïve CTLs encounter the pMHC-I complexes presented by professional APCs, cells with unique co-stimulatory capability able to prime naïve T cells. Upon recognition of a pMHC-I complex the CTLs become active dividing cells able to kill infected cells outside the lymphoid organs (Santana and Esquivel-Guadarrama 2006). An important characteristic of CTL activity is that it is pMHC-I restricted, giving that it only recognizes the peptide antigen in the context of a certain MHC-I molecule. Also, the pMHC-I is only recognized if it reaches and remains on the cell surface of the APC. If the pMHC-I disintegrates along the maturation and transport to, or while staying at, the cell surface it will never be available for CTL scrutiny. These criteria impose serious requirements to the intricate MHC-I maturation processes inside the cell as we shall describe in this chapter.

2. The mature MHC-I binds only certain peptides in its binding groove

Before we delve deep into the MHC-I maturation in the cell, we first introduce the reader to the final product - the mature pMHC-I complex and some of its important properties. MHC-I molecules are found on most nucleated cells in the body. The MHC-I in humans is called human leukocyte antigen class I (HLA-I) and is grouped into A, B and C based on the genetic locus. Because the protein products, the allomorphs, of the alleles occupying the HLA-A, -B and -C loci are all co-dominantly expressed and chromosomes exist in pairs, one from the paternal and one from the maternal side, usually six different allomorphs are expressed in each human. To date (2011), over 5,000 different alleles and over 3,000 different allomorphs have been identified and sequence information is freely available from the HLA Informatics Group (http://www.anthonynolan.com/HIG/data.html). As seen in figure 1 the final pMHC-I complex consists of a MHC-I heavy chain (HC) that is folded into three α-domains; the α_1- and α_2-domains are intertwined making up the membrane distal peptide binding groove, whereas the membrane proximal α_3-domain has an Ig-like structure that supports binding of the MHC-I light chain, β_2-microglobulin (β_2m). In addition, β_2m stabilizes from below the anti-parallel β-sheets and α–helices allowing these structural elements to create a large, but tight, peptide binding groove containing six peptide amino acid binding pockets.

These pockets are very important in determining the peptide binding specificity of any particular MHC-I allomorph. The MHC-I residues in each binding pocket determine, which peptide residues are compatible enough to bind in the pocket, and thus determine the requirement for particular residues at particular positions in the binding peptide. This is the MHC-I peptide binding specificity, and it turns out that only a few residue positions in the peptide are the major determinants of peptide binding specificity. Thus, only a small fraction of the entire peptide universe will be allowed to bind to any particular MHC-I allomorph, and it is this knowledge that is one important key to allow us to design peptide-based vaccines that are highly specific, cheap and easy to disseminate. In this respect, it is important to understand MHC-I maturation and the underlying criteria.

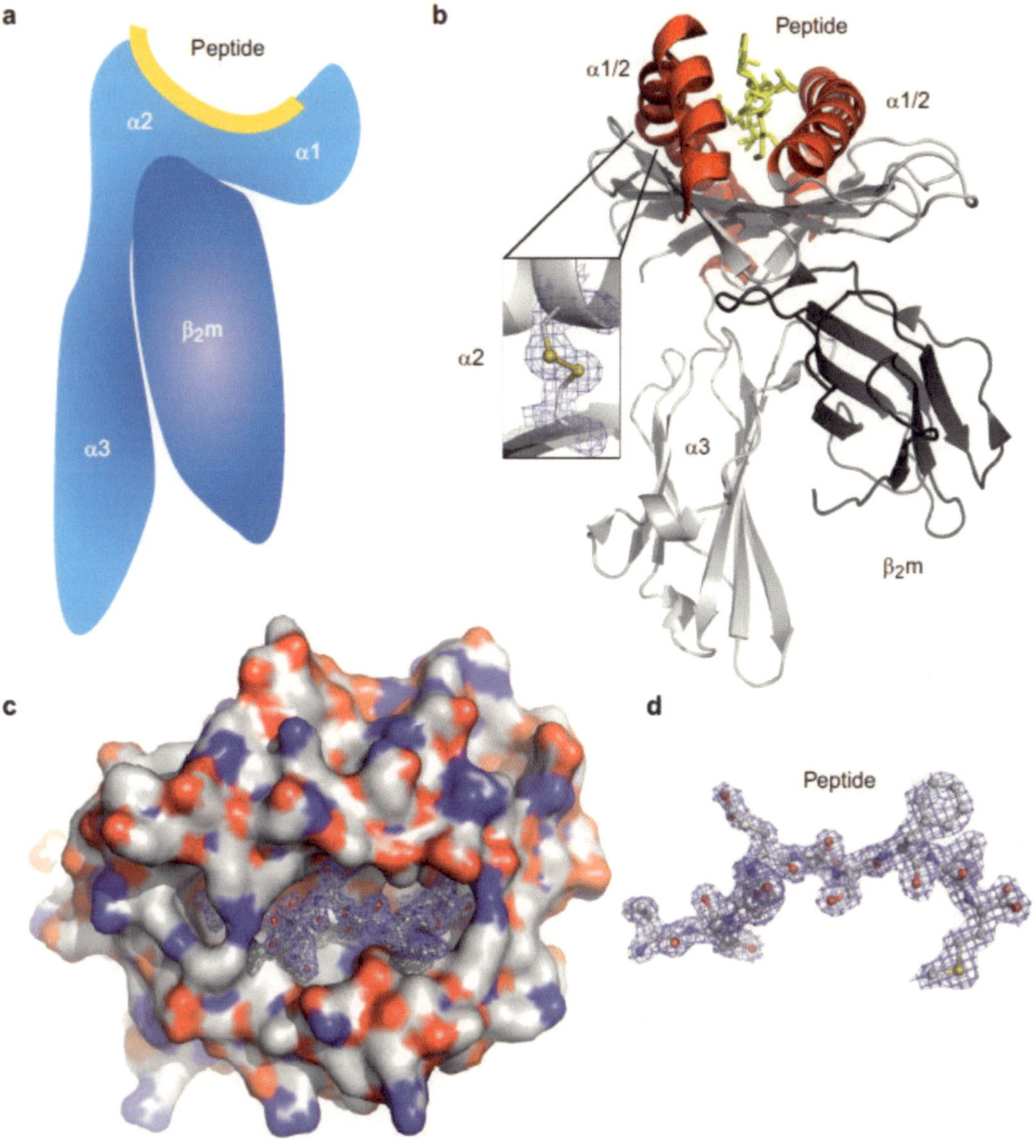

Fig. 1. The MHC-I protein structure allows short peptides to bind tightly in the peptide binding groove spanning the MHC-I α_1/α_2-domains. A) Schematic structure of MHC-I, which consists of a HC with 3 α-domains (light blue) and β_2m (dark blue). In the peptide binding groove (at the top) the MHC-I has bound a peptide (yellow). B) The protein crystal structure of HLA-B*15:01. The HC is colored light grey and β_2m is colored dark grey. The peptide binding groove is located at the top between two encapsulating α-helices (red). The peptide (yellow) is seen from the C-terminal. The electron density of the Cys101-Cys164 disulfide bond in the peptide binding groove is shown in the inset. C) Top down view of the MHC-I peptide binding groove. D) The electron density of the peptide (LEKARGSTY). Shown from the α_2-helix the peptide N-terminal is at the left.

3. MHC-I matures and is loaded with peptide inside the cell

The maturation of MHC-I and ultimate generation of pMHC-I complexes initially involves two different processes that later merge into one common maturation process. Firstly, the HC and β_2m have to be produced separately and translocated into the endoplasmic reticulum (ER). At the same time, the peptide that will later bind to the MHC-I has to be produced and transported into the lumen of the ER. The entire MHC-I antigen processing machinery (APM) process is illustrated in figure 2 showing the accessory proteins and chaperones involved in the stepwise processes ultimately resulting in a fully mature pMHC-I complex that is exported to and situated on the cell surface.

Several APM components are involved in the MHC-I quality control cycle, and regulates the sequential maturation process of MHC-I (Paulsson and Wang 2004). The HC undergoes co-translational glycosylation while being translocated into the ER lumen in a nascent unfolded state. Inside the ER the HC instantly interacts with BiP, the Hsp90 protein, and soon also with calnexin, a general ER lectin chaperone. Calnexin binds to newly synthesized proteins with mono-glycosylated N-linked glycans, and in line with this also to early folding stages of the N-glycosylated HC (Ware, Vassilakos et al. 1995). This initial chaperoning of the HC prevents it from collapse and aggregation, and also sets the HC in a conformation that allows mature β_2m to bind the HC forming the MHC-I heterodimer. Calnexin interacts with ERp57, a member of the protein disulfide isomerase (PDI) family, and is thought to involve in the correct formation of disulfide bonds within the HC (Oliver, Roderick et al. 1999). These intramolecular disulfide bonds strengthen the structural integrity and stability of the final pMHC-I complex. The newly formed MHC-I heterodimer is inherently unstable, but might be partly stabilized by binding a suboptimal peptide that later dissociates from the MHC-I. During these maturation steps calnexin dissociates from MHC-I and is immediately replaced by calreticulin, its soluble homologue.

At this stage the MHC-I might not be further matured due to the following reasons: 1) The MHC-I has acquired a peptide that induces final MHC-I maturation, 2) the particular MHC-I allomorph is inherently less prone to, or binds a peptide not inducing full maturation but inducing a structure not able to integrate into the peptide-loading complex (PLC), or 3), the MHC-I integration into the PLC is prohibited by viral interference (Roder, Geironson et al. 2008). However, for most HLA-I allomorphs the majority of MHC-I molecules are integrated into the PLC through binding to tapasin, where the late-stage maturation of the pMHC-I complex takes place. Tapasin has been ascribed many functions besides integrating MHC-I into the PLC. One of the most important functions, but also difficult to study, is to edit - and thereby optimize - the peptide loaded onto the MHC-I in the PLC with the purpose of generating stable pMHC-I complexes. In the PLC, which at least consists of the transporter associated with antigen processing (TAP), tapasin, calreticulin and ERp57, the MHC-I finally matures into a stable pMHC-I complex. ERp57 has proven important in the PLC, because it forms a disulfide conjugate with tapasin (Peaper, Wearsch et al. 2005). The tapasin-ERp57 disulfide conjugate has been suggested to significantly boost the efficiency, whereby tapasin edits the MHC-I bound peptide repertoire (Wearsch and Cresswell 2007).

So far, we have discussed the production and initial folding of the MHC-I. The generation and supply of peptides is equally important in the maturation of the final pMHC-I complex, and it all starts in the cytosol. Here, proteins are produced by the ribosome, but sometimes the production fails, resulting in defective ribosomal products (DRiPs). The DRiPs are targeted for degradation by the cytosolic *proteasome,* and it is from this cleavage process that peptides are generated. It has been proposed that a large fraction of the MHC-I binding peptides derive from DRiPs (Yewdell, Anton et al. 1996). Other cytosolic proteases, such as TPPII, may assist in trimming the proteasome processed peptides.

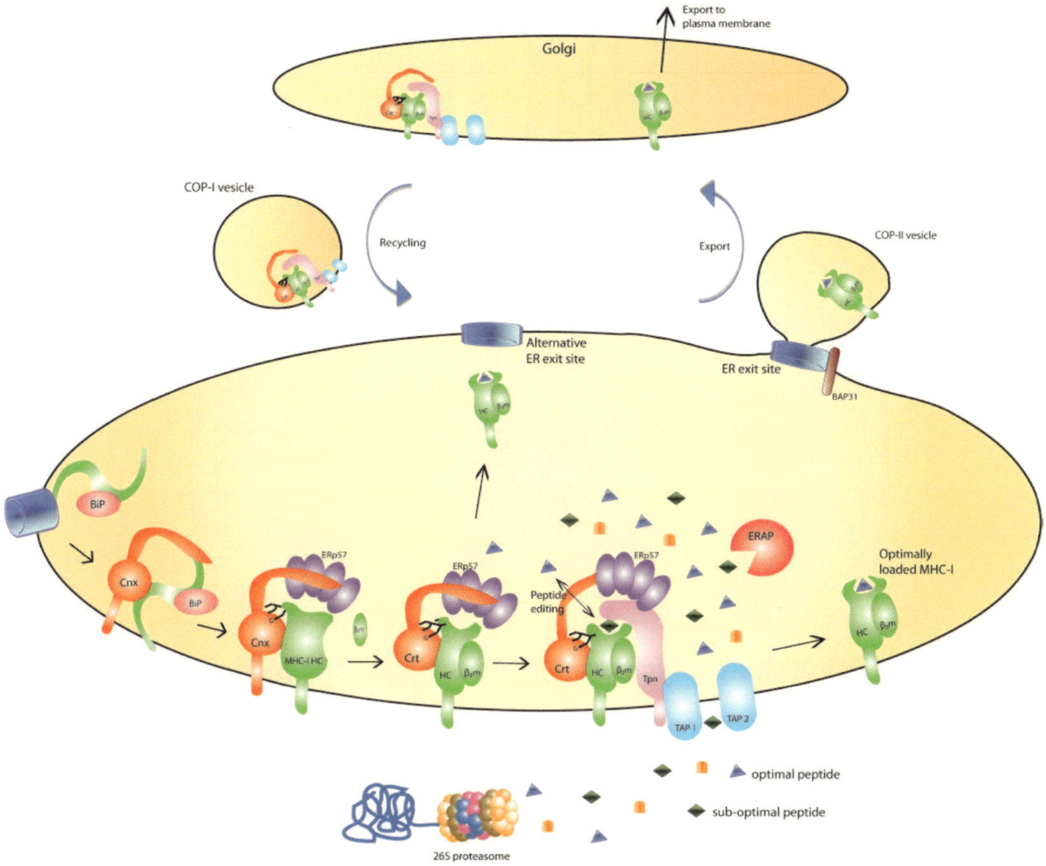

Fig. 2. An array of APM components present in the ER and the cytosol is involved in the sequential maturation and peptide loading of MHC-I. Early folding stages of MHC-I are promoted by BiP and then calnexin, which recruits ERp57. Subsequently, the MHC-I HC associates with β_2m, and calnexin is replaced by calreticulin. Most of the MHC-I molecules are recruited into the PLC, which consists of ERp57, calreticulin, tapasin and TAP, where the folding of the mature MHC-I conformation as well as peptide loading is facilitated. Peptides are generated in the cytosol by the proteasome and trimmed in the ER to MHC-I optimal lengths by ERAP1. MHC-I molecules loaded with optimal peptides become stable and can exit the ER and be transported via the Golgi network to the cell surface, possibly, between ER and Golgi, through transport in COP-II vesicles. Loading of an optimal peptide can also occur before recruitment into PLC. The stable pMHC-I complex can the exit the ER through alternative ER exit sites for transport to the cell surface. Sub-optimally loaded MHC-I molecules can escape the ER but are the recycled in COP-I vesicles recruited by tapasin, which recycles the MHC-I molecule back to the ER for optimal loading.

An essential part of the PLC is the heterodimeric TAP, which is composed of the TAP1 and TAP2 subunits, both containing an N-terminal transmembrane domain and a C-terminal cytosolic nucleotide-binding domain. Situated in the ER membrane TAP actively translocates the cytosolic peptides into the ER in a multistep process, which begins with association of peptides, usually 8-16 amino acid long with TAP (van Endert, Tampe et al. 1994). Peptide binding to TAP is followed by an isomerization of the TAP complex that triggers an ATP-dependent peptide translocation across the ER membrane (Neefjes, Momburg et al. 1993). Many of the peptides that are transported by TAP into the ER lumen are still too long to bind firmly in the MHC-I peptide binding groove. These peptides are then further trimmed by the ER aminopeptidases ERAP1 and ERAP2 at the extended N-terminus to 8-10 amino acids, which is the appropriate length for association with MHC-I (York, Chang et al. 2002; Tanioka, Hattori et al. 2003).

We define an *optimal* MHC-I binding peptide as a peptide binding to MHC-I resulting in a stable pMHC-I complex. Thus, as a general rule, an optimal peptide has to bind firmly in the MHC-I peptide binding pockets. When a stable pMHC-I is formed, it is released from the PLC and transported to the cell surface. This underscores the importance of PLC-mediated pMHC-I quality control. pMHC-I complexes that consists only of suboptimal peptides are (per definition) unstable, and are not released from the PLC. This ensures the release of only stable pMHC-I complexes to the cell surface, which is vital for the subsequent CTL scrutiny. The pMHC-I transportation to the cell surface has been suggested to start with packaging of the pMHC-I complexes in COPII vesicles, which then migrate to the Golgi apparatus, and then further on to the cell surface (Paquet, Cohen-Doyle et al. 2004). The following sections discuss the MHC-I maturation, and peptide supply in much more detail.

4. The MHC-I maturation is facilitated by multi-protein complexes in the ER

In this section we go through the details of the HC production and folding in the ER involving APM components such as calnexin, calreticulin, ERp57 and tapasin. The chaperone BiP, known to interact cotranslationally with the nascent HC before other chaperones will not be further discussed. The following interactions of HC with each APM component are discussed in the maturation sequence as it is thought to occur.

4.1 Calnexin and calreticulin shape the initial MHC-I heterodimer

Both calnexin and its soluble homologue calreticulin are part of the general ER protein folding machinery, and bind to mono-glucosylated proteins. Despite overlapping substrate specificities, they also have distinct preferences, which can be explained by: 1) the positions and numbers of the glycosylation sites on the target protein (High, Lecomte et al. 2000), and 2) the membrane anchoring of calnexin versus the soluble calreticulin. The latter was shown to be a major determinant, since an experiment with soluble calnexin demonstrated that the glycoprotein association pattern for soluble calnexin resembles the pattern for calreticulin (Danilczyk, Cohen-Doyle et al. 2000). Similarly, calreticulin expressed with an ER membrane anchor binds to a set of glycoproteins resembling those proteins normally bound to calnexin (Wada, Imai et al. 1995).

4.1.1 Calnexin and calreticulin bind differently to MHC-I around the glycosylation site

As alluded to in the previous section, the location of the glycosylation sequon in the MHC-I determines its binding to calnexin and calreticulin, which would then be reflected in the sequential maturation of MHC-I. Human MHC-I HCs have a single N-linked glycosylation site at Asn86, whereas mouse HC possess glycosylation sequons at additional sites (Maloy 1987). To support this notion, experiments have shown that introduction of a second glycosylation site in the human HC at the same position as in mouse HC, resulted in a maturation process that more resembled the mouse HCs with respect to calnexin and calreticulin association (Zhang and Salter 1998). In the human, the HC glycosylation sequon is located close to the ER membrane during translocation into the ER, calnexin first gains access to this site. Calnexin induces β_2m binding to the HC, which brings the glycosylation sequon away from the membrane allowing the soluble calreticulin to replace calnexin (Solheim, Carreno et al. 1997).

In the β_2m deficient human cell line Daudi, there is little or no association of MHC-I HC with calreticulin, suggesting that calreticulin only binds the MHC-I heterodimer, but not the single HC (Solheim, Harris et al. 1997; Tector, Zhang et al. 1997). In mice the situation is somewhat different, because calnexin not only binds to free HC but also to the HC heterodimer (Nossner and Parham 1995). Furthermore, it was shown that calnexin is associated with assembled mouse MHC-I even after peptide loading and dissociation from the PLC (Suh, Mitchell et al. 1996). Mouse HCs are able to bind to TAP also in the β_2m deficient mouse cell line S3, and calnexin is present in this complex. Interestingly, also the fully folded human HLA-B*27 heterodimer has been shown to bind calnexin in human cells when using sensitive experimental systems, this is however outside the PLC (Carreno, Solheim et al. 1995). This shows, that the calnexin and calreticulin binding to MHC-I is not only species specific but also HC allomorph specific.

4.1.2 Glycosylation and the calnexin/calreticulin cycle

During the folding process, the MHC-I go through several rounds of dynamic binding, release and re-binding of calnexin/calreticulin in what is referred to the glycoprotein quality-control cycle (Helenius and Aebi 2004). The cycle is part of the general protein folding machinery in the ER, and is here illustrated in figure 3 in the context of MHC-I maturation. When bound calnexin or calreticulin is released from the HC, its glycosyl moiety becomes available for de-glucosylation by glucosidase II. Subsequently, the MHC-I folding status is evaluated by the soluble enzyme UDP-glucose glycosyl transferase (UGGT). If MHC-I is incorrectly folded the HC will be re-glycosylated and re-enter the glycoprotein quality control cycle (Helenius and Aebi 2004).

During translation and the BiP assisted folding the Asn86 of the MHC-I HC is N-glycosylated resulting in attachment of a $Glc_3Man_9GlcNAc_2$ oligosaccharide moiety (Kornfeld and Kornfeld 1985). The two outer glucose residues are then removed by glycosidase I and II leaving the MHC-I HC mono-glucosylated ($Glc_1Man_9GlcNAc_2$) at this step in the maturation process (Elbein 1991). This enables subsequent interaction of HC with the lectin chaperones, calnexin and calreticulin (Hebert, Foellmer et al. 1995; Ware, Vassilakos et al. 1995).

Both calnexin and calreticulin bind mono-glucosylated substrates (Hammond, Braakman et al. 1994; Peterson, Ora et al. 1995). In addition they both interact with unfolded

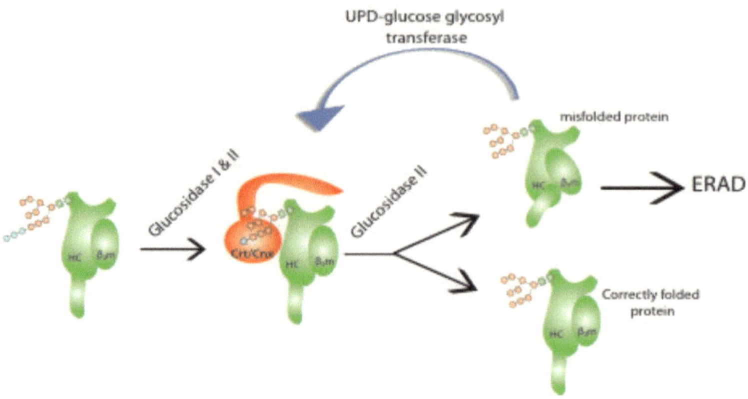

Fig. 3. The glycoprotein quality control cycle. Following the cotranslational glycosylation of MHC-I during translocation into the ER, glucosidase I and II remove the two outer glucoses immediately. When calnexin/calreticulin releases MHC-I the third glucose is removed and the folding status is evaluated by UDP-glucose glycosyl transferase. Incorrectly folded proteins will be re-glycosylated and re-enter the glycoprotein quality cycle whereas terminally misfolded proteins are degraded in the ER associated degradation (ERAD) pathway.

non-glucosylated proteins (Ihara, Cohen-Doyle et al. 1999; Saito, Ihara et al. 1999). As the newly synthesized MHC-I HC enters the ER via the translocon it is subjected to N-linked glycosylation of the sequon Asn-X-Ser/Thr (Bause, Muller et al. 1983). The glycosylation adds three glucose residues to the protein. The presence of a glycosylation site within the first 50 amino acids of a protein entering the ER through the translocon allows the interaction with calnexin and calreticulin to begin cotranslationally (Molinari and Helenius 2000). Inhibition of glycosylation results in many cases in misfolded, aggregated and dysfunctional proteins (Hickman, Kulczycki et al. 1977; Konig, Ashwell et al. 1988; Williams and Enns 1991). After trimming by glucosidase I and glucosidase II, mono-glucosylated HC is generated (Parodi 2000). The mono-glucosylated HC will then bind to calnexin for oxidative folding (Nossner and Parham 1995). Sequentially, the immature HC will create a heterodimer with the stabilising polypeptide β_2m. As this occurs, calnexin is replaced by calreticulin, which then recruits the immature heterodimer into the PLC where it can be loaded with high affinity peptides (Wearsch, Peaper et al. 2011).

It has been shown that the glycosylation of the MHC-I molecules in the ER is highly regulated. Nearly all monoglycosylated HC found in human cells are incorporated into the PLC and if deglycosylation is inhibited, their interaction with the PLC is significantly prolonged (Radcliffe, Diedrich et al. 2002; Wearsch, Peaper et al. 2011). A study using *in vitro* methods showed that glucosidase II could only trim free monyglycosylated HC and not those that were bound to the PLC (Wearsch, Peaper et al. 2011). This indicates that the glucose residues of the monoglycosylated MHC-I molecule become accessible to the glucosidase II first after its release from the PLC. After the last glucose residues has been removed, the MHC-I molecule can no longer associate with the PLC as its recruitment is dependent on the interaction with calreticulin which only binds to monoglycosylated proteins (Wearsch, Peaper et al. 2011). However, it has been proposed that if a deglycosylated MHC-I molecule is loaded with suboptimal peptide it can be rescued back into the PLC via the soluble enzyme UDP-glucose glycoprotein glucosyltransferase 1

(UGT1) (Zhang, Wearsch et al. 2011). The UGT1 can selectively reglycosylate the suboptimally loaded/incorrectly folded MHC-I molecule, and after trimming by glucosidase I and glucosidase II the monoglycosylated MHC-I molecule can ones again enter the PLC, this what is called the calnexin/calreticulin cycle. After the MHC-I molecule has become correctly folded and loaded with an optimal peptide it will be deglycosylated and released from the calnexin/calreticulin cycle for transport from the ER to the cell surface for presentation (Radcliffe, Diedrich et al. 2002). The time spent in the calnexin-calreticulin cycle can range from a few minutes to several hours, the more complex the folding of a protein, the more time it needs to spend. If a protein fails to reach mature conformation it is destined for ERAD (Klausner and Sitia 1990). Also for degradation tags the trimming of N-linked glycans has been shown to be of importance and calnexin has been implicated in the sequestering of proteins tagged for degradation (Liu, Choudhury et al. 1997).

4.1.3 Lack of calreticulin, but not calnexin, diminishes MHC-I quality control

In normal human cells the PLC consist of calreticulin, tapasin, ERp57, TAP, maturing MHC-I (Sadasivan, Lehner et al. 1996; Peaper, Wearsch et al. 2005). Ten years ago the hypothesis was that the abundant ERp57 found in the PLC was a consequence of its interaction with calreticulin or possibly calnexin (Oliver, Roderick et al. 1999). However, co-immunoprecipitation from K42 cells (a calreticulin deficient embryonic mouse fibroblast cell line) showed complexes of calnexin together with ERp57, tapasin and HC suggesting an alternative PLC constellation lacking calreticulin (Gao, Adhikari et al. 2002). Co-immunoprecipitation in lysates of K42 cells showed that ERp57 was associated with TAP, but that no calnexin could be detected in these precipitates, suggesting that neither calnexin nor calreticulin are essential for recruitment of ERp57 to the PLC (Suh, Mitchell et al. 1996; Gao, Adhikari et al. 2002). More recently it has been shown that ERp57 is directly disulfide conjugated to tapasin in the PLC (Peaper, Wearsch et al. 2005).

Calnexin deficient mice are viable and they show no discernible effects on other systems, including the immune system, possible because calreticulin effectively replaces the calnexin function even at the earlier MHC-I HC maturation stages. In contrast, calreticulin deficiency negatively impacts both trafficking and localization of MHC-I molecules. In the absence of calreticulin the MHC-I molecules are not retained in the ER, and the transport of immature MHC-I to the cell surface is accelerated. In K42 cells, many MHC-I molecules would be loaded with suboptimal peptides, due to lack of calreticulin in the MHC-I quality control, and the pMHC-I complexes would fall apart either before or on the cell surface (Gao, Adhikari et al. 2002). It was shown that the peptide-receptive MHC-I molecules were not found in the *cis*-Golgi or ER as they would be in wild type cells; instead they were found in endosomes and lysosomes. Under these circumstances the suboptimally loaded MHC-I molecules are transported to the cell surface, where the pMHC-I complexes almost instantly disintegrate, and are readily endocytosed ultimately leading to a significant reduction in MHC-I mediated antigen presentation (Howe, Garstka et al. 2009).

4.2 ERp57 oxidizes the MHC-I heavy chain and supports tapasin function

ERp57 is a multifunctional protein belonging to the thioredoxin family of proteins (Khanal and Nemere 2007). The protein structure is made up of four domains *a, b, a′* and *b′* (Ferrari and Soling 1999; Silvennoinen, Myllyharju et al. 2004). ERp57 is mainly, but not exclusively, an ER resident protein (Turano, Coppari et al. 2002) with a C-terminal Gln-Glu-Asp-Leu (QEDL) retention signal (Urade, Oda et al. 1997) and two thioredoxin domains with CGHC motifs shared with ERp72, protein disulfide isomerase (PDI) and other members of the thioredoxin family. Not only have many names been designated to this protein but several different functions of ERp57 have also been suggested including thiol-dependent oxidoreductase (Bourdi, Demady et al. 1995; Hirano, Shibasaki et al. 1995), cysteine protease (Urade and Kito 1992; Urade, Nasu et al. 1992), carnitine palmitoyl transferase (Wada, Imai et al. 1995), a hormone induced protein of the brain (Mobbs, Fink et al. 1990; Mobbs, Fink et al. 1990) and in combination with calnexin and/or calreticulin as a chaperone for N-glycosylated proteins in the ER (Oliver, van der Wal et al. 1997).

In the ER, ERp57 has been shown to be associated with the PLC where it plays a critical role in the MHC-I maturation (Dong, Wearsch et al. 2009). It has also been shown to be involved in the quality control of other newly synthesized glycoproteins (Urade, Okudo et al. 2004; Khanal and Nemere 2007). In the PLC, ERp57 is covalently bound to tapasin via a disulfide bond between Cys95 of tapasin and Cys57 of ERp57, however the structural characterisation of the complex indicates that the heterodimer is also stabilised by non-covalent interactions between tapasin and the *a* and *a'* domains of ERp57 (Dong, Wearsch et al. 2009). Calnexin and calreticulin, which both bind to ERp57 associate at the *b* and *b'* domains of the protein (Russell, Ruddock et al. 2004; Kozlov, Maattanen et al. 2006). It has been suggested that the binding to calnexin and calreticulin is required for the recruitment of ERp57 into the PLC (Oliver, van der Wal et al. 1997; Oliver, Roderick et al. 1999). However, in more recent studies it has been proposed that ERp57 also on its own can recognize and bind some newly synthesized proteins such as MHC-I HC in the absence of calnexin and calreticulin (Zhang, Kozlov et al. 2009). An important function of ERp57 is its thiol-dependent reductase activity that catalyse the formation of protein disulide-bonds during the folding of glycoproteins in the ER (Tector and Salter 1995). However, in contrast, it has been shown that in the PLC and during the maturation of MHC-I, ERp57 has a more structural role by stabilising tapasin and the PLC (Garbi, Tanaka et al. 2006). The heterodimer of tapasin and ERp57 has also been shown to have a peptide editing function thereby playing a key role in the generation of mature and stable pMHC-I complexes that are to be presented on the cell surface (Wearsch and Cresswell 2007).

An ubiquitous deletion of the ERp57 gene in mouse results in death in utero. To study the effects of ERp57 deficiency this problem was circumvented by generating a tissue specific deletion in the B cell compartment that resulted in B cells lacking the expression of ERp57 (Garbi, Tanaka et al. 2006). The development and survival of the ERp57 deficient B cells were not affected nor was there any indication that the folding of glycoproteins such as the immunoglobulin, CD25, CD1d, CD19, CD23, CD72, CD40, CD80 and CD86 was reduced. This suggests that ERp57 is not essential for the basic B cell functions and glycoprotein folding in these mouse cells (Garbi, Tanaka et al. 2006). However, in another study the folding of specific glycoprotein substrates was shown to be reduced in the absence of ERp57 (Jessop, Chakravarthi et al. 2007). Even though the general glycoprotein folding was not shown to be affected in the ERp57 deficient B cells there was a significantly lower surface expression of MHC-I molecules (H-2K^b showing a reduction of 50% whereas H-2D^b was only slightly reduced) compared to non-B cells expressing wild type amounts of ERp57

(Garbi, Tanaka et al. 2006). This further confirms the importance of ERp57 as a key player in generation of stable mature MHC-I molecules.

4.3 Tapasin optimizes the MHC-I peptide repertoire by releasing only stable pMHC-I

Tapasin (TAP associated glycoprotein) was discovered more than a decade ago and has during the years been assigned a central role in the loading aspects of the MHC-I quality control (Sadasivan, Lehner et al. 1996). In 1994, the description of the human lymphoblastoid B-cell line, termed LCL-721.220, marked the beginning of the discovery of tapasin. The LCL-721.220 did not have any HLA-A or HLA-B and only minor expression of HLA-C, and were devoid of full-length tapasin (Copeman, Bangia et al. 1998). The HLA-I cell surface expression of different HLA-I transfectants was monitored and found to be dependent on the particular HLA-I allomorph (Greenwood, Shimizu et al. 1994). For example, HLA-A*1 and HLA-B*8 were reduced to 21% of the expression in a normal cell having tapasin, whereas HLA-A*2, HLA-A*3 and HLA-B*7 were reduced. The HLA-I cell surface expression was restored when LCL-721.220 was fused with either LCL-721.174 or Daudi; cell lines having tapasin. Thus, LCL-721.220 lacked one or several unknown mechanisms responsible for the maturation of MHC-I (Grandea, Androlewicz et al. 1995). At the same time, a 48 kDa protein with a yet unknown function was shown to co-immunoprecipitate with TAP in a wild type cell line (Ortmann, Androlewicz et al. 1994). In 1996, this 48 kDa protein was named tapasin (Sadasivan, Lehner et al. 1996), and it was shown by western blot to be absent in LCL-721.220 possibly explaining the defect in MHC-I maturation (Copeman, Bangia et al. 1998). Later, expression of tapasin in LCL-721.220 restored MHC-I cell surface expression and confirmed this hypothesis (Ortmann, Copeman et al. 1997). At that time, the true identity of tapasin was not known. The following year, the cDNA of the TAP-associated protein corresponding to tapasin was cloned, and it was found that tapasin is a 428 amino acid large, type-I transmembrane glycoprotein with a short cytoplasmic tail (Li, Sjogren et al. 1997; Ortmann, Copeman et al. 1997).

In 1997, it was proposed that tapasin is a member of the Ig superfamily containing an IgC1-SET domain (Ortmann, Copeman et al. 1997; Herberg, Sgouros et al. 1998). Subsequently, it was suggested that amino acids 284 - 401 mostly originating from exon 5 has an Ig-like structure (Mayer and Klein 2001). This was further elaborated on using homology modeling suggesting that 287 - 401 has an Ig-like fold (Turnquist, Petersen et al. 2004). After many crystallization attempts, the first protein crystal structure was reported of tapasin in a stable disulfide conjugate with ERp57 (Dong, Wearsch et al. 2009). ERp57 has been proposed to stabilize tapasin when covalently associated through a disulfide bond (Peaper, Wearsch et al. 2005). The structure reveals that tapasin has two ER luminal domains. Domain-1 is the N-terminal domain spanning residues 1-269, and domain-2 spans the remaining residues 270-381 in the luminal part of tapasin.

To this date, it has not been possible to predict the structure of tapasin based on the amino acid sequence. This could be attributed to the fact that tapasin has a unique amino acid sequence especially within the now recognized domain-1. Related to the unique amino acid sequence the structure of tapasin domain-1 also has a unique 3-dimensional fold compared to other proteins. This domain consists mainly of anti-parallel beta-sheets. Interestingly, there are several ways to describe the structure of this domain. The most obvious regions within this domain are two beta-barrel-like structures that are tightly bound to each other. The stretch spanning the residues 77-102 contains a small alpha-helix (residues 83-90), but does not otherwise contain any secondary structure elements. The stretch contains the cysteine at position 95 and might serve as an extension from tapasin towards ERp57.

4.3.1 Tapasin only integrates β_2m-associated MHC-I HC into the PLC

Tapasin directly interacts with at least three components inside the PLC; it bridges MHC-I and TAP, and is simultaneously covalently bound to ERp57 thereby serving as an important structural component in the PLC. Tapasin does only interact with β_2m-associated MHC-I HC supported by observations showing that the MHC-I HC cannot be co-immunoprecipitated together with tapasin in Daudi cells, a β_2m negative cell line (Paulsson, Wang et al. 2001). Furthermore, the PLC is not assembled in Daudi cells, strongly suggesting that the MHC-I maturation takes place in successive stages inside the ER, and that β_2m is required for interaction with tapasin and integration into the PLC (Lewis and Elliott 1998). A contrasting study reported that tapasin directly interacts with MHC-I in the absence of β_2m (Rizvi and Raghavan 2006). In the absence of other cellular components it was shown that recombinant tapasin directly interacts with MHC-I HC alone or the MHC-I heterodimer. The study also showed that sufficient β_2m would effectively disrupt the tapasin-MHC-I interaction. In this regard, it may be speculated that in this *in vitro* system sufficient amounts of β_2m may stabilize MHC-I to such an extent, that it is no longer unstable and is therefore not able to interact with tapasin.

4.3.2 In the PLC, tapasin keeps MHC-I peptide-receptive

Exactly how MHC-I gets loaded with (the right) peptide in the ER is controversial. MHC-I incorporation into the PLC is mediated by tapasin structurally bridging MHC-I and TAP (Li, Sjogren et al. 1997; Ortmann, Copeman et al. 1997). In addition to serving as a structural component in the PLC, tapasin has also been suggested to facilitate peptide loading, edit the MHC-I peptide cargo, retain and recycle sub-optimally loaded pMHC-I complexes (Grandea, Lehner et al. 1997; Paulsson, Kleijmeer et al. 2002; Zarling, Luckey et al. 2003; Paulsson, Jevon et al. 2006). Here, we will describe what is currently known about the role of tapasin in MHC-I quality control within the PLC.

To describe the chaperone and peptide-editor function of tapasin it is necessary to accurately define these terms. A *chaperone* is a protein that assists the folding of a target protein. Regarding tapasin, the only target protein identified is MHC-I, and the chaperone function of tapasin is to facilitate the folding of MHC-I. During MHC-I maturation, tapasin has been found to facilitate the assembly of MHC-I in the ER ultimately resulting in increased cell surface expression (Lauvau, Gubler et al. 1999; Zarling, Luckey et al. 2003; Everett and Edidin 2007). To support this notion, a study using recombinant tapasin and HLA-I showed that tapasin facilitates folding of HLA-I in the absence of other PLC proteins (Chen and Bouvier 2007). We have recently shown that tapasin has chaperone function, and that at least part of this chaperone function is located within the first 87 amino acids of tapasin ($Tpn_{1\text{-}87}$) (Roder, Geironson et al. 2009; Roder, Geironson et al. 2011). A cell-free assay was developed to study the $Tpn_{1\text{-}87}$ chaperone function on folding HLA-I under controllable conditions. We observed that $Tpn_{1\text{-}87}$ facilitated the folding of HLA-I, and the extend of the folding could be directly, but inversely, correlated with the intrinsic stability of the pMHC-I complex. Based on these observations a model for the tapasin chaperone function can be constructed in which, tapasin chaperones the MHC-I heterodimer by keeping it in a peptide-receptive state. A suboptimal peptide that only confers a low-stability pMHC-I complex will either not release bound tapasin (and thus be retained in the ER), or the pMHC-I will quickly disintegrate, and tapasin will instantly re-associate to the MHC-I heterodimer. Only optimal peptides will confer a highly stable pMHC-I complex and cause the release of tapasin.

Regarding the aforementioned *peptide-editor* function, it is here defined as tapasin catalyzing the exchange of peptides on MHC-I. More specifically, tapasin directly interacts with the MHC-I thereby keeping it in a peptide-receptive conformational state. Only when an optimal peptide is loaded onto the MHC-I will tapasin release the MHC-I as shown in a study using recombinant proteins (Rizvi and Raghavan 2006). Tapasin and ERp57 are disulfide linked in the PLC, and it was shown this tapasin-ERp57 disulfide conjugate catalyzes MHC-I peptide-exchange (Peaper, Wearsch et al. 2005). Interestingly, both tapasin chaperone and peptide-editor function can be thought of as consequences of the same underlying tapasin mechanism, which is tapasin assisted stabilization of MHC-I. Tapasin arrests the MHC-I in a conformation preventing the MHC-I from aggregation and degradation, the chaperone function. The same conformation also keeps the MHC-I in a peptide-receptive state, allowing the association and dissociation of peptides. Only an optimal peptide binding to the MHC-I is able to change the MHC-I conformation causing the release of MHC-I from tapasin. Taken together, chaperone and peptide-editor functions of tapasin could be considered the mere consequences of its interaction with the MHC-I.

One consequence of keeping the MHC-I in a peptide-receptive conformation is giving an increasing diversity of peptides a chance to bind to the MHC-I. Of course, in the ER most of these peptides will be of suboptimal nature. In this line of reason, tapasin is expected to alter the pool of peptides presented by MHC-I. This was observed in one study that reported a reduced number of peptides presented on HLA-A*02:01 in the absence of tapasin (Barber, Howarth et al. 2001). This observation supports the theory presented here, because in the absence of tapasin suboptimal peptides will out-compete the optimal peptide for binding to HLA-A*02:01, and the suboptimal pMHC-I complexes will still be transported to the cell surface, because tapasin is not present to retain them in the ER.

4.3.3 Tapasin mediates recycling of unstable pMHC-I back to the ER

Assurance of mature and highly stable pMHC-I complexes on the cell surface in wild-type cells has generally been attributed to ER retention of immature MHC-I. The established theory arises from different experimental systems showing that tapasin retains MHC-I molecules in the ER until loaded with optimal peptides, i.e. peptides binding to MHC-I and resulting in stable pMHC-I complexes (Schoenhals, Krishna et al. 1999; Grandea, Golovina et al. 2000).

In addition, a recycling mechanism of MHC-I from late secretory compartments back to the ER has been suggested to exist based on evidence from several studies (Hsu, Yuan et al. 1991; Bresnahan, Barber et al. 1997; Park, Lee et al. 2001; Paulsson, Kleijmeer et al. 2002). Shown in figure 2 are COP-I coated vesicles that recognize and bind to C-terminal KKXX-motifs in membrane proteins thereby functioning as ER retrieval signals for proteins (Cosson and

Letourneur 1994). The findings that tapasin contains a C-terminal KKXX-motif and has been shown to have prolonged association with sub-optimally loaded pMHC-I complexes led to the investigation of tapasin involvement in COP-I transport (Paulsson, Kleijmeer et al. 2002). Tapasin was demonstrated to bind to COP-I via its KKXX-motif (Paulsson, Jevon et al. 2006). In cells expressing tapasin with the KKXX-motif mutated to AAXX, neither tapasin nor MHC-I were detected in association with COP-I, indicating a direct role for the tapasin KKXX-motif in mediating the MHC-I transport by COP-I coated vesicles. In the same cells, cell surface expression of MHC-I molecules was significantly increased, but MHC-I degradation was also increased suggesting escape to the cell surface of immature MHC-I. Thus, immature pMHC-I complexes having accidentally escaped the ER before being loaded with an optimal peptide, can be returned to the PLC in the ER for another round of peptide cargo optimization before being exported to the cell surface as mature and stable pMHC-I complexes.

4.3.4 The maturation of different MHC-I allomorphs depends differently on tapasin

A frequently used concept in the tapasin literature is *tapasin dependency* associated with each MHC-I allomorph. There has been a lack of previous consensus of this concept, and the use of *dependency* has been used referring to several types of distinct observations. In its strict sense, the dependency is how the cell surface expression of MHC-I depends on the presence of tapasin inside the cell. Thus, cell surface expression of HLA-I allomorphs that are highly dependent on tapasin will then be dramatically reduced in the absence of tapasin and vice versa. In this sense, HLA-I antigen presentation is controlled by tapasin to an extent depending on the HLA-I allomorph. To further investigate this dependency, we recently quantified the ability of $Tpn_{1\text{-}87}$ to chaperone different pMHC-I complexes, see figure 4. HLA-B*44:02 has been shown to be almost completely dependent on tapasin, since HLA-B*44:02 steady-state surface expression level is reduced by more than 90% in the tapasin deficient LCL-721.220 human cell line compared to the transfected homologues (Peh, Burrows et al. 1998). The same study also showed that HLA-B*27:05 surface expression was only slightly dependent on tapasin, whereas HLA-B*08:01 in this and another study was shown to be intermediate dependent on tapasin (Zarling, Luckey et al. 2003).

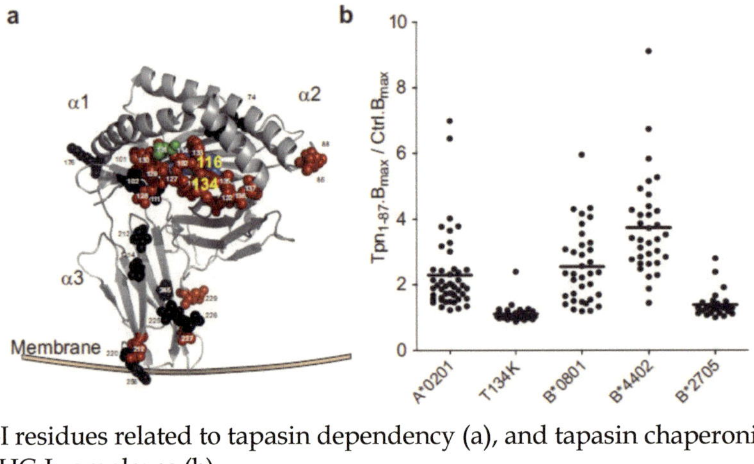

Fig. 4. MHC-I residues related to tapasin dependency (a), and tapasin chaperoning of different pMHC-I complexes (b).

Regarding the specificity of the tapasin-MHC-I interaction, several reports have shown that entire regions and single residues on MHC-I and tapasin that are important in their interaction and function. The most well-studied single mutation was in HLA-A*02:01 where a threonine at position 134 was mutated to a lysine (T134K) (Lewis, Neisig et al. 1996; Peace-Brewer, Tussey et al. 1996). The HLA-A*02:01-T134K mutant allomorph is unable to interact with tapasin, and this mutation can thus be used as a negative control in experiments studying the tapasin- MHC -I interaction.

Notoriously, it is the amino acid sequence that makes MHC-I allomorph distinct. The amino acid at position 114 of HLA-B*44:02 and HLA-B*27:05 has been shown to be of crucial importance regarding tapasin dependence, the higher the acidity of this amino acid the higher the tapasin dependence (Park, Lee et al. 2003). HLA-B*27:05 and HLA-B*44:02 (D114H) both have histidine at position 114, and are both tapasin-independent, while HLA-B*44:02 and HLA-B*35:01 have aspartic acid at residue 114 and are demonstrated to be dependent on tapasin (Peh, Burrows et al. 1998; Park, Lee et al. 2003). It is very interesting that a single residue (in certain HLA-I allomorphs) can completely change tapasin dependency, and it is especially interesting that residue 114 has this effect since it is not surface exposed, but buried deep down in the peptide binding groove close to the apex of the F-pocket. The tapasin interaction site on MHC-I is thought to be the surface exposed loop where the much discussed residue 134 is situated, and thus residue 114 is distal to the proposed tapasin interaction site, but is even though a strong determinant of tapasin dependence.

4.3.5 Tapasin stabilizes TAP and increases peptide transport efficiency

Tapasin binds directly to MHC-I, and form together with TAP the core of the PLC. The TAP-tapasin complex interacts with MHC-I, calreticulin and ERp57 to form a fully functional PLC capable of loading peptides into the peptide-receptive MHC-I binding groove (Garbi, Tan et al. 2000; Gao, Adhikari et al. 2002; Williams, Peh et al. 2002; Garbi, Tanaka et al. 2006), see figure 2. The precise binding site to TAP has not yet been mapped, but it has been suggested that the first N-terminal transmembrane helix of TAP binds to the transmembrane domain of tapasin (Koch, Guntrum et al. 2006), supported by the fact that soluble human tapasin variants are defective in TAP association, also resulting in MHC-I that does not bind to TAP (Sadasivan, Lehner et al. 1996). As we will go in more detail with in a later section, TAP transports cytosolic peptides into the ER lumen. TAP exists as a TAP1/2 heterodimer, which was shown to be stabilized by tapasin (Garbi, Tiwari et al. 2003). Furthermore, tapasin was shown to increase the peptide transport throughput by TAP (Li, Paulsson et al. 2000). Thus, in addition to localizing MHC-I close to the source of peptide transportation, tapasin also structurally bridges the PLC together while at the same time interacts with and keeps the MHC-I in a peptide-receptive conformation.

5. The MHC-I binding peptide has been processed by many proteases

5.1 The proteasome generates long peptides from degradable proteins

Large multicatalytic protease complexes named proteasomes are located in the cytosol and degrade proteins as part of normal cellular turnover. The proteasome is essential for MHC-I antigen presentation, and inhibitors of the proteasome reduce the generation of peptides presented on MHC-I molecules (Rock, Gramm et al. 1994). Defective ribosomal products

(DRiPs) are polypeptides that never reach a functional state owing to errors in translation or folding. They are rapidly ubiquitylated during translation and have been shown to be a major source of peptides presented by MHC-I (Reits, Vos et al. 2000; Schubert, Anton et al. 2000). The use of these newly translated proteins, facilitates rapid recruitment of effector cells to virally infected cells, resulting in a more efficient withdrawal of the infection.

The proteasome contains IFN-γ-inducible subunits. Under conditions of IFN-γ induction the β1, β2 and β5 subunits are replaced by immunosubunits, low-molecular-mass polypeptide 2 (LMP2), multi-catalytic endopeptidase complex-like 1 (MECL-1) and LMP7 respectively, resulting in assembly of new proteasomes called immunoproteasome (Loukissa, Cardozo et al. 2000; Jamaluddin, Wang et al. 2001). Immunoproteasomes are concentrated around the ER, whereas constitutive proteasomes are distributed evenly in the cytoplasm and in the nucleus (Brooks, Murray et al. 2000). Immunoproteasomes, compared to constitutive proteasomes, have an increased capacity to cleave peptides after hydrophobic and basic residues but reduced capacity to cleave after acidic amino acids (Gaczynska, Rock et al. 1993; Gaczynska, Rock et al. 1994). Furthermore, immunoproteasomes generate peptides with an extended N-terminal sequence that will facilitate transport into the ER (Cascio, Hilton et al. 2001; Knuehl, Spee et al. 2001). Even though immunoproteasomes favour the production of peptides presented by MHC-I molecules, they are not an absolute requirement (Arnold, Driscoll et al. 1992; Yewdell, Lapham et al. 1994), and some antigenic peptides are even efficiently produced by the constitutive proteasomes only (Chapiro, Claverol et al. 2006).

5.2 TAP transports cytosolic peptides into the ER and supports MHC-I quality control

An essential part of the PLC is the heterodimeric TAP composed of the TAP1 and TAP2 subunits, both containing an N-terminal transmembrane domain and a C-terminal cytosolic nucleotide-binding domain. TAP1 and TAP2 have 10 and 9 transmembrane helices, respectively, where the 6 C-terminal helices from each subunit build together to form the so called 6+6 TM core complex which has been shown to be essential and sufficient for ER targeting, assembly of the heterodimer, binding of peptide and peptide translocation (Koch, Guntrum et al. 2004). The translocation is a multistep process, beginning with association of peptides with TAP in an ATP-independent manner (Androlewicz, Anderson et al. 1993; van Endert, Tampe et al. 1994; Neumann and Tampe 1999). Peptides with a length of 8-16 amino acids are preferentially bound to TAP (van Endert, Tampe et al. 1994). Peptides with 8-12 amino acids are transported most efficiently, although peptides longer than 40 amino acids are also transported, albeit with a lower efficiency (Androlewicz, Anderson et al. 1993; Koopmann, Post et al. 1996). The C-terminal amino acid and the first three N-terminal residues of the peptide have been shown to play a key role in TAP recognition (Scholz and Tampe 2005). Peptides with basic or hydrophobic amino acids at the C-terminus are particularly preferred by human TAP. Peptide binding to TAP is followed by a slow isomerization of the TAP complex that triggers an ATP-dependent peptide translocation across the ER membrane (Neefjes, Momburg et al. 1993; Shepherd, Schumacher et al. 1993; Scholz and Tampe 2005).

5.3 Calreticulin and calnexin bind peptides – part of the peptide relay system

As has been previously described both calnexin and calreticulin are multifunctional proteins. In addition to playing a key role in the maturation of MHC-I molecules via the calnexin/calreticulin cycle it has also been shown that they are able to bind peptides. Neefjes and colleagues have shown that both the chaperones calnexin and calreticulin bind peptides *in vitro* (Spee and Neefjes 1997; Spee, Subjeck et al. 1999). Calreticulin has also been shown to bind peptides *in vivo* (Nair, Wearsch et al. 1999). Many other heat shock proteins have also been demonstrated to bind peptide and a model of peptide transfer along a line of chaperones from the cytosol to the lumen of the ER - the *peptide relay system* - has been suggested to be responsible for directing peptides towards MHC-I presentation (Srivastava, Udono et al. 1994). The complexes formed when chaperones bind peptide have been suggested to bind to heat shock protein receptors on the surface of professional APCs, which leads to en internalization of the complex. The peptide from the complex is then presented by the MHC-I resulting in the elicitation of a CTL response. It has also been shown that chaperone-peptide complexes can stimulate the APCs to secrete certain cytokines (Srivastava, Menoret et al. 1998).

5.4 ERAP aminopeptidases trim ER peptides to fit the MHC-I peptide binding groove

After the peptides have been transported by TAP into the ER they may be further trimmed by aminopeptidases such as ER aminopeptidases 1 and 2 (ERAP1 and ERAP2) (Saric, Chang et al. 2002; Serwold, Gonzalez et al. 2002; Saveanu, Carroll et al. 2005). Although both are members of the M1 family of zinc metolloproteases (Rawlings, Barrett et al. 2010) ERAP1 and ERAP2 show striking differences in their substrate preferences. ERAP1 has a preference for large hydrophobic residues while ERAP2 prefers basic residues (Hattori, Kitatani et al. 2000; Tanioka, Hattori et al. 2003; Saveanu, Carroll et al. 2005). In contrast to most other aminopeptidases, that are more or less restricted to cleaving peptides shorter than four residues, ERAP1 shows a strong increase in cleaving activity towards peptides that are between 10-16 residues long (York, Chang et al. 2002). As ERAP1 and ERAP2 cleave substrates with different preferential for the N-terminal residues ERAP1 and ERAP2 have been suggested to work in concert for trimming of MHC-I binding peptides (Saveanu, Carroll et al. 2005).

The mechanism by with ERAP1 recognizes and cleaves peptides of a specific length has been debated. The crystal structure of ERAP1 (bound to bestatin) reveals a large cavity that would explain the preference for longer substrates compared to most other aminopeptidases (Nguyen, Chang et al. 2011). In this large cavity a catalytic site is found to which the N-terminal part of the peptide binds. It has been proposed that in close proximity to this catalytic site a regulatory site is found to which the C-terminal part of the peptide is bound, this "double binding" ensures a closed conformation of the ERAP1 molecule resulting in effective cleaving of the peptide. However, if the peptide is too short the C-terminal will not reach the regulatory site and the "double binding" will not be achieved resulting in an ineffective cleaving of the peptide (Nguyen, Chang et al. 2011).

The preference for longer immature antigenic peptide precursors supports the role of ERAP1 in the processing of antigenic peptides that are to be presented on MHC-I molecules, which preferentially bind peptides of eight to ten amino acid residues. It has been shown that over expression of ERAP1 enhances the presentation of antigenic peptides by MHC-I, confirming the importance of ERAP1 for MHC-I antigen presentation.

In agreement with this is the finding from ERAP1 siRNA knock down studies that showed a reduction in antigenic peptides presented by the MHC-I molecules (York, Chang et al. 2002). In mice ERAP1 deficiency gives a significantly reduced MHC-I expression on the cell surface (Yan, Parekh et al. 2006). ERAP1 is IFN-γ inducible as is many important APM components, putting ERAP1 in the same category (York, Chang et al. 2002).

6. Perspectives

Understanding the antigen processing and quality control of pMHC-I complexes is likely to significantly help us understand the criteria for why some MHC-I binding peptides are presented while others are not, and also why some peptides are able, and others are unable to function as CTL epitopes. The stability of pMHC-I complexes is likely to influence both positive and negative selection of responding CTLs implicating pMHC-I quality control as important in both autoimmune disease and as tumour antigens. Moreover, expression of many APM components is altered in many tumours and certain virus alter APM component activity and/or expression, and as a consequence change the MHC-I presented peptide pool both qualitatively and quantitatively. In conclusion further study of the APM and quality control of MHC-I will improve the identification of epitopes involved in both malignant neoplasms, viral diseases and in autoimmune diseases.

7. References

Androlewicz, M. J., K. S. Anderson, et al. (1993). "Evidence that transporters associated with antigen processing translocate a major histocompatibility complex class I-binding peptide into the endoplasmic reticulum in an ATP-dependent manner." *Proceedings of the National Academy of Sciences of the United States of America* 90(19): 9130-9134.

Arnold, D., J. Driscoll, et al. (1992). "Proteasome subunits encoded in the MHC are not generally required for the processing of peptides bound by MHC class I molecules." *Nature* 360(6400): 171-174.

Barber, L. D., M. Howarth, et al. (2001). "The quantity of naturally processed peptides stably bound by HLA-A*0201 is significantly reduced in the absence of tapasin." *Tissue antigens* 58(6): 363-368.

Bause, E., T. Muller, et al. (1983). "Synthesis and characterization of lipid-linked mannosyl oligosaccharides in Volvox carteri f. nagariensis." *Archives of biochemistry and biophysics* 220(1): 200-207.

Bourdi, M., D. Demady, et al. (1995). "cDNA cloning and baculovirus expression of the human liver endoplasmic reticulum P58: characterization as a protein disulfide isomerase isoform, but not as a protease or a carnitine acyltransferase." *Archives of biochemistry and biophysics* 323(2): 397-403.

Bresnahan, P. A., L. D. Barber, et al. (1997). "Localization of class I histocompatibility molecule assembly by subfractionation of the early secretory pathway." *Human immunology* 53(2): 129-139.

Brooks, P., R. Z. Murray, et al. (2000). "Association of immunoproteasomes with the endoplasmic reticulum." *The Biochemical journal* 352 Pt 3: 611-615.

Carreno, B. M., J. C. Solheim, et al. (1995). "TAP associates with a unique class I conformation, whereas calnexin associates with multiple class I forms in mouse and man." *Journal of immunology* 155(10): 4726-4733.

Cascio, P., C. Hilton, et al. (2001). "26S proteasomes and immunoproteasomes produce mainly N-extended versions of an antigenic peptide." *The EMBO journal* 20(10): 2357-2366.

Chapiro, J., S. Claverol, et al. (2006). "Destructive cleavage of antigenic peptides either by the immunoproteasome or by the standard proteasome results in differential antigen presentation." *Journal of immunology* 176(2): 1053-1061.

Chen, M. and M. Bouvier (2007). "Analysis of interactions in a tapasin/class I complex provides a mechanism for peptide selection." *The EMBO journal* 26(6): 1681-1690.

Copeman, J., N. Bangia, et al. (1998). "Elucidation of the genetic basis of the antigen presentation defects in the mutant cell line .220 reveals polymorphism and alternative splicing of the tapasin gene." *European journal of immunology* 28(11): 3783-3791.

Cosson, P. and F. Letourneur (1994). "Coatomer interaction with di-lysine endoplasmic reticulum retention motifs." *Science* 263(5153): 1629-1631.

Danilczyk, U. G., M. F. Cohen-Doyle, et al. (2000). "Functional relationship between calreticulin, calnexin, and the endoplasmic reticulum luminal domain of calnexin." *The Journal of biological chemistry* 275(17): 13089-13097.

Dong, G., P. A. Wearsch, et al. (2009). "Insights into MHC class I peptide loading from the structure of the tapasin-ERp57 thiol oxidoreductase heterodimer." *Immunity* 30(1): 21-32.

Elbein, A. D. (1991). "Glycosidase inhibitors: inhibitors of N-linked oligosaccharide processing." *The FASEB journal : official publication of the Federation of American Societies for Experimental Biology* 5(15): 3055-3063.

Everett, M. W. and M. Edidin (2007). "Tapasin increases efficiency of MHC I assembly in the endoplasmic reticulum but does not affect MHC I stability at the cell surface." *Journal of immunology* 179(11): 7646-7652.

Ferrari, D. M. and H. D. Soling (1999). "The protein disulphide-isomerase family: unravelling a string of folds." *The Biochemical journal* 339 (Pt 1): 1-10.

Gaczynska, M., K. L. Rock, et al. (1993). "Gamma-interferon and expression of MHC genes regulate peptide hydrolysis by proteasomes." *Nature* 365(6443): 264-267.

Gaczynska, M., K. L. Rock, et al. (1994). "Peptidase activities of proteasomes are differentially regulated by the major histocompatibility complex-encoded genes for LMP2 and LMP7." *Proceedings of the National Academy of Sciences of the United States of America* 91(20): 9213-9217.

Gao, B., R. Adhikari, et al. (2002). "Assembly and antigen-presenting function of MHC class I molecules in cells lacking the ER chaperone calreticulin." *Immunity* 16(1): 99-109.

Garbi, N., P. Tan, et al. (2000). "Impaired immune responses and altered peptide repertoire in tapasin-deficient mice." *Nature immunology* 1(3): 234-238.

Garbi, N., S. Tanaka, et al. (2006). "Impaired assembly of the major histocompatibility complex class I peptide-loading complex in mice deficient in the oxidoreductase ERp57." *Nature immunology* 7(1): 93-102.

Garbi, N., N. Tiwari, et al. (2003). "A major role for tapasin as a stabilizer of the TAP peptide transporter and consequences for MHC class I expression." *European journal of immunology* 33(1): 264-273.

Grandea, A. G., 3rd, M. J. Androlewicz, et al. (1995). "Dependence of peptide binding by MHC class I molecules on their interaction with TAP." *Science* 270(5233): 105-108.

Grandea, A. G., 3rd, T. N. Golovina, et al. (2000). "Impaired assembly yet normal trafficking of MHC class I molecules in Tapasin mutant mice." *Immunity* 13(2): 213-222.

Grandea, A. G., 3rd, P. J. Lehner, et al. (1997). "Regulation of MHC class I heterodimer stability and interaction with TAP by tapasin." *Immunogenetics* 46(6): 477-483.

Greenwood, R., Y. Shimizu, et al. (1994). "Novel allele-specific, post-translational reduction in HLA class I surface expression in a mutant human B cell line." *Journal of immunology* 153(12): 5525-5536.

Hammond, C., I. Braakman, et al. (1994). "Role of N-linked oligosaccharide recognition, glucose trimming, and calnexin in glycoprotein folding and quality control." *Proceedings of the National Academy of Sciences of the United States of America* 91(3): 913-917.

Hattori, A., K. Kitatani, et al. (2000). "Characterization of recombinant human adipocyte-derived leucine aminopeptidase expressed in Chinese hamster ovary cells." *Journal of biochemistry* 128(5): 755-762.

Hebert, D. N., B. Foellmer, et al. (1995). "Glucose trimming and reglucosylation determine glycoprotein association with calnexin in the endoplasmic reticulum." *Cell* 81(3): 425-433.

Helenius, A. and M. Aebi (2004). "Roles of N-linked glycans in the endoplasmic reticulum." *Annual review of biochemistry* 73: 1019-1049.

Herberg, J. A., J. Sgouros, et al. (1998). "Genomic analysis of the Tapasin gene, located close to the TAP loci in the MHC." *European journal of immunology* 28(2): 459-467.

Hickman, S., A. Kulczycki, Jr., et al. (1977). "Studies of the mechanism of tunicamycin in hibition of IgA and IgE secretion by plasma cells." *The Journal of biological chemistry* 252(12): 4402-4408.

High, S., F. J. Lecomte, et al. (2000). "Glycoprotein folding in the endoplasmic reticulum: a tale of three chaperones?" *FEBS letters* 476(1-2): 38-41.

Hirano, N., F. Shibasaki, et al. (1995). "Molecular cloning of the human glucose-regulated protein ERp57/GRP58, a thiol-dependent reductase. Identification of its secretory form and inducible expression by the oncogenic transformation." *European journal of biochemistry / FEBS* 234(1): 336-342.

Howe, C., M. Garstka, et al. (2009). "Calreticulin-dependent recycling in the early secretory pathway mediates optimal peptide loading of MHC class I molecules." *The EMBO journal* 28(23): 3730-3744.

Hsu, V. W., L. C. Yuan, et al. (1991). "A recycling pathway between the endoplasmic reticulum and the Golgi apparatus for retention of unassembled MHC class I molecules." *Nature* 352(6334): 441-444.

Ihara, Y., M. F. Cohen-Doyle, et al. (1999). "Calnexin discriminates between protein conformational states and functions as a molecular chaperone in vitro." *Molecular cell* 4(3): 331-341.

Jamaluddin, M., S. Wang, et al. (2001). "IFN-beta mediates coordinate expression of antigen-processing genes in RSV-infected pulmonary epithelial cells." *American journal of physiology. Lung cellular and molecular physiology* 280(2): L248-257.

Jessop, C. E., S. Chakravarthi, et al. (2007). "ERp57 is essential for efficient folding of glycoproteins sharing common structural domains." *The EMBO journal* 26(1): 28-40.

Khanal, R. C. and I. Nemere (2007). "The ERp57/GRp58/1,25D3-MARRS receptor: multiple functional roles in diverse cell systems." *Current medicinal chemistry* 14(10): 1087-1093.

Klausner, R. D. and R. Sitia (1990). "Protein degradation in the endoplasmic reticulum." *Cell* 62(4): 611-614.

Knuehl, C., P. Spee, et al. (2001). "The murine cytomegalovirus pp89 immunodominant H-2Ld epitope is generated and translocated into the endoplasmic reticulum as an 11-mer precursor peptide." *Journal of immunology* 167(3): 1515-1521.

Koch, J., R. Guntrum, et al. (2004). "Functional dissection of the transmembrane domains of the transporter associated with antigen processing (TAP)." *The Journal of biological chemistry* 279(11): 10142-10147.

Koch, J., R. Guntrum, et al. (2006). "The first N-terminal transmembrane helix of each subunit of the antigenic peptide transporter TAP is essential for independent tapasin binding." *FEBS letters* 580(17): 4091-4096.

Konig, R., G. Ashwell, et al. (1988). "Glycosylation of CD4. Tunicamycin inhibits surface expression." *The Journal of biological chemistry* 263(19): 9502-9507.

Koopmann, J. O., M. Post, et al. (1996). "Translocation of long peptides by transporters associated with antigen processing (TAP)." *European journal of immunology* 26(8): 1720-1728.

Kornfeld, R. and S. Kornfeld (1985). "Assembly of asparagine-linked oligosaccharides." *Annual review of biochemistry* 54: 631-664.

Kozlov, G., P. Maattanen, et al. (2006). "Crystal structure of the bb' domains of the protein disulfide isomerase ERp57." *Structure* 14(8): 1331-1339.

Lauvau, G., B. Gubler, et al. (1999). "Tapasin enhances assembly of transporters associated with antigen processing-dependent and -independent peptides with HLA-A2 and HLA-B27 expressed in insect cells." *The Journal of biological chemistry* 274(44): 31349-31358.

Lewis, J. W. and T. Elliott (1998). "Evidence for successive peptide binding and quality control stages during MHC class I assembly." *Current biology : CB* 8(12): 717-720.

Lewis, J. W., A. Neisig, et al. (1996). "Point mutations in the alpha 2 domain of HLA-A2.1 define a functionally relevant interaction with TAP." *Current biology : CB* 6(7): 873-883.

Li, S., K. M. Paulsson, et al. (2000). "Tapasin is required for efficient peptide binding to transporter associated with antigen processing." *The Journal of biological chemistry* 275(3): 1581-1586.

Li, S., H. O. Sjogren, et al. (1997). "Cloning and functional characterization of a subunit of the transporter associated with antigen processing." *Proceedings of the National Academy of Sciences of the United States of America* 94(16): 8708-8713.

Liu, Y., P. Choudhury, et al. (1997). "Intracellular disposal of incompletely folded human alpha1-antitrypsin involves release from calnexin and post-translational trimming of asparagine-linked oligosaccharides." *The Journal of biological chemistry* 272(12): 7946-7951.

Loukissa, A., C. Cardozo, et al. (2000). "Control of LMP7 expression in human endothelial cells by cytokines regulating cellular and humoral immunity." *Cytokine* 12(9): 1326-1330.

Maloy, W. L. (1987). "Comparison of the primary structure of class I molecules." *Immunologic research* 6(1-2): 11-29.

Mayer, W. E. and J. Klein (2001). "Is tapasin a modified Mhc class I molecule?" *Immunogenetics* 53(9): 719-723.

Mobbs, C. V., G. Fink, et al. (1990). "HIP-70: a protein induced by estrogen in the brain and LH-RH in the pituitary." *Science* 247(4949 Pt 1): 1477-1479.

Mobbs, C. V., G. Fink, et al. (1990). "HIP-70: an isoform of phosphoinositol-specific phospholipase C-alpha." *Science* 249(4968): 566-567.

Molinari, M. and A. Helenius (2000). "Chaperone selection during glycoprotein translocation into the endoplasmic reticulum." *Science* 288(5464): 331-333.

Nair, S., P. A. Wearsch, et al. (1999). "Calreticulin displays in vivo peptide-binding activity and can elicit CTL responses against bound peptides." *Journal of immunology* 162(11): 6426-6432.

Neefjes, J. J., F. Momburg, et al. (1993). "Selective and ATP-dependent translocation of peptides by the MHC-encoded transporter." *Science* 261(5122): 769-771.

Neumann, L. and R. Tampe (1999). "Kinetic analysis of peptide binding to the TAP transport complex: evidence for structural rearrangements induced by substrate binding." *Journal of molecular biology* 294(5): 1203-1213.

Nguyen, T. T., S. C. Chang, et al. (2011). "Structural basis for antigenic peptide precursor processing by the endoplasmic reticulum aminopeptidase ERAP1." *Nature structural & molecular biology* 18(5): 604-613.

Nossner, E. and P. Parham (1995). "Species-specific differences in chaperone interaction of human and mouse major histocompatibility complex class I molecules." *The Journal of experimental medicine* 181(1): 327-337.

Oliver, J. D., H. L. Roderick, et al. (1999). "ERp57 functions as a subunit of specific complexes formed with the ER lectins calreticulin and calnexin." *Molecular biology of the cell* 10(8): 2573-2582.

Oliver, J. D., F. J. van der Wal, et al. (1997). "Interaction of the thiol-dependent reductase ERp57 with nascent glycoproteins." *Science* 275(5296): 86-88.

Ortmann, B., M. J. Androlewicz, et al. (1994). "MHC class I/beta 2-microglobulin complexes associate with TAP transporters before peptide binding." *Nature* 368(6474): 864-867.

Ortmann, B., J. Copeman, et al. (1997). "A critical role for tapasin in the assembly and function of multimeric MHC class I-TAP complexes." *Science* 277(5330): 1306-1309.

Paquet, M. E., M. Cohen-Doyle, et al. (2004). "Bap29/31 influences the intracellular traffic of MHC class I molecules." *Journal of immunology* 172(12): 7548-7555.

Park, B., S. Lee, et al. (2003). "A single polymorphic residue within the peptide-binding cleft of MHC class I molecules determines spectrum of tapasin dependence." *Journal of immunology* 170(2): 961-968.

Park, B., S. Lee, et al. (2001). "The truncated cytoplasmic tail of HLA-G serves a quality-control function in post-ER compartments." *Immunity* 15(2): 213-224.

Parodi, A. J. (2000). "Role of N-oligosaccharide endoplasmic reticulum processing reactions in glycoprotein folding and degradation." *The Biochemical journal* 348 Pt 1: 1-13.

Paulsson, K. M., M. Jevon, et al. (2006). "The double lysine motif of tapasin is a retrieval signal for retention of unstable MHC class I molecules in the endoplasmic reticulum." *Journal of immunology* 176(12): 7482-7488.

Paulsson, K. M., M. J. Kleijmeer, et al. (2002). "Association of tapasin and COPI provides a mechanism for the retrograde transport of major histocompatibility complex (MHC) class I molecules from the Golgi complex to the endoplasmic reticulum." *The Journal of biological chemistry* 277(21): 18266-18271.

Paulsson, K. M. and P. Wang (2004). "Quality control of MHC class I maturation." *The FASEB journal : official publication of the Federation of American Societies for Experimental Biology* 18(1): 31-38.

Paulsson, K. M., P. Wang, et al. (2001). "Distinct differences in association of MHC class I with endoplasmic reticulum proteins in wild-type, and beta 2-microglobulin- and TAP-deficient cell lines." *International immunology* 13(8): 1063-1073.

Peace-Brewer, A. L., L. G. Tussey, et al. (1996). "A point mutation in HLA-A*0201 results in failure to bind the TAP complex and to present virus-derived peptides to CTL." *Immunity* 4(5): 505-514.

Peaper, D. R., P. A. Wearsch, et al. (2005). "Tapasin and ERp57 form a stable disulfide-linked dimer within the MHC class I peptide-loading complex." *The EMBO journal* 24(20): 3613-3623.

Peh, C. A., S. R. Burrows, et al. (1998). "HLA-B27-restricted antigen presentation in the absence of tapasin reveals polymorphism in mechanisms of HLA class I peptide loading." *Immunity* 8(5): 531-542.

Peterson, J. R., A. Ora, et al. (1995). "Transient, lectin-like association of calreticulin with folding intermediates of cellular and viral glycoproteins." *Molecular biology of the cell* 6(9): 1173-1184.

Radcliffe, C. M., G. Diedrich, et al. (2002). "Identification of specific glycoforms of major histocompatibility complex class I heavy chains suggests that class I peptide loading is an adaptation of the quality control pathway involving calreticulin and ERp57." *The Journal of biological chemistry* 277(48): 46415-46423.

Rawlings, N. D., A. J. Barrett, et al. (2010). "MEROPS: the peptidase database." *Nucleic acids research* 38(Database issue): D227-233.

Reits, E. A., J. C. Vos, et al. (2000). "The major substrates for TAP in vivo are derived from newly synthesized proteins." *Nature* 404(6779): 774-778.

Rizvi, S. M. and M. Raghavan (2006). "Direct peptide-regulatable interactions between MHC class I molecules and tapasin." *Proceedings of the National Academy of Sciences of the United States of America* 103(48): 18220-18225.

Rock, K. L., C. Gramm, et al. (1994). "Inhibitors of the proteasome block the degradation of most cell proteins and the generation of peptides presented on MHC class I molecules." *Cell* 78(5): 761-771.

Roder, G., L. Geironson, et al. (2008). "Viral proteins interfering with antigen presentation target the major histocompatibility complex class I peptide-loading complex." *Journal of virology* 82(17): 8246-8252.

Roder, G., L. Geironson, et al. (2009). "The outermost N-terminal region of tapasin facilitates folding of major histocompatibility complex class I." *European journal of immunology* 39(10): 2682-2694.

Roder, G., L. Geironson, et al. (2011). "Tapasin discriminates peptide-human leukocyte antigen-A*02:01 complexes formed with natural ligands." *The Journal of biological chemistry* 286(23): 20547-20557.

Russell, S. J., L. W. Ruddock, et al. (2004). "The primary substrate binding site in the b' domain of ERp57 is adapted for endoplasmic reticulum lectin association." *The Journal of biological chemistry* 279(18): 18861-18869.

Sadasivan, B., P. J. Lehner, et al. (1996). "Roles for calreticulin and a novel glycoprotein, tapasin, in the interaction of MHC class I molecules with TAP." *Immunity* 5(2): 103-114.

Saito, Y., Y. Ihara, et al. (1999). "Calreticulin functions in vitro as a molecular chaperone for both glycosylated and non-glycosylated proteins." *The EMBO journal* 18(23): 6718-6729.

Santana, M. A. and F. Esquivel-Guadarrama (2006). "Cell biology of T cell activation and differentiation." *International review of cytology* 250: 217-274.

Saric, T., S. C. Chang, et al. (2002). "An IFN-gamma-induced aminopeptidase in the ER, ERAP1, trims precursors to MHC class I-presented peptides." *Nature immunology* 3(12): 1169-1176.

Saveanu, L., O. Carroll, et al. (2005). "Concerted peptide trimming by human ERAP1 and ERAP2 aminopeptidase complexes in the endoplasmic reticulum." *Nature immunology* 6(7): 689-697.

Schoenhals, G. J., R. M. Krishna, et al. (1999). "Retention of empty MHC class I molecules by tapasin is essential to reconstitute antigen presentation in invertebrate cells." *The EMBO journal* 18(3): 743-753.

Scholz, C. and R. Tampe (2005). "The intracellular antigen transport machinery TAP in adaptive immunity and virus escape mechanisms." *Journal of bioenergetics and biomembranes* 37(6): 509-515.

Schubert, U., L. C. Anton, et al. (2000). "Rapid degradation of a large fraction of newly synthesized proteins by proteasomes." *Nature* 404(6779): 770-774.

Serwold, T., F. Gonzalez, et al. (2002). "ERAAP customizes peptides for MHC class I molecules in the endoplasmic reticulum." *Nature* 419(6906): 480-483.

Shepherd, J. C., T. N. Schumacher, et al. (1993). "TAP1-dependent peptide translocation in vitro is ATP dependent and peptide selective." *Cell* 74(3): 577-584.

Silvennoinen, L., J. Myllyharju, et al. (2004). "Identification and characterization of structural domains of human ERp57: association with calreticulin requires several domains." *The Journal of biological chemistry* 279(14): 13607-13615.

Solheim, J. C., B. M. Carreno, et al. (1997). "Are transporter associated with antigen processing (TAP) and tapasin class I MHC chaperones?" *Journal of immunology* 158(2): 541-543.

Solheim, J. C., M. R. Harris, et al. (1997). "Prominence of beta 2-microglobulin, class I heavy chain conformation, and tapasin in the interactions of class I heavy chain with calreticulin and the transporter associated with antigen processing." *Journal of immunology* 158(5): 2236-2241.

Spee, P. and J. Neefjes (1997). "TAP-translocated peptides specifically bind proteins in the endoplasmic reticulum, including gp96, protein disulfide isomerase and calreticulin." *European journal of immunology* 27(9): 2441-2449.
Spee, P., J. Subjeck, et al. (1999). "Identification of novel peptide binding proteins in the endoplasmic reticulum: ERp72, calnexin, and grp170." *Biochemistry* 38(32): 10559-10566.
Srivastava, P. K., A. Menoret, et al. (1998). "Heat shock proteins come of age: primitive functions acquire new roles in an adaptive world." *Immunity* 8(6): 657-665.
Srivastava, P. K., H. Udono, et al. (1994). "Heat shock proteins transfer peptides during antigen processing and CTL priming." *Immunogenetics* 39(2): 93-98.
Suh, W. K., E. K. Mitchell, et al. (1996). "MHC class I molecules form ternary complexes with calnexin and TAP and undergo peptide-regulated interaction with TAP via their extracellular domains." *The Journal of experimental medicine* 184(2): 337-348.
Tanioka, T., A. Hattori, et al. (2003). "Human leukocyte-derived arginine aminopeptidase. The third member of the oxytocinase subfamily of aminopeptidases." *The Journal of biological chemistry* 278(34): 32275-32283.
Tector, M. and R. D. Salter (1995). "Calnexin influences folding of human class I histocompatibility proteins but not their assembly with beta 2-microglobulin." *The Journal of biological chemistry* 270(33): 19638-19642.
Tector, M., Q. Zhang, et al. (1997). "Beta 2-microglobulin and calnexin can independently promote folding and disulfide bond formation in class I histocompatibility proteins." *Molecular immunology* 34(5): 401-408.
Turano, C., S. Coppari, et al. (2002). "Proteins of the PDI family: unpredicted non-ER locations and functions." *Journal of cellular physiology* 193(2): 154-163.
Turnquist, H. R., J. L. Petersen, et al. (2004). "The Ig-like domain of tapasin influences intermolecular interactions." *Journal of immunology* 172(5): 2976-2984.
Urade, R. and M. Kito (1992). "Inhibition by acidic phospholipids of protein degradation by ER-60 protease, a novel cysteine protease, of endoplasmic reticulum." *FEBS letters* 312(1): 83-86.
Urade, R., M. Nasu, et al. (1992). "Protein degradation by the phosphoinositide-specific phospholipase C-alpha family from rat liver endoplasmic reticulum." *The Journal of biological chemistry* 267(21): 15152-15159.
Urade, R., T. Oda, et al. (1997). "Functions of characteristic Cys-Gly-His-Cys (CGHC) and Gln-Glu-Asp-Leu (QEDL) motifs of microsomal ER-60 protease." *Journal of biochemistry* 122(4): 834-842.
Urade, R., H. Okudo, et al. (2004). "ER-60 domains responsible for interaction with calnexin and calreticulin." *Biochemistry* 43(27): 8858-8868.
van Endert, P. M., R. Tampe, et al. (1994). "A sequential model for peptide binding and transport by the transporters associated with antigen processing." *Immunity* 1(6): 491-500.
Wada, I., S. Imai, et al. (1995). "Chaperone function of calreticulin when expressed in the endoplasmic reticulum as the membrane-anchored and soluble forms." *The Journal of biological chemistry* 270(35): 20298-20304.
Ware, F. E., A. Vassilakos, et al. (1995). "The molecular chaperone calnexin binds Glc1Man9GlcNAc2 oligosaccharide as an initial step in recognizing unfolded glycoproteins." *The Journal of biological chemistry* 270(9): 4697-4704.

Wearsch, P. A. and P. Cresswell (2007). "Selective loading of high-affinity peptides onto major histocompatibility complex class I molecules by the tapasin-ERp57 heterodimer." *Nature immunology* 8(8): 873-881.

Wearsch, P. A., D. R. Peaper, et al. (2011). "Essential glycan-dependent interactions optimize MHC class I peptide loading." *Proceedings of the National Academy of Sciences of the United States of America* 108(12): 4950-4955.

Williams, A. M. and C. A. Enns (1991). "A mutated transferrin receptor lacking asparagine-linked glycosylation sites shows reduced functionality and an association with binding immunoglobulin protein." *The Journal of biological chemistry* 266(26): 17648-17654.

Williams, A. P., C. A. Peh, et al. (2002). "Optimization of the MHC class I peptide cargo is dependent on tapasin." *Immunity* 16(4): 509-520.

Yan, J., V. V. Parekh, et al. (2006). "In vivo role of ER-associated peptidase activity in tailoring peptides for presentation by MHC class Ia and class Ib molecules." *The Journal of experimental medicine* 203(3): 647-659.

Yewdell, J., C. Lapham, et al. (1994). "MHC-encoded proteasome subunits LMP2 and LMP7 are not required for efficient antigen presentation." *Journal of immunology* 152(3): 1163-1170.

Yewdell, J. W., L. C. Anton, et al. (1996). "Defective ribosomal products (DRiPs): a major source of antigenic peptides for MHC class I molecules?" *Journal of immunology* 157(5): 1823-1826.

York, I. A., S. C. Chang, et al. (2002). "The ER aminopeptidase ERAP1 enhances or limits antigen presentation by trimming epitopes to 8-9 residues." *Nature immunology* 3(12): 1177-1184.

Zarling, A. L., C. J. Luckey, et al. (2003). "Tapasin is a facilitator, not an editor, of class I MHC peptide binding." *Journal of immunology* 171(10): 5287-5295.

Zhang, Q. and R. D. Salter (1998). "Distinct patterns of folding and interactions with calnexin and calreticulin in human class I MHC proteins with altered N-glycosylation." *Journal of immunology* 160(2): 831-837.

Zhang, W., P. A. Wearsch, et al. (2011). "A role for UDP-glucose glycoprotein glucosyltransferase in expression and quality control of MHC class I molecules." *Proceedings of the National Academy of Sciences of the United States of America* 108(12): 4956-4961.

Zhang, Y., G. Kozlov, et al. (2009). "ERp57 does not require interactions with calnexin and calreticulin to promote assembly of class I histocompatibility molecules, and it enhances peptide loading independently of its redox activity." *The Journal of biological chemistry* 284(15): 10160-10173.